*To my family and friends*
*And to nurses and their clients*

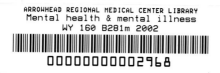

# Mental Health & Mental Illness

## SEVENTH EDITION

**Patricia D. Barry, PhD, APRN, CS**
Clinical Nurse Specialist in Consultation/Liaison
    Psychiatry
Psychotherapist in Private Practice
Nursing Consultant
Hartford, Connecticut

**CONSULTANT AND CONTRIBUTOR**
**Suzette Farmer, RN, MS, PhD Candidate**
Assistant Professor
Practical and Associate Degree Nursing
Utah Valley State College
Orem, Utah

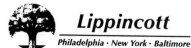

**Lippincott**
*Philadelphia · New York · Baltimore*

*Acquisitions Editor:* Lisa Stead
*Managing Editor/Development:* Karin McAndrews
*Senior Production Editor:* Tom Gibbons
*Senior Production Manager:* Helen Ewan
*Art Director:* Carolyn O'Brien
*Cover Design:* B.J. Crim
*Manufacturing Manager:* William Alberti
*Indexer:* Ellen Brennan
*Compositor:* LWW
*Printer:* R.R. Donnelley

7th Edition

9  8  7  6  5  4  3  2

Library of Congress Cataloging-in-Publication Data
Barry, Patricia D.
    Mental health and mental illness/Patricia D. Barry ; consultant and contributor, Suzette Farmer.—7th ed.
      p. ; cm
    Includes bibliographical references and index.
    ISBN 0-7817-3138-0 (paper : alk. paper)
    1. Psychiatry. 2. Mental health. 3. Psychiatric nursing. I. Farmer, Suzette. II. Title.
    [DNLM: 1. Mental Disorders—Nurses' Instruction. 2. Mental Health—Nurses' Instruction. 3. Psychiatric Nursing—Nurses' Instruction. WY 160 B281m 2002]
    RC454.4 .B372 2002
    616.89—dc21

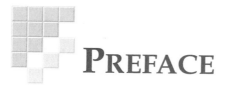# PREFACE

It is a pleasure to introduce you to the seventh edition of *Mental Health and Mental Illness*. There are many exciting new changes in this text that make it user friendly and an improved resource for the psychiatric nursing student. There are new features in every chapter. They include:

- Key terms listed at the beginning of the chapter to alert the student to the importance of the term in reading the chapter and in self-learning activities
- Self awareness activities that encourage the student's self-reflection relating to the content of the chapter
- Key points described in a table format at the conclusion of each chapter
- Key points described in a table format at the conclusion of each chapter to reiterate important points in the text.

In addition, there are several new features that have been included in each clinical chapter in Unit 4. They are:

- A case example based on the clinical criteria presented in the chapter
- A series of nursing diagnosis statements based on the clinical example
- Patient/family teaching guidelines for nurses
- Websites that describe community resources for the specific types of clinical conditions in each chapter. Websites are also included for Chapter 28, Psychopharmacology and Electroconvulsive Treatment of Mental Disorders.

This book is written for nurses everywhere who are attending to persons with mental distress and mental disorders. Usually, this textbook is most frequently used by nurses who are training in the field of mental health and psychiatric nursing. In addition, the concepts in these pages are also intended to be used in all clinical settings where clients are experiencing mental health disorders or distress. These clinical settings include inpatient, community, and home health physical care settings; long-term care facilities; prison populations; and wherever nurses practice nursing. In physical illness settings, the nursing care principles used with clients with mental disorders work equally well when physically ill clients are experiencing emotional or mental distress.

Insurance cost-containment measures have markedly altered the environment in which mental health care is delivered. Mental health admissions that used to be 4 weeks in length a decade or two ago have now been shortened to only a few days. Patients and staff alike are under more stress as they struggle to effect change in a very brief period of time, often before medications are able to modify the distressing emotions and behavior that necessitated admission. The need for high-quality psychiatric nursing care has never been greater.

## OVERVIEW OF CONTENT IN THIS TEXT

This book is written to provide the most up-to-date information for nurses training in the field of psychiatric and mental nursing. All units include updated information about the most frequently occurring mental disorders and the most effective nursing care approaches for each type of disorder.

**Unit 1—Patterns of Mental Health Care** discusses the current and evolving trends in mental health care, including the current care options for a client experiencing a mental health crisis. The differences in mental health nursing care in inpatient treatment settings, community settings, and the home care setting are discussed. The changing professional, legal, and ethical issues of nurses in the mental health setting are also included in this unit.

**Unit 2—Foundations of the Therapeutic Relationship** presents the clinical foundations of mental health nursing, beginning with therapeutic communication skills, the primary theories about the formation of the human personality, and the important effects of family and socio-cultural environment on the developing child

**Unit 3—Foundations of Decision Making in the Mental Health Setting** describes the various bases on which clinical decisions are based in the mental health setting. These bases include the use of the nursing process, the understanding of human emotions and information about effective and ineffective types of responses to stress. The unit concludes with the various criteria used to assess mental status.

**Unit 4—Nursing the Client With a Mental Disorder** includes the mental disorders most frequently seen in mental health treatment settings. These disorders are described in the fourth edition of the Diagnostic and Statistical Mental Disorders, the source of diagnostic information used in the field of mental health. Three new chapters are included, reflecting the increasing prevalence of these conditions in the society at large.

The new information on suicide assessment and nursing care is relevant in all clinical settings with people of all ages and with all types of mental and physical conditions. Clinical information about eating disorders in adolescents is presented, as well as a new chapter about the increasing numbers of children and adolescents with different types of learning disorders. The new chapters are italicized in the list below. The chapters in Unit 4 include:

- The Client With a Mood Disorder

- The Client With an Anxiety Disorder

- The Client With an Anxiety Disorder

- The Client With Delirium, Dementia, and other Cognitive Disorder: With Schizophrenia and Other Psychotic Disorders

- *The Client Who Is Contemplating Suicide*

- The Client With a Substance Related Mental Disorder

- The Client With a Personality Disorder

- *The Client With an Eating Disorder*

- *The Infant, Child or, Adolescent With a Developmental Disorder*

**Unit 5—Intervention and Treatment of Mental Disorders** includes information on crisis intervention, milieu and group therapy, care of the older adult with a mental disorder and psychopharmacology and electroconvulsive treatment of mental disorders. There is also new content on the use of complementary therapies in mental health settings.

Throughout the writing of this text, it has been my fervent hope that this information will make a difference in the way that every nurse who reads this text will administer care with every mental health client he or she meets. In addition, with the new section on self-awareness activities in each chapter, the reader has an opportunity to examine his or her own personal reactions to the mental health environment. Perhaps a kinder and gentler self-view will be the result. One of the opportunities in the field of mental health is the possibility of developing increased personal insights about one's own view of self and of the world

My best wishes to all,
*Pat Barry, PhD, APRN*

# ACKNOWLEDGMENTS

I want to thank the nursing faculty who select this text for their students. I wrote this new edition with your needs and those of your students in mind. My goal in preparing the seventh edition of *Mental Health and Mental Illness* is to provide you with the information you and your students need to provide compassionate nursing care to individuals whose quality of life is deeply affected by mental illness.

I also want to thank two editors at Lippincott, Williams & Wilkins for their important assistance in the preparation of this text. Margaret Zuccarini has been the nursing editor who has overseen this text for several editions. When she and I began to plan for changes and updates in the seventh edition, her vision was to add new chapters that would provide students with information about topics that are increasing societal concern, as well as increase their knowledge about the psychiatric nursing care of these conditions. Margaret also wanted to add new features that would make all of the chapter content more meaningful and easier to learn. We spent several months creating the revision plan. At the same time that the plan was completed, Margaret's role at Lippincott Williams & Wilkins changed. I was sorry that Margaret wasn't going to actively participate in the writing and production phases of this book—and to oversee the development of her vision.

Lisa Stead became the new editor of the text. It has been a delight to work with her. Her support was ever present and rapidly available. Whenever I asked Lisa for information that was needed in order to move forward in the writing, she was a constant support and always responsive. Her assistant, Karin McAndrews, was an important support for me also and was a pleasure to work with. Karin also was the managing editor for this edition. The managing editor plays a very important role in the production of the book and in implementing the author's work. So, in addition. I am grateful to Karin for her excellent assistance in reviewing the manuscript and preparing it for production. In addition, thanks to Tom Gibbons, Senior Production Editor, who oversaw all aspects of the production process.

In order to provide you with the most current information in the field of psychiatric and mental health nursing. I asked Suzette Farmer,

RN, MS, PhD Candidate, to assist in the preparation of the new edition. Suzette Farmer, RN, MS, PhD Candidate, to assist in the preparation of the new edition. Suzette participated in all phases of the revision plan. She carefully reviewed and made thoughtful and excellent suggestions regarding all content in the new edition to ensure that it would meet the needs of nursing students in today's educational and mental health environments. In addition, Suzette wrote Chapter 6, Professional, Legal and Ethical Issues in Mental Health Nursing, and Chapter 28, Psychopharmacology and Electroconvulsive Treatment of Mental Disorders. Her revisions of these important chapters add significantly to the updating of information in this edition of *Mental Health and Mental Illness*.

Thanks also to Dr. Connie Weiskopf, PhD, APRN, Program Manager of Accreditation at the University of Connecticut Health Center in Farmington, Connecticut, for generously sharing the information from her doctoral research and thesis that is included in Chapter 2 in the section on nursing care of the mentally disordered person in prison settings.

Beth Richards provided invaluable assistant in the preparation of this edition by bringing her exceptional editing and educational skills to the review and revision of the behavioral objectives and key terms in each chapter, as well as the updating of the glossary. It was a pleasure to work with her.

In conclusion, as this new edition moves into its printed reality, I am happy to have been able to prepare it for you and am grateful to all who participated with me in its preparation.

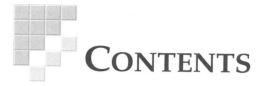

# CONTENTS

# Unit 3 ◆ Foundations of Decision Making in the Mental Health Setting **121**

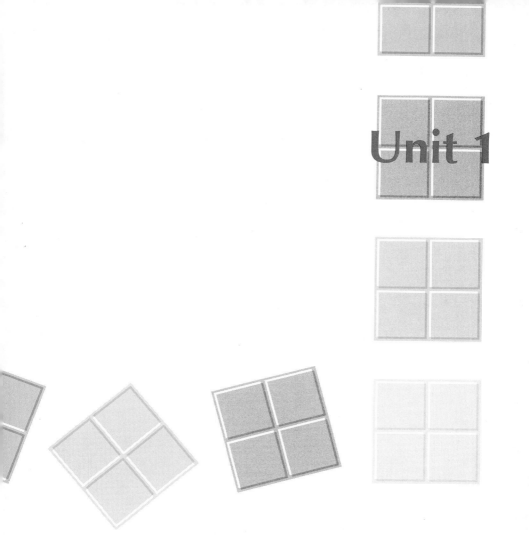

# Unit 1

# PATTERNS OF MENTAL HEALTH CARE

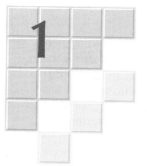

# Current and Evolving Patterns of Mental Health Care

## Behavioral Objectives

*After reading this chapter the student will be able to:*

- Name the three major forces that have caused changes in mental health care since the 1940s.
- Explain how each of those forces is continuing to cause changes in mental health care services.
- Explain the shift from inpatient to community-based mental health services that began in the late 1950s.
- Describe the current economic factors that have affected the availability of mental health care services.
- List three of the major plans designed to decrease mental health care costs.

## Key Terms

- Biological psychiatry
- Capping
- Continuum of care
- Deinstitutionalization
- Diagnostic related groups (DRGs)
- Quality assurance programs
- Sheltered environment
- Triage

## ◆ HISTORY OF MENTAL HEALTH CARE

The treatment of mental disorders has gone through many stages of development during the past 100 years. The guiding principle throughout has been to move the mentally disordered person from his or her normal family, social, and community surroundings to a sheltered environment. During the past 20 years, the **sheltered environment** has shifted from one that was primarily custodial in an institution to one that is dynamically oriented toward community-based rehabilitation of the person with a mental disorder. This philosophical change in treatment is evident from the preadmission through the active treatment and postdischarge phases of mental health care.

## HISTORY OF THE SHIFT FROM INPATIENT TO COMMUNITY-BASED MENTAL HEALTH SERVICES

The original change in philosophy from inpatient to outpatient care of seriously mentally disordered individuals began in the late 1950s and early 1960s. This change was the result of a number of factors:

- Research on psychiatric disorders was increasingly demonstrating that environmental and social factors contributed strongly to the development of mental illness.
- An increase in the incidence of mental illness in the community can be inferred by the incidence of mental disorders in inductees into the armed services. During the preinduction process of U.S. citizens in World War II, 1,875,000 men were found to be emotionally unfit for service and 850,000 (40% of *all* discharges) were released from active service because of mental illness.
- The introduction of phenothiazines in the mid-1950s, new and effective tranquilizers for persons with major psychiatric disorders, followed by "second" and "third" generations of more effective medications in the 1990s that reduced the incidence of active psychotic episodes in people with schizophrenia and other types of psychotic mental disorders. The use of these psychotropic medications has been the primary contributing factor in the cost reduction of mental health care in the United States.
- Studies in state mental institutions revealed that clients were living under poor conditions.

As a result of these findings, many government agencies were eager to develop community-based programs in which formerly state-supported mental health clients could receive care as outpatients in their home communities.

The premise of community psychiatry is that custodial, institution-based care should be reserved only for acutely ill individuals; thus, many people formerly treated in long-term residential care centers should be returned to their home environments. Community psychiatry also focuses on prevention, using community-based programs.

These findings and related recommendations are at the heart of the concept of deinstitutionalization. **Deinstitutionalization** is the act of transferring formerly institutionalized individuals to sheltered community environments or homes in the community. The philosophy of deinstitutionalization is viewed as the primary cause of the increased incidence of homeless mentally ill individuals throughout the United States.

## ◆ CHANGING PATTERNS OF MENTAL HEALTH CARE DELIVERY

The delivery of health care is changing rapidly, driven by health insurance and government reform of its payment systems. Nurses often are important buffers and interpreters of those changes. When an individual becomes ill, there is a profound effect on that person and his or her loved ones. The role of the nurse includes assisting the patient to understand the cause and nature of the illness and the means of restoring health. These important nursing values can be expressed regardless of the site where care is administered.

The guiding principle of nursing care continues to be the nursing process. The openness and flexibility of the nursing process allows it to be used in all settings. Many treatment settings have been developed to provide adequate care levels to clients and their families as a response to the variety of needs affecting health care decision making today.

### DETERMINING FACTORS THAT CONTRIBUTE TO A CONTINUUM OF CARE

The time frame of the health care decision-making process is often influenced by the overriding expectation of providing the most cost-effective care in a succession of settings ranging from acute inpatient care to community-based partial hospitalization and, finally, to home care. This succession of care settings is known as a **continuum of care.** When a client requires medical care, the primary medical caregiver examines the options available.

Large urban centers usually have a greater variety of home care, community, partial hospitalization, and inpatient hospitalization sites available. The concept of a continuum of care is more likely to be put into practice in these urban centers and their surrounding suburbs. The availability of a continuum of services, ranging from home to inpatient care options, depends primarily on the vision of the leaders of the community health institutions and agencies in medium-sized and rural communities. Have those leaders recognized the rapidly changing trends and planned accordingly?

Government funding to assist community health care planners is another important factor that contributes to the availability of a range of services. Government funds include those from federal, state, and local community resources. Often the federal government provides grants for innovative health care programs whose effectiveness has been documented by research. Federal grants usually require that state and local communities also provide funds from their own treasuries as evidence of their involvement with and commitment to the successful implementation of a new program.

## SELECTING THE APPROPRIATE CARE SITE

**Triage** is the process by which an individual with a health problem is assessed by a health care provider, usually a physician or nurse specialist, in order to determine what type(s) of illness are occurring and what type of immediate health care is needed by the individual. The triage process determines the level of care as well as the appropriate site for care. An important consideration in triage is the selection by a knowledgeable health care provider of the settings that can most efficiently and economically provide care. The triage decision also includes assessment of the state of the client, his or her family or home environment, the availability of community resources, and the financial resources for different levels of care.

The most important considerations that guide decision making are:

1. The state of the client
2. The site where care can be provided most effectively in order to promote stabilization and well being

These factors can be determined by considering the following:

- Is the client's life at risk from a mental or physical disorder?
- Is there a life-threatening physical disorder that must be stabilized?
- Is there a mental disorder that poses a threat to the life of the client or another?
- Are there services necessary to stabilize the client that can be provided only in an inpatient setting?
- Is there an unstable home environment that is inadequate to provide safe care to the client?
- Are there no supportive community services available that can provide the care required to stabilize the client?
- If the client has insurance, will the insurance company approve financial reimbursement for one site rather than another?

Whenever the answer to one of these questions is yes, the choices then become focused around that factor in identifying the appropriate environment, out of the options available in the individual's community that provide the safest and most cost-effective care. Ideally, the following services are available:

1. Outpatient clinic or private treatment options
2. Home care
   a. Crisis assessment and intervention
   b. Family therapy consultation
3. Partial hospitalization programs
4. Residential programs
5. Inpatient settings (information about inpatient settings is found in Chapter 3, Inpatient Hospitalization: The Mental Health Treatment Team and the Therapeutic Milieu, with an overview of the role of the nurse in each of these settings)

A significant outcome of health care policy making in the past decade is that clients are rapidly moved from one treatment setting and focus to another. These rapid changes can be further unsettling to a client and family when they occur during a time of emotional crisis.

As individuals move from one treatment setting to another, their care providers often change as well. The effectiveness of communication between care sites is an important aspect of the "seamlessness" of a continuum of care. Nurses often provide the bridge of understanding about the specific needs of a patient from one setting to another.

## ◆ CHANGES IN INPATIENT MENTAL HEALTH TREATMENT

Many forces have shaped these changes. The most significant influences have been the following:

- *Economic forces that do not support long-term psychiatric care.* Funding emphasis has shifted from chronic inpatient care to community models of outpatient care.
- *Development of medications that significantly decrease the major symptoms of psychiatric disorders, psychosis, and depression.* These medications, when properly used, can allow those who formerly required long-term institutionalization to return to outpatient community care.
- *Advent of a variety of mental health disciplines that train individuals to work with different aspects of a mental health client's psychological and social functioning in both inpatient and community care settings.* With their combined skills, these individuals comprise a treatment team that utilizes a comprehensive mental health care approach.

The economic forces that are shaping the changing patterns of mental health care in the United States are addressed elsewhere in this chapter. A discussion of the medications used to treat various symptoms of mental disorders can be found in Unit 5, Interventions and

Treatment of Mental Disorders. The mental health treatment team and its approaches to therapeutic care are presented in Chapter 3, Inpatient Hospitalization: The Mental Health Treatment Team and the Therapeutic Milieu.

## ◆ IMPORTANCE OF ECONOMIC FACTORS IN DECISION MAKING ABOUT MENTAL HEALTH TREATMENT

During the 1980s, the cost of health care in the United States increased at a greater rate than any other cost of living factor in our national economy. Accordingly, these costs were addressed in both the public and private sectors during the late 1980s and early 1990s. Mental health care costs were targeted for major changes and strategic planning regarding the delivery of both inpatient and outpatient care. The results of these changes were:

- Increased emphasis on biological psychiatry, the use of new and more effective medications to manage the effects of serious mental disorders that once required inpatient hospitalization for symptom stabilization
- Deinstitutionalization of seriously mentally disordered individuals in public-funded mental health care
- Community versus inpatient mental health care for individuals with acute mental health disturbances
- Changes in payment mechanisms by private insurers for both inpatient and outpatient care
- Use of DRGs by federal and state funding agencies to create guidelines for lengths of hospital stay. **Diagnostic related groups** are the categories of mental disorders listed with the guidelines for normal days expected for inpatient hospitalization.
- Quality assurance programs mandated by public and private agencies to ensure the quality of health care to all people, regardless of whether their care is paid by the individual, public funding, or insurance

These factors have brought about many changes in current mental health treatment and will continue to be important forces in the future. The reasons are described in the following.

### BIOLOGICAL PSYCHIATRY

**Biological psychiatry** is the use of biological means to treat mental disorders. There is a strong emphasis on the use of psychopharmacology to produce rapid results in treating acute mental states because the majority of mental disorders show that there are changes in the laboratory findings of normal patterns of neurochemistry. Increasingly, health maintenance organizations that are overseeing managed mental health services disallow ongoing psychotherapy services and urge the primary use of medication to manage mental health symptoms.

## DEINSTITUTIONALIZATION

Rather than serving as centers for chronic care, federal and state-funded, long-term psychiatric care institutions were adapted to treat people in crisis or with serious mental disorders requiring acute (7 days or less) and midterm (usually 7 to 21 days) treatment. The effects of deinstitutionalization on mental health care are discussed in Chapter 4, Community-Based Treatment Settings for Mental Disorders. Alternative, community-based mental health treatment programs are intended to provide ongoing treatment for the chronically mentally ill individual.

## CHANGES IN PAYMENT MECHANISMS USED BY PRIVATE INSURERS FOR MENTAL HEALTH CARE

Stringent limits were set for both inpatient and outpatient mental health treatment because mental health care costs were escalating faster than general physical health care costs. The limit on inpatient care costs resulted in a more aggressive treatment process during acute "crisis" admissions, usually 7 days or less in duration. Longer-term admissions are becoming increasingly rare because of the stringent criteria used to justify inpatient hospitalization.

The emphasis on short lengths of inpatient admissions is being driven by a policy known as "capping." **Capping** is the practice of allowing a limited dollar amount for lifetime psychiatric care. For example, an insurance company may set a limit of $50,000 on the amount that it will reimburse to a person during his or her lifetime for any type of psychiatric care, whether in the hospital or community. A person with a chronic psychiatric disorder such as schizophrenia can exhaust the "lifetime" psychiatric benefit before the age of 30 with the cost of standard outpatient care and two or three brief hospital admissions.

## USE OF DIAGNOSTIC RELATED GROUPS BY FEDERAL AND STATE FUNDING AGENCIES

Diagnostic related groups are being used to establish guidelines for appropriate lengths of stay in another effort to reduce unnecessary hospital costs. Hospitals are permitted to charge for a specific number of days of treatment using these guidelines. The approved number of days can be extended only when there are unusual complications that meet previously defined criteria. Payments for Medicaid and Medicare admissions cut off after the DRG deadline is reached. Accordingly, short-term aggressive treatment that discharges clients as soon as they are reasonably able to leave the hospital is rewarded. On the other hand, if hospitals lag in discharging a significant number of their clients, they can quickly encounter major financial difficulties.

## QUALITY ASSURANCE PROGRAMS MANDATED BY PUBLIC AND PRIVATE AGENCIES

**Quality assurance programs** are designed to monitor the quality of health care delivered in hospitals and communities. The services of all health care providers, including nurses, are reviewed, whether in inpatient or outpatient settings and publicly or privately funded health care. Using quality assurance guidelines, the following aspects of health care are evaluated:

- Assessment
- Accuracy of diagnosis
- Rationale for diagnostic testing
- Effectiveness of care planning
- Evaluation of outcomes

The quality assurance programs in hospitals actively review the care planning of nurses in the psychiatric setting. Good quality inpatient and outpatient mental health care is strongly dependent on the effective use of the nursing process by psychiatric nurses. The nursing process is described in Unit 3, Foundations of Decision Making in the Mental Health Setting.

KEY   POINTS

---

- Three significant forces have shaped the treatment of mental disorders:
  —Development of medications that decrease major symptoms of mental disorders
  —Shifts in economic focus
  —Development of a range of mental health disciplines to treat clients
- Beginning in the late 1950s and early 1960s, many seriously mentally disordered people were transferred from inpatient settings to outpatient or community-based care. This shift is known as deinstitutionalization.
- Community mental health treatment uses social and environmental measures to prevent mental illness and to treat and care for those who develop mental disorders.
- To reduce the rising cost of mental health care, fewer clients are treated in inpatient settings, spending limits are set on lifetime care, and length and quality of client care are closely monitored.

■ Quality assurance programs actively review the care plans of all mental health providers, including those of psychiatric nurses.

During the next week listen or watch for the terms health management organization (HMO) or managed care company in the news media. Notice what is being said in each report.

- Does the report mention whether the public is satisfied or dissatisfied with this approach to managing health care costs?
- Is the report describing the financial state of a particular managed care company that is operating in your area? What is being said about the financial state?
- Is your health insurance a managed care or HMO plan? What do you like or dislike about this form of health insurance?

## QUESTIONS

1. The major forces that have changed mental health care since the 1940s are
   a. an increased emphasis on institution-based care and greater funding for psychiatric hospitals.
   b. significant government support of inpatient and outpatient mental health care.
   c. more clinical psychologists available for consultations.
   d. development of medications, shift in funding emphasis from inpatient to outpatient, and increased variety of people trained to care for mental health clients.
2. Deinstitutionalization increases the likelihood that a nurse will
   a. not be able to find a job.
   b. work with the mentally ill only in institutional settings.
   c. work with the mentally ill in any care setting.
   d. not need to be involved in discharge planning.
3. The *highest* priority consideration involved in the triage process is
   a. Is the client's life at risk from a mental or physical disorder?
   b. Will the insurance company approve financial reimbursement for one site over another?
   c. Are supportive community services available that can provide the care required to stabilize the client?
   d. Are there services necessary to stabilize the client that can be provided only in an inpatient setting?

**4.** The purpose of DRGs is to
   a. group similar mental health caregivers for greater efficiency.
   b. make organized lists of client diagnoses.
   c. create a monopoly of services.
   d. create guidelines for length of hospital stay.

## BIBLIOGRAPHY

Boyd, M., & Nihart, M. (1998). *Psychiatric nursing: Contemporary practice.* Philadelphia: Lippincott Williams & Wilkins.

Goldman, H. (1999). Justifying mental health care costs. *Health Affairs, 18*(2), 94–95.

Grazier, K., & Eselius, L. (1999). Mental health carve-outs: Effects and implications. *Medical Care Research and Review, 56*(Suppl 2), 37–59.

Leslie, D., & Rosenbeck, R. (1999). Changes in inpatient mental health utilization and costs in a privately insured population. *Medical Care, 37*(5), 457–468.

Leslie, D., & Rosenbeck, R. (1999). Inpatient treatment of comorbid psychiatric and substance abuse disorders. *Administration and Policy in Mental Health, 26* (4), 253–268.

Rydman, R., Trybus, D., Butki, N., Kampe, L., & Marley, J. (1999). Outcome of case management and comprehensive support services following policy changes in mental health care delivery. *Journal of Medical Systems, 23*(4), 309–323.

Sadock, B., & Kaplan, H. (1998). *Synopsis of psychiatry: Behavioral sciences/Clinical psychiatry.* Philadelphia: Lippincott Williams & Wilkins.

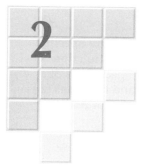

# 2

# The Roles of the Nurse in Different Mental Health Settings

## Behavioral Objectives

*After reading this chapter the student will be able to:*

- Explain the concepts of nursing and the four themes of nursing practice.
- Explain the role of nursing in addressing a client's psychosocial needs.
- Define nursing scope of practice.
- Identify the types of problems that the mental health nurse addresses.
- Explain the three major nursing roles in mental health settings.
- Explain the role of the LPN/LVN in three different practice settings.

## Key Terms

- Biopsychosocial
- Case manager/team leader
- Clinical nurse specialist
- Correctional nurse
- Environment
- Function
- Health
- Holistic
- Home health aide
- Job description
- Nursing
- Nursing Practice Standards of the Licensed Practical/Vocational Nurse
- Person
- Psychopathology
- Psychotropic medications
- Role
- Scope of practice

The word **role** describes the expected behaviors of a person engaged in a particular activity. It is used in the world of work to define the expectations of persons working in particular types of occupations. Within a particular type of occupation or occupational role, there are specific functions that make up the types of activities in that role. A **function** is a specific type of activity that belongs within the role expectations of a particular occupation. In order to understand the roles and functions of the LPN/LVN it is important to be aware of the concepts that underlie nursing practice.

## ◆ CONCEPTS OF NURSING PRACTICE

Nursing is an art and a science that combines and integrates the theories and practices of many different fields: social sciences, such as psychology and sociology; basic sciences, such as anatomy, physiology, microbiology, and biochemistry; and medical science, the diagnosing and treating of illness. Nursing is a biopsychosocial science—that is, in assessing and planning care for the human responses to illness, nursing draws on knowledge of human biology, psychology, and the human social systems of family, friends, and community as the foundations of its practice. This approach to assessment is called a **holistic** model of care.

### FOUR THEMES OF NURSING

Many nursing scientists have developed theoretical models about the concepts of nursing practice. As a whole, nursing models generally address four critical aspects or themes of nursing.

#### Person

The nurse views a **person** as a human being composed of biological, psychological, and social functions or domains. These functions or domains are blended in a complex system that results in a unique individual.

#### Nursing

**Nursing** is a role that includes the following dimensions of person-centered care: comfort (including physical and emotional care) and the monitoring and maintenance of safety and hygiene.

#### Environment

**Environment** includes all the internal and external forces that affect the well being of the person. These forces include biological, psychological, and social dynamics, as well as the external physical surroundings.

#### Health

**Health** is a state of physical and mental functioning. It can exist in a continuum that ranges from wellness to death.

The functions of a psychiatric mental health nurse in providing nursing care in the mental health setting are shown in Table 2-1.

TABLE 2–1. **Functions of Nurses in the Psychiatric-Mental Health Setting**

| | |
|---|---|
| Health promotions and health maintenance | Health teaching |
| Intake screening and evaluation | Crisis intervention |
| Case management | Counseling |
| Milieu therapy | Home visit community action |
| Self-care activities | Advocacy |
| Psychobiologic interventions | |

Adapted with permission from Boyd, M., & Nihart, M. (1998). *Psychiatric nursing: Contemporary practice.* Philadelphia: Lippincott Williams & Wilkins.

The concept of what constitutes health can be affected by a person's value judgments. What is subjectively viewed as "good" or "bad" health by one person may be viewed differently by another. The perception of what constitutes good health by health care professionals may depend on the professional discipline of the caregiver, for example, nursing, medicine, psychology, or social work.

## THE ROLE OF NURSING IN ADDRESSING PSYCHOSOCIAL NEEDS

According to the prior definition of nursing practice, the nurse assesses the whole person using knowledge of normal and pathologic physical, psychological, and social functioning. In psychiatric-mental health nursing the whole-person focus continues, so that all aspects of a client's functioning are assessed. The primary cause of admission to a mental health setting, however, is some form of mental disorder or psychopathology that has caused a temporary incapacity in the client's ability to function in his or her normal social environment. **Psychopathology** is defined as disease of the mind. The medical approach to caregiving is based on a model of curing pathology or disease, whether physical or mental. Using this approach, there is usually a specific focus on curing the identified disease.

Nursing, on the other hand, views the disease process as the cause of distress to the whole person. The distress resulting from disease affects the person's overall sense of well being—physical, mental, and social. Nursing care involves assessing each of these functional domains. Care planning intervenes directly with the disease process using physicians' orders when necessary, as well as the guiding principles of nursing practice described in the preceding. In addition, the nurse assesses, plans, and implements care and continually evaluates the outcomes of care as measured by client responses in the physical, mental, and social domains. This assessment process uses the same holistic principles whether the person has a mental or physical disorder.

In the mental health setting the primary focus is on the cause of the admission. The client has a mental disorder that has changed his or her mental functioning. When mental functioning is disordered, it results in behavioral changes that affect social relationships. The major goals of nursing care planning and intervention are to work collaboratively with other mental health disciplines to set a cohesive set of therapeutic goals that support the client's recovery and return to psychosocial adaptation.

## ◆ ROLES AND FUNCTIONS OF THE LICENSED PRACTICAL AND VOCATIONAL NURSE

The role and functions of the LPN/LVN are based on many different standards and state regulations. The **Nursing Practice Standards of the Licensed Practical/Vocational Nurse** are developed by the National Federation of Licensed Practical Nurses. Each state in the United States has a board of nursing that makes recommendations to the state legislature and attorney general's office. These governing groups then write the statutes and regulations that define the specific **scope of practice** for the LPN/LVN. Scope of practice is the set of functions performed by a person working in a particular occupational role. All scope of practice rules and regulations are voted on by a state governing body before they are passed into law. Nursing practice standards of the LPN are discussed in Chapter 6, Professional, Legal, and Ethical Issues in Mental Health Nursing.

Each institution that employs the LPN/LVN has its own official protocols and procedures that further clarify the expected role of the LPN/LVN in that institution. The expected functions within that role are included in the LPN/LVN job description. A job description is a formal document that defines the expected work functions of the LPN/LVN in that institution. The job description also describes the limits of that role and the role of the supervisor who evaluates the quality of the work of the LPN/LVN.

The American Nurses Association is the organization that overviews the general climate of nursing in the United States. The organization developed the *Statement of Psychiatric-Mental Health Clinical Nursing Practice* and *Standards of Psychiatric-Mental Health Nursing Practice* in order to clarify the focus and scope of mental health nurses. Table 2-2 describes the types of problems that the mental health nurse addresses in all practice settings.

As described, the word role is a general term that refers to the functions customarily performed in a certain type of position. Within the field of nursing the term is used to describe two different perspectives on the functions of the nurse. They are (1) the different levels of

---

**TABLE 2–2. Clinical Problems Addressed by Psychiatric Mental Health Nurses**

---

Actual or potential mental health problems of clients pertaining to:

- The maintenance of optimal health and well-being and the prevention of psychobiologic illness
- Self-care limitations or impaired functioning related to mental and emotional distress
- Deficits in the functioning of significant biologic, emotional, and cognitive systems
- Emotional stress or crisis components of illness, pain, and disability
- Self-concept changes, developmental issues, and life process changes
- Problems related to emotions such as anxiety, anger, sadness, loneliness, and grief
- Physical symptoms that occur along with altered psychological functioning
- Alterations in thinking, perceiving, symbolizing, communicating, and decision making
- Difficulties in relating to others
- Behaviors and mental states that indicate the client is a danger to self or others or has a severe disability
- Interpersonal, systemic, sociocultural, spiritual, or environmental circumstances or events that affect the mental and emotional well-being of the individual, family, or community
- Symptom management, side effects/toxicities associated with psychopharmacologic intervention and other aspects of the treatment regimen

---

American Nurses Association, American Psychiatric Nurses Association, Association of Child and Adolescent Psychiatric Nurses, Society for Education and Research in Psychiatric-Mental Health Nursing. (1994). *Statement of psychiatric-mental health clinical nursing practice and standards of psychiatric-mental health clinical nursing practice.* Washington, DC: American Nurses Publishing.

Adapted with permission from Boyd, M., & Nihart, M. (1998). *Psychiatric nursing: Contemporary practice.* Philadelphia: Lippincott Williams & Wilkins.

---

nursing roles as determined by the educational preparation of the nurse, and (2) the customary functions or responsibilities that are within the practice guidelines for each level of nursing.

## ◆ TYPES OF NURSING ROLES IN MENTAL HEALTH SETTINGS

### LICENSED PRACTICAL/VOCATIONAL NURSE

Licensed practical/vocational nurses (LPN/LVNs) are employed in all mental health settings. Their functions within each type of mental health setting are related to the list of mental health client problems listed in Table 2-1. The registered nurse or other health team leader delegates the functions of the LVN. The delegated functions are described in the *Nursing Practice Standards for the Licensed Practical/Vocational Nurse.* These standards are related to promoting and maintaining mental health, preventing disease and disability, caring for and rehabilitating individuals who are experiencing an altered health state, and contributing to the ultimate quality of life until death.

### Registered Nurse

Registered nurses (RNs) have Associate's (ADN) or Bachelor's (BSN) Degrees in Nursing. In mental health settings registered nurses assess, create nursing diagnoses, and plan nursing care. Registered nurses are prepared to work with individuals, families, groups, and communities. They administer medications and evaluate outcomes of medications, including side effects of those medications. Registered nurses work under the authority of the physician who heads the mental health team, as well as the team leader or clinical coordinator overseeing clinical care.

### Clinical Nurse Specialist

**Clinical nurse specialists** (CNSs) are registered nurses with masters' or doctoral degrees in nursing. Most CNSs have completed board certification as specialists in mental health nursing by meeting the requirements of the American Nurses' Credentialing Center, the testing arm of the American Nurses Association. Clinical nurse specialists have broad clinical experience in planning, administering, and evaluating patient care in inpatient and outpatient mental health settings, including home care. They serve as team leaders on teams in inpatient settings, directing the care of clients by registered and licensed vocational nurses. Clinical nurse specialists also have clinical training in psychotherapy. Clinical nurse specialists in the inpatient setting work under the authority of the physician who heads the clinical unit. They have the skills and training to serve as the team leader or clinical coordinator overseeing clinical care in the mental health setting.

In most states the CNS is eligible to prescribe medications administered in the mental health setting, provided that he or she meets the requirements to obtain a special license. The license to prescribe medications is obtained after completing a master's or doctoral degree and requires additional training in the knowledge and management of psychotropic medications. Psychotropic medications are the pharmaceuticals used to treat psychiatric disorders. Each state has different requirements that a CNS must meet to obtain a medication-prescribing license. When this license is obtained the CNS uses the title Advanced Practice Registered Nurse (APRN) or a similar derivation of the name.

## ◆ THE ROLE OF THE LPN/LVN IN DIFFERENT SETTINGS

*Inpatient Setting.* Only a small percentage of individuals with mental disorders are treated in hospital settings because of the high cost of inpatient mental health treatment. A client is admitted when there is a need for structure and safety that cannot be provided at home or in the community. Often, one of the primary goals of inpatient admission is to stabilize the client's acute mental symptoms by using psychotropic medications, psychotherapy, group therapy, and the therapeutic milieu.

Licensed practical/vocational nurses are active care providers, performing many functions in the inpatient care setting. The scope of those functions is determined by the specific policies of a hospital, community treatment center, or home care agency. The RN is responsible for assigning specific patient care assignments to the LPN/LVN, including explaining the guidelines for administering care and performing nursing care activities. All nursing care in mental health settings is planned within the context of the mental health interdisciplinary team goals for discharge.

*Outpatient Clinic.* Many individuals are able to obtain community treatment in clinic or private clinical therapy settings. Registered nurses are often adjunctive care providers in outpatient clinic settings. They give medications and monitor the clinical environment. Licensed practical/ vocational nurses employed in these settings work in supportive roles to those of the RN.

*Home Care.* The home care setting offers the client the opportunity to be in his or her natural environment and test new ways of coping; this is the environment that offers the highest degree of control to the client. The RN is the **case manager** or **team leader** in the home responsible for the coordination of care. He or she supervises and assigns the functions of the LPN/LVN in home care settings. The primary need of the client is to have a plan with structure that will augment and strengthen his or her normal coping methods. If the admission was coordinated by a crisis assessment home care team, the recommendations and orders derived from the crisis assessment will direct the initial nursing care and structure of the home care setting.

Another important need of the client is to have support from his immediate family or others who live in the home. The LPN/LVN is in a good position to observe the quality and nature of these relationships; in addition, the nurse can assist the client to interpret and respond to others in an adaptive manner. The nurse is also in an important position to interpret the behavior and needs of the client with his or her family or those in the home environment.

The steps of the nursing process are in a dynamic state in the home because events that can affect the client are more likely to occur than when he or she is in a protected hospital environment. Family therapy consultation can be considered in order to provide a more supportive and adaptive home environment when events in the home appear to have a direct impact on the stability of the client.

The client participates in all aspects of assessment, planning, implementation, and evaluation. The discussions among the LPN/LVN, client, and home caregiver can become the model for communication in the family. Reviewing daily activities and events that are most challenging or threatening for the client can assist in supporting decision making and effective coping. The home care nurse communicates and coordinates care with other members of the home care team.

Another important member of the team is the **home health aide**; an individual who has received special training in the basic skills required to provide support to clients in the type of care setting where he or she is employed. The home health aide follows the directions of the RN or LPN/LVN in knowing the specific types of care required by a client. The nurse communicates with and provides supervision to the home health aide. The communication supports the nursing care plan addressing specific behaviors or problems.

*Correctional/Prison Facilities.* Nearly 2,000,000 persons are incarcerated in the U.S. Between 1980 and 1995 the population of prisoners in state and federal prisons nearly tripled, primarily due to the escalating federal War on Drugs program. As a result, there was significant overcrowding in prisons and a corresponding need for health services. Because prisoners are often from lower socioeconomic circumstances, this population experiences a wide range of health problems. A nurse who works with prison populations is called a **correctional nurse**.

Weiskopf reports that these health problems include both physical and mental disorders. The National Commission on Correctional Health Care reported in 1997 that between 6% and 14% of the prison population might have a psychiatric disorder. Of this number, approximately 72% have a *dual diagnosis*—a combination of more than one major psychiatric disorder, one of which is a substance use disorder. It has been reported that 82.2% of persons in the general prison population use drugs or alcohol or both. Because of the history of drug abuse before incarceration, many prisoners have serious mental and physical health problems. Alzheimer's disease and other types of dementia/cognitive mental disorders are prevalent in aging prison populations. Drug and alcohol disorders are important pre-existing conditions in many prisoners and are important contributing factors to the high incidence of dementia in older prisoners.

Weiskopf further suggests that nurses who work in correctional settings are challenged by the contrasts between the cultures of nursing and imprisonment. The caring culture of nursing includes the goals of promoting the health and well being of the patient and not inflicting harm or punishment. On the other hand, the goals of incarceration are retribution to society for criminal behavior, protection of society, reformation of the criminal, and deterrence of future crimes.

K E Y   P O I N T S

■ The word role describes the expected behaviors of a person engaged in a particular activity.

■ A function is a specific type of activity that belongs within the role expectations of a particular occupation.

■ *The Nursing Practice Standards of the Licensed Practical/Vocational Nurse* were developed by the National Federation of Licensed Practical Nurses.

■ Scope of practice is the set of functions performed by a person working in a particular occupational role.

■ A job description is a formal document that defines the expected work functions of an individual working in a specific occupational role in an institution.

■ A CNS is a registered nurse with a master's or doctoral degree in nursing who has completed board certification as a specialist in mental health nursing by passing a test that meets the requirements of the American Nurses Association.

■ Psychotropic medications are the pharmaceuticals used to treat psychiatric disorders.

■ The case manager or team leader supervises and assigns the functions of the LPN/LVN in mental health care settings.

### SELF-AWARENESS ACTIVITY

- Did you envision yourself as a nurse before you began your training as an LPN/LVN?

- What is that vision like?

- How do you look in that vision?

- What are you doing?

- Where are you?

- How do you feel as you experience that vision?

- As you have that vision in your mind, you are probably seeing yourself performing a particular nursing function within the role of the LPN/LVN. This is potentially an important image for you. It is the type of image that serves as a motivating force as you continue to learn more of the underlying knowledge on which the functions and different potential roles of the LPN/LVN are based.

## Q U E S T I O N S.

1. A scope of practice
   a. is the legally mandated set of functions performed by a person working in a particular occupational role.
   b. is established by an employing agency and provides a basis for evaluation.
   c. is a formal document that defines the expected work functions of the nurse in an institution.
   d. refers to suggested guidelines from the American Nurses Association.
2. Nursing models have identified four critical aspects or themes of nursing, including
   a. Person, Function, Holism, and Happiness.
   b. Biology, Psychology, Social Systems, and Practice.
   c. Person, Nursing, Environment, and Health.
   d. Assessment, Planning, Intervention, and Evaluation.
3. The role of the LPN/LVN in mental health settings
   a. is the same as that of the RN.
   b. includes caring for clients and prescribing medications.
   c. is the same as that of the home health aide.
   d. includes actions that promote and maintain mental health.
4. A nurse working in a correctional facility
   a. should not promote health and well being among his or her clients.
   b. rarely works with clients who have mental illness.
   c. will likely work with clients with more than one psychiatric diagnosis.
   d. is not held to the same legal standards as nurses in other facilities.

### BIBLIOGRAPHY

American Nurses Association, American Psychiatric Nurses Association, Association of Child and Adolescent Psychiatric Nurses, Society for Education and Research in Psychiatric Mental Health Nursing. (1994). *Statement of psychiatric mental health clinical nursing practice and standards of psychiatric mental health clinical nursing practice.* Washington, D.C.: American Nurses Publishing.

American Nurses Association. (1985). *Code for nurses with interpretive statements.* Washington, D.C.: American Nurses Association.

American Nurses Association. (1994). *Statement on the scope and standards of psychiatric-mental health clinical nursing practice.* Washington, D.C.: American Nurses Association.

Boyd, M. & Nihart, M. (1998). *Psychiatric nursing: Contemporary practice.* Philadelphia: Lippincott-Raven.

National Federation of Licensed Practical Nurses. (1996). *Nursing practice standards for the Licensed Practical Nurse.* Garner, NC: National Federation of Licensed Practical Nurses.

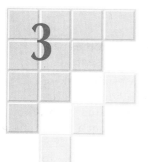

# 3

# Inpatient Hospitalization: The Mental Health Treatment Team and the Therapeutic Milieu

## Behavioral Objectives

*After reading this chapter the student will be able to:*

- Name the conditions that precede admission to an inpatient mental health treatment setting.
- Explain two benefits to the use of critical paths.
- Describe six members of the inpatient mental health treatment team and the clinical roles they fill.
- List three characteristics that contribute to effective mental health team communication.
- Describe the meaning of the concept *therapeutic milieu*.
- List the characteristics of a therapeutic environment.
- Describe the objectives of a therapeutic treatment team.

## Key Terms

- Clinical director
- Clinical psychologist
- Critical path
- Expressive therapist
- Head nurse/unit manager
- Licensed practical or vocational nurse
- Medication technician
- Mental status
- Occupational therapist
- Orderly
- Psychiatric aide
- Psychiatric social worker
- Psychiatrist
- Registered nurse
- Team communication
- Therapeutic milieu

Inpatient hospitalization of clients with mental disorders becomes necessary when one or more of the following conditions are present:

1. There is a change in mental status that increases the risk of harm to self or others so that safety must be provided. Admission can be voluntary or court ordered. **Mental status** is the state of mental functioning a person is demonstrating at a given time.

2. The normal social environment of the individual is not able to continue the emotional, physical, or financial support of the vulnerable, mentally disabled person.

3. There is a self-perception that the emotionally vulnerable individual is unable to cope effectively. The mental status of the individual must then meet the admission criteria of an inpatient psychiatric unit.

The average number of inpatient hospitalization days continues to decrease because of legislation supporting outpatient mental health care, plus increasingly stringent mental health care reimbursement mechanisms. Clients once regularly treated on an inpatient basis now often receive outpatient treatment or a combination of inpatient intervention and outpatient follow-up. See Chapter 4, Community-Based Treatment Settings for Mental Disorders, for more information.

Thus, when inpatient care is indicated, it must be planned in an aggressive manner designed to restore a person's effective coping ability as soon as possible. Such an objective requires rapid preadmission assessment; this includes selection of the appropriate inpatient setting to meet the particular needs of the person with a mental disorder. For example, a person with a substance-related disorder sometimes can be effectively treated in a partial hospitalization drug program. Certain characteristics of the client's history may indicate that he or she would be better suited to inpatient hospitalization in a local drug treatment center, whereas another person would be recommended to a residential drug treatment program in a different location.

## ◆ PRELIMINARY CARE PLANNING IN THE INPATIENT TREATMENT SETTING

Care planning for a newly admitted person with a mental disorder ideally begins before he or she is admitted. Consultation between the **clinical director,** usually a physician, and the **head nurse** or **unit manager** can assist in assigning an incoming client to a particular location on the unit that will provide a proper level of safety. In addition, the clinical director often preassigns the newly admitted person to a particular treatment team. The clinical leader of the team is called the team leader. He or she usually begins to consider treatment options before the newly admitted person arrives on the unit.

# ◆ CRITICAL PATHS

Quality assurance mechanisms track the most effective client care outcomes and cost-effective approaches in mental health settings. As data are assembled, patterns emerge indicating that certain types of care, when paired with specific diagnoses, produce better outcomes than others. These data are used to identify the most effective care for individuals with specific types of diagnoses. A **critical path** is the use of a specific care protocol for individuals with specific diagnoses. Examples of the types of diagnoses included in the critical path protocols include:

- Major depression
- Cognitive mental disorder
- Schizophrenia
- Chemical dependency
- Bipolar disorder

The advantage of using critical paths is that interventions can be predictably sequenced and planned; discharge planning within a specific number of days can occur more reliably. In addition, all members of the mental health team are working with a very specific treatment protocol. Integration of the goals of all members of the multidisciplinary team is more assured. The primary goal of inpatient hospitalization is to stabilize the client in a short period of time, so that a more rapid return to his or her normal environment can occur.

# ◆ THE MENTAL HEALTH TREATMENT TEAM

The ability to provide rapid and aggressive assessment and treatment in the inpatient setting requires a cohesive team of clinicians with comprehensive skills in assessing and treating mental disorders in a secure and supportive environment. These team members are named in the following with a brief description of their roles.

The clinical director of an inpatient unit is usually a psychiatrist. A **psychiatrist** is a physician who has attended medical school and completed at least 4 years of residency training as a psychiatrist. The care of inpatients is his or her ultimate responsibility. In addition to the clinical director, other inpatient staff psychiatrists usually assist in the care of clients by providing overall direction in assessment and care planning, provision of safety, and prescription of appropriate medications to ensure a therapeutic treatment outcome.

The head nurse or unit manager, usually a registered nurse, manages the physical environment and resources of the unit. He or she also supervises other registered nurses and nursing personnel on the unit.

The **registered nurse** in the psychiatric setting uses the nursing process to plan and implement the care of his or her assigned clients.

The philosophy and scope of practice of psychiatric nursing are presented in Chapter 7, Communicating in the Therapeutic Relationship. The nursing process is presented in Chapter 10, Nursing Process in the Mental Health Setting. The role of the registered nurse (RN) on the mental health team is to assess collaboratively the client's current problems and personal resources and develop a nursing care plan that provides for the safety and hygiene needs of the client as well as the other inpatients and the mental health team. The safety of all individuals on the unit, whether clients or staff members, is a major priority in nursing care. The nurse may also coordinate the therapeutic milieu (discussed elsewhere in this chapter) in inpatient settings. The administration of medications is a nursing function on most psychiatric units. Some units, however, have **medication technicians,** supervised by hospital pharmacists, who prepare and deliver medications to clients.

Other aspects of the nurse's role depend on a client's specific symptoms, the level of expertise of the nurse, and the particular norms of the unit regarding the functions of nurses. Other nursing personnel who work under the direction of the RN include the licensed practical or vocational nurse, psychiatric aide, and orderly.

The role of the **licensed practical or vocational nurse** (LPN/LVN) is to assist in the implementation of the nursing care plan, including assessing, implementing, and evaluating the client's current status. These observations are reported to the registered nurse, who uses the new data to evaluate the current nursing plan and modify nursing interventions to achieve the desired outcomes. Licensed practical or licensed vocational nurses also may be asked to prepare and deliver medication on psychiatric units.

The **psychiatric aide** is a member of the therapeutic team who receives his or her training in programs developed by the psychiatric institution. Usually this job category is found in large psychiatric institutions. Typically, general hospital psychiatric units do not have the inservice training capability to develop such a position. The psychiatric aide in most instances develops good assessment and intervention skills and is a valuable asset to the nursing team.

The **orderly** may be a permanently assigned member of the psychiatric team, depending on the size and resources of the psychiatric unit. This individual's presence is most important during critical incidents on the unit, when numbers of physically strong personnel are needed as a deterrent to loss of control in a client or group of clients.

Another member of the mental health team is the **clinical psychologist.** A clinical psychologist has attended 4 years of graduate school beyond college and usually 1 or 2 years of postdoctoral training. He or she is trained to administer psychological tests that can identify the specific causes of a person's mental dysfunction. Such information can be used to design strategic, symptom-related intervention. In addition, targeting the cause of symptoms usually assists physicians in selecting appropriate medications for reducing the symptoms.

Another important member of the mental health treatment team is the **psychiatric social worker.** He or she brings knowledge of community resources that can assist in the recovery of the person with mental illness. A psychiatric social worker is knowledgeable about the effect of family on the development, course, and treatment of mental disorders. He or she meets with family members during periods of hospitalization to obtain information about the client's family history and the context of the client's current need for hospitalization.

**Expressive therapists** are trained to use a special medium, such as art, music, drama, or other creative modalities, to allow expression of the emotional conflict that has caused the client's need for hospitalization. The client may be able to express the underlying conflict using one of these modalities, even though he or she may not have an intellectual understanding of the cause of his or her conflict. By using the insights gained through expressive work, an expressive therapist can assist clients in reaching a deeper understanding of why he or she became ill and how to address the resulting problems.

The **occupational therapist** is another important contributor to the treatment team. He or she designs activities in conjunction with clients that provide structured outlets for emotional or physical tensions. These activities also test the client's abilities to solve problems, set goals, maintain concentration, and perform purposeful tasks. The inability to participate in one or more of these functions can provide information to the team about the client's current clinical status and rate of improvement.

## ◆ COMMUNICATION WITHIN THE TREATMENT TEAM

The goals of inpatient treatment are to

- rapidly identify the symptoms that caused the need for hospitalization
- develop a treatment plan that will modify the symptoms
- identify the effective coping behaviors necessary to meet discharge requirements

Skilled mental health clinicians work as a team to assess and intervene in the comprehensive range of ineffective client behaviors that indicate mental disorder. The inherent factor that contributes to cohesive teamwork is mutual trust. Mutual trust can occur in an environment where there is general respect for the unique role and skills of each clinical discipline.

**Team communication** is the essence of effective care planning. Each discipline includes skills that can be used to evaluate specific aspects of behavior and functioning: mental status, social skills, cognitive status, vocational capacities, and so on. When the observations and identified client care goals of each discipline are discussed, the result can be a comprehensive plan designed to meet the unique and specific needs of each client.

An important consideration in team communication is that the unit management and members of the team recognize the value of ongoing evaluation of the team communication process. For example, does the team take the time to discuss and evaluate its own communication patterns? Does it recognize conflict? Does it provide a mechanism to work through the conflict? Does it take time away from the unit for a "day away" or "retreat" to evaluate its current status, ongoing goals, and deterrents to achieving those goals? Most teams find that prioritizing such questions allows for a higher level of professional performance and job satisfaction for each member of the team. Effective communication within the team supports the concept of the therapeutic milieu.

## ◆ THE THERAPEUTIC MILIEU

The term "milieu" is derived from the French words *ma*, meaning "my," and *lieu*, meaning "place." The phrase "my place" signifies a trusted environment where one can be real and authentic and respected for these qualities. The concept of the **therapeutic milieu** is based on the premise that an individual's "here and now" behavior is a reflection of his or her current reality and normal social interactions. This reflection offers insights about why the individual is having difficulty in his or her internal reality or social interactions with others. The treatment team can be most effective by assessing these "here and now" behaviors and designing interventions to modify them so that therapeutic client insights and outcomes can be realized.

In 1989 Jack identified several characteristics of a therapeutic milieu:

- Every interaction is an opportunity for therapeutic intervention.
- Clients must assume responsibility for their own behavior.
- Problem solving is achieved by discussion, negotiation, and consensus, rather than by a few authority figures.
- Community meetings exist to discuss information and interactions that apply to all staff and clients.
- Peer pressure is a useful and powerful tool.
- Inappropriate behaviors are dealt with as they occur.
- Communication is open and direct between the staff and clients.
- Clients are encouraged to participate actively in their own treatment and decision making on the unit.

- The unit remains in close contact with the community, and there is frequent communication with family and significant members of the client's social network.
- Usually the unit's door is unlocked, and the clients have access to areas beyond the unit.

The activities that promote open communication in the therapeutic milieu are shown in Table 3-1.

## ◆ THERAPEUTIC TEAM TREATMENT

By using these "here and now" therapeutic milieu concepts, the treatment team is able to develop a comprehensive list of the mental status symptoms, social interactive style, and behaviors that caused the client to be hospitalized. Therapeutic team treatment includes the following objectives:

1. Developing a team treatment plan to modify specific ineffective coping and social behaviors
2. Naming the objectives or goals of inpatient treatment for each of these ineffective behaviors
3. Describing the intervention plan for each member of the mental health treatment team with the client
4. Listing the mental status and coping criteria necessary for discharge
5. Describing the outpatient discharge recommendations of the team

---

**TABLE 3–1. Communication Strategies That Enhance the Therapeutic Milieu**

Leader of the team is known to clients

Roles of unit staff that interact with the client are known to client

Rules and norms of behavior on the unit are given to client

All issues raised by a client are addressed

Purpose of each meeting that client is expected to attend is told to client

All attendees in meeting introduce themselves

Keep meetings brief

Purpose of meeting, agenda, and topics to be addressed are announced at beginning of meeting

Questions that arise in meeting are recorded and addressed after the meeting, with follow-up communication as indicated

Extraneous discussion by others while the meeting is in progress is avoided

Difficult issues are openly and actively addressed

The most therapeutic inpatient hospitalizations are ensured when team planning occurs as described in the preceding. Well-synchronized team planning is the result of good clinical leadership and professional participation by each member of the team. Such planning and therapeutic outcomes can contribute significantly to the ongoing job satisfaction of each team member.

## K E Y    P O I N T S

- Inpatient hospitalization of a person with a mental disorder is necessary when
  - —a change in mental status increases the risk of harm to self and others.
  - —the individual's normal environment cannot support him or her.
  - —the individual's self-perception is that he or she cannot cope effectively.
- Therapeutic team treatment includes five objectives:
  - —Develop a team treatment plan to modify ineffective behaviors and coping devices.
  - —Name objectives or goals in the treatment for these behaviors.
  - —Describe the plan and role of each team member to the client.
  - —List the mental status and coping criteria necessary for discharge.
  - —Describe the team's recommendations for outpatient discharge.
- Communication and mutual trust are essential for effective functioning of a mental health treatment team.
- The concept of the therapeutic milieu focuses on addressing current client behavior, assessing how it reflects the client's inadequate coping or relational skills, and determining interventions to modify the ineffective behaviors.

### SELF-AWARENESS ACTIVITY

- Before you entered nursing, what was your opinion about individuals who have mental disorders?
- Have you ever known a family member or friend who was hospitalized with a mental disorder?
- How did you feel at the time this person was hospitalized?
- Why do you think this person was hospitalized?
- What do you think it would be like to be a patient on a psychiatric unit?
- What do you think it would be like to be a nurse on a psychiatric unit?

# QUESTIONS

1. The treatment team member who generally assesses client problems, develops a care plan for inpatient client safety and hygiene needs, and administers medication is the
   a. clinical psychologist.
   b. psychiatric social worker.
   c. registered nurse.
   d. orderly.
2. A critical path
   a. is used for clients whose condition is considered critical.
   b. is used only by nursing professionals.
   c. is developed for every psychiatric diagnosis.
   d. provides guidelines for interventions related to specific diagnoses.
3. When working in a therapeutic milieu, the nurse
   a. makes treatment decisions for the client.
   b. deals with inappropriate behaviors as they occur.
   c. ignores inappropriate behaviors so as not to reinforce them.
   d. encourages the client to rely on the treatment team for resolution of conflicts.
4. The factors that contribute *most* to cohesive teamwork on the treatment team are
   a. shared philosophies on therapeutic milieu and behavior.
   b. adequate certification and experience of all team members.
   c. abilities to avoid conflict and set treatment timetables.
   d. mutual trust and communication.

## BIBLIOGRAPHY

Boyd, M., & Nihart, M. (1998). *Psychiatric nursing: Contemporary practice.* Philadelphia: Lippincott Williams & Wilkins.

Cleary, M., Edwards, C., & Meehan, T. (1999). Factors influencing nurse–patient interactions in the acute psychiatric setting: An exploratory investigation. *Australian New Zealand Journal of Mental Health Nursing, 8*(3), 109–116.

Jack, L.W. (1989). Use of milieu as a problem-solving strategy in addiction treatment. *Nursing Clinics of North America, 24,* 69–80.

Jones, A. (1999). Pathways of care in the inpatient treatment of schizophrenia: An experimental project. *Mental Health Care, 2*(6), 194–197.

Jones, A., & Kamath, P. (1998). Issues for the development of care pathways in mental health services. *Journal of Nursing Management, 6*(2), 87–95.

Sadock, B., & Kaplan, H. (1998). *Synopsis of psychiatry: Behavioral sciences/clinical psychiatry.* Philadelphia: Lippincott Williams & Wilkins.

Thomas, S. (1999). Some challenges for mental health nurses in 1999. *Issues in Mental Health Nursing, 20*(1), 1–3.

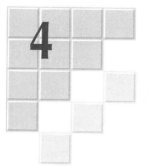

# Community-Based Treatment Settings for Mental Disorders

## Behavioral Objectives

*After reading this chapter the student will be able to:*

- Name three different groups of individuals who are outpatient mental health care consumers.
- List the different types of payment mechanisms used for community mental health services.
- Describe the five basic mental health services of a community mental health center.
- Explain two benefits of partial hospitalization programs.
- Name the three most common problems of the homeless mentally ill.
- Describe the differences between the services offered by community mental health centers and the assertive community treatment model of mental health care.

## Key Terms

- Assertive Community Treatment (ACT)
- Catchment area
- Community case manager
- Comprehensive community mental health center
- Dual diagnosis
- Medicaid
- Medicare
- Social breakdown syndrome

Active planning was implemented to treat people with mental disorders in their communities in order to decrease all health care costs. There are three major populations of individuals who may be community-based or outpatient mental health care consumers:

1. *The physically disabled or elderly infirm who require home services for mental health care.* These individuals use a variety of payment options that affect the quality and duration of their care at home. The first two payment options, Medicare and Medicaid, which are sponsored by the federal and state governments, are the most common options for individuals in this category. **Medicare** is a health insurance program offered by the federal government to persons who are over 65 years of age. It reimburses physicians and hospitals for care to elderly persons. This insurance is often supplemented by private health insurance by those who can afford it. **Medicaid** is a health insurance program funded by both the federal and state governments. It covers health care costs for adults under age 65 and children who are eligible for public aid programs.

    In addition to Medicare and Medicaid, health care costs are funded by private health insurance, health maintenance organizations, or self-pay. The clinical options open to these individuals include contracting for mental health services from visiting nurse associations, other public or private mental health caregiver groups, or private practitioners. Currently, it is estimated that there are 40,000,000 people with no health insurance in the United States. It is believed that this number is growing rapidly because of the increasing numbers of middle-class Americans who cannot afford to pay health insurance premiums.

2. *Individuals with nondisabling mental disorders who are able to continue working and fulfilling their normal social roles.* The ability of such individuals to continue their normal roles is supported by the use of psychotropic medications. Psychotropic medications alter the neurochemistry of the brain so that brain chemistry approaches more normal levels. Disabling mental symptoms are reduced to more comfortable levels. Outpatient individual or group therapy augments pharmacotherapy.

    Funding options for outpatient therapy and medications include partial funding by private health insurance, limited numbers of therapy sessions funded by health maintenance organizations, very restricted numbers of sessions funded by Medicaid and Medicare, or self-payment by those who have adequate resources. The individual who lacks financial or insurance resources will most often function at a borderline disabled level. This type of disabled mental functioning usually increases the risks not only to the individual, but also to his or her family members.

3. *Individuals who are psychiatrically disabled.* There is a growing percentage of people with chronic, disabling mental disorders

because of the decreasing public and private support for mental health services. This segment of the population is particularly affected by the current crisis in health care costs. The Community Mental Health Act legislated by the U.S. Congress in the 1960s was originally designed to provide a range of mental health care options to all people. Inadequate funding and lack of comprehensive policy planning left woeful gaps in care, particularly when accompanied by the national trend of deinstitutionalization. Currently, the most commonly used treatment option open to the chronically mentally ill client is the community mental health center.

## ◈ COMMUNITY MENTAL HEALTH CENTERS

The Community Mental Health Act states that a community mental health center should be accessible to the community it serves and that it should provide five basic services:

1. Inpatient treatment
2. Outpatient treatment
3. Partial hospitalization (day or night programs)
4. Emergency services on a 24-hour basis
5. Consultation and education services to community agencies, groups, and individuals

Five additional services, although not mandatory, are desirable in order to assist in the functioning, implementation, and continuity of the five basic services listed in the preceding:

1. Diagnostic services
2. Rehabilitation
3. Precare and aftercare
4. Training programs for professionals and nonprofessionals
5. Research and evaluation

A center is known as a **comprehensive community mental health center** when it offers all 10 of these services and is fully operational.

The Community Mental Health Act specifies that such a center must serve a specific area with a population between 75,000 and 200,000. This geographic area is known as a **catchment area.** In a densely populated urban area, such a maximum population may be found in fewer than 100 square blocks; in some remote rural areas, the minimum population may be scattered over hundreds of square miles. Therefore, the community mental health center is not always near the area of residents wanting or needing services. Nonetheless, travel time to the center should not exceed 1 hour if at all possible.

Of the delivery modalities within the community mental health system, two have enjoyed outstanding growth and appear to have permanently changed the face of psychiatric practice. They are crisis intervention and partial hospitalization or day-treatment programs. Almost all private and public mental hospitals have both partial hospitalization and crisis intervention services. Community-based home crisis intervention programs and community-based home care are described in Chapter 5, Home Care Setting: Client and Family Issues.

*Partial Hospitalization and Day or Evening Treatment Programs.* These programs are designed to meet the needs of two types of clients:

1. Those who were recently discharged from acute care institutions but require an overview by mental health professionals to continue their rehabilitation
2. Mentally ill individuals who are currently living at home or are homeless and who require stabilization in order to avoid inpatient hospitalization

Partial hospitalization programs are designed to meet the needs of their clients. They provide a structured environment that can avert inpatient hospitalization. These programs are designed to accommodate the schedules of clients who are employed; these individuals usually attend partial evening programs.

In an evening program, clients have an opportunity to discuss their coping concerns about work and family and find support from staff members and fellow attendees. Other clients who require supportive care during the day, when their family members may be out of the home at work or school, attend partial daytime programs.

*Assessment in a Partial Day or Evening Program.* The assessment of an individual newly admitted to a partial mental health program is comprehensive. It includes a review of the following factors:

- Physical health
- Psychosocial functioning
- Emotions
- Behavior
- Recreation
- Vocation
- Legal circumstances
- Nutrition

As each of these factors is assessed and addressed in the partial program, it is possible to plan interventions that support the individual in his or her normal social environment. Interventions that are based on daily reports of the individual's coping challenges can provide strong support for a successful return to his or her pre-crisis level of functioning.

# ◆ THE HOMELESS AND MENTAL ILLNESS

The political decision to deinstitutionalize people with chronic mental illness began with the active use of phenothiazine medications in the 1960s. These medications dramatically reduced the psychosis-induced instability of many individuals with serious mental disorders. Legislators at both the state and federal levels looked at the high cost of long-term psychiatric hospitalization. Social scientists assured them that community-based care would be in the best interests of all concerned, the mentally ill and the general tax-paying public.

It was believed that chronically mentally ill people who were institutionalized for extensive periods developed a social breakdown syndrome. The **social breakdown syndrome** includes the following characteristics: lack of initiative, submission to authority, withdrawal, and excessive dependence on the institution.

Although deinstitutionalization was humane in its original philosophy, the actual implementation of the concept has been seriously undermined by the lack of good community alternatives. It has been widely recognized that the largest group of users of public community mental health services are the poor. At this time, a large proportion of the individuals using community mental health treatment services are the "homeless" poor.

Nearly half of the homeless population is chronically mentally ill. The types of mental disorders experienced by the homeless are similar to those of persons across all social levels. They include mood disorders, anxiety disorders, schizophrenia, substance abuse, organic brain syndrome, personality disorders, post-traumatic stress disorders, developmental delays, and disabilities. It is the high incidence of these disorders in the homeless that continues to challenge the resources of community mental health programs and their staff members. The chronically mentally ill may frequently experience the dual diagnosis of functional mental illness, such as schizophrenia and addiction disorders. A **dual diagnosis** is the presence of two major types of mental disorder in one individual.

Chronic mentally ill individuals are often alienated from their families and are socially isolated. They avoid contact with social structures, such as community mental health treatment centers. Because of these factors they often discontinue their medications, become psychotic and disorganized, and begin to live on the street. Their lives are seriously endangered by their disordered mental states.

As noted, community-based crisis intervention and partial hospitalization programs are the most important deterrents to inpatient hospitalization. Two intervention models are currently offering these two types of outpatient care: community mental health centers, described earlier, and assertive community treatment, described below.

It is currently recognized that many homeless mentally ill individuals are resistant to the outreach of community mental health resources. Many homeless persons avoid contact with any type of health caregiver. Accordingly, by the time the homeless enter the health care system they are often acutely ill and their recovery is complicated by their delay in accessing care. Table 4-1 shows the types of comprehensive health services required by a homeless person who is in poor health.

### ◆ ASSERTIVE COMMUNITY TREATMENT

Community mental health professionals recognized the importance of **assertive community treatment** (ACT), an intervention model that uses assertive, active outreach to the homeless mentally ill and others who avoided coming to community mental health centers (CMHCs). Table 4-2 compares the differences in approach of these two major intervention models.

Early research on the cost-effectiveness of these two programs indicates that clients who are participating in ACT programs have fewer hospitalizations on an annual basis than those using CMHCs. The cost of the ACT program is higher on a per-client basis than that of the CMHC. The higher cost is offset by the higher psychiatric hospitalization patterns of CMHC clients or, more important, the higher psychiatric hospitalization patterns of the mentally ill who do not customarily use the CMHC services.

In contrast to the CMHC model, which requires that clients seek out services at the mental health center, the direct searching out of mentally ill people in the community ensures that a larger percentage of potential clients are reached. Additionally, the ACT model uses a case manager. The **community case manager** is the member of the mental health team who oversees all aspects of support, including direct mental health services, housing, physical care, and so on. The case manager is also the clinician providing direct care.

A case manager's ideal case load is around 10 to 12 clients, and allows for more active support of the client during precrisis periods. Government financial support for community mental health services for the indigent continues to be cut, however; accordingly, the numbers of clients managed by many community mental health case managers is increasing to a level that can cause a breakdown in the delivery system of such care.

An important component of the ACT care model is ongoing training in activities of daily living, such as communication, problem solving, and coping skills. Other important aspects of the case manager approach are medication overview and support regarding adequate housing and physical care. More detailed research on the ACT model

## TABLE 4-1. Essential Elements in a Comprehensive System of Health Care for the Homeless Mentally Ill

| Element | Rationale |
|---|---|
| Assertive outreach | • The effectiveness of this approach lies in addressing patients and their needs on their own turf. |
| | • Nurses who go out into the community to actively seek out those in need of care get to see first-hand how homeless people live; thus, obstacles to the wellness of the homeless are no longer merely academic. |
| Integrated case management | • Allows for coordination of multiple facets of care. |
| | • Primary goals are to: Identify the patient's needs Provide for continuity of care *after* discharge Ensure that care and services provided are effective |
| Safety | • Recuperative powers may depend on ability to escape the corrosive physical and psychological stresses associated with homelessness. |
| | • A secure shelter affords a measure of privacy that may foster recuperation. |
| Treatment of mental illness | • Accurate diagnosis and treatment of mental illness are important to increase the possibility of breaking the cycle of poverty. |
| | • Treatment often involves long-term follow-up care and, in many cases, psychotherapy. |
| Housing | • Must be secure and afford privacy but be linked to other supportive services. |
| | • Many persons need help with basic tasks such as managing a household and budget and meal preparation. |
| Alcohol and drug abuse treatment | • Must meet the need for detoxification, treatment, and support through recovery. |
| | • Substance abuse is a big problem among the homeless population. |
| Health care | • The harsh conditions of homelessness put tremendous stress on the human body and can shorten the life span. |
| | • Provision of adequate health care helps reduce this risk. |
| Income support and benefit | This includes advising homeless persons of their eligibility for and assisting them in gaining access to: |
| | • Supplemental Security Income (SSI) |
| | • Social Security Disability Insurance (SSDI) |
| | • Aid to Families with Dependent Children |
| | • Food stamps |
| | • State and local welfare programs |
| | • Veterans' benefits |

*(continues)*

### TABLE 4-1. Essential Elements in a Comprehensive System of Health Care for the Homeless Mentally Ill *(Continued)*

| Element | Rationale |
|---|---|
| Rehabilitation, vocational training, and employment assistance | • Provide access to rehabilitation measures that will support the homeless mentally ill person in establishing and maintaining interpersonal relationships, including those in the realm of employment.<br>• Teach a range of skills—from general interpersonal skills to more specific skills that prepare them to obtain and maintain gainful employment. |
| Consumer and family involvement | • With supportive counseling, estranged families, which are a generally overlooked resource, can be engaged to help homeless persons regain their equilibrium.<br>• Homeless persons and their families must be helped to understand and exercise their rights as consumers and taught how to access reliable supportive services. |
| Legal protection | • Assist in obtaining legal protection to help manage financial difficulties, both *before* and *after* the onset of homelessness.<br>• Recognize the need to interface with the criminal justice system when necessary and gain access to a range of other rights of which they might otherwise be unaware. |
| Improved service delivery | • Advocate ongoing research and community education.<br>• Advocate the timely re-education of service providers. |

and its cost effectiveness can support its use and increased availability to the chronically mentally ill, who are the primary users of community psychiatry services.

K E Y   P O I N T S

- Three major populations are treated in community-based or outpatient settings:
  —Physically disabled or elderly individuals needing mental health care
  —Individuals with nondisabling mental disorders
  —Individuals who are psychiatrically disabled
- Insurance reimbursement for mental health services is derived from a number of sources: Medicaid, Medicare, private health insurance, and managed care organizations.
- It is estimated that 40,000,000 Americans have no health insurance.
- Community mental health centers should be accessible to the community and provide inpatient and outpatient services, day or night

**TABLE 4–2. Comparison of Characteristics of Assertive Community Treatment (ACT) and Community Mental Health Center (CMHC) Programs**

| Characteristic | ACT | CMHC |
|---|---|---|
| Treatment base | Predominantly in the community | In the community, but predominantly in the clinic |
| Staffing | Clinical staff-to-client ratio of around 1:10 | Clinical staff-to-client ratio of around 1:30–50 |
| Frequency of contact | Daily in most cases | Usually once every 1 or 2 weeks |
| Frequency of contact with family or support structure | Average of once a week | Occasional |
| Medication | Responsibility of staff; can be administered by staff daily if needed | Responsibility of client or family |
| Physical health | Monitored by program staff | Therapist and case manager encourage a healthy lifestyle |
| After-hours service | Monitored by program staff; team on call | Provided by therapist or case manager during day hours, emergency room or mobile team otherwise |
| Occupational rehabilitation | Actual job placement or volunteer job | Psychosocial programs |
| Housing arrangement | Responsibility of staff | Varies, but usually responsibility of client and family |
| Continuity of care | Team follows case through hospitalization; maintains legal, health system, and other contacts | Responsibility of therapist and case manager |
| Staff structure | Team structure: integration of clinical and case management roles | Individual staff model: therapist and case manager are different individuals |

From *Hospital and Community Psychiatry, 41*(6), p. 643, 1990. Copyright 1990, the American Psychiatric Association. Reprinted by permission.

programs (partial hospitalization), 24-hour emergency services, and consultation/education services.

■ Nearly half the homeless population is chronically mentally disordered, and the homeless poor are a large proportion of those using community mental health services.

■ Assertive community treatment focuses on direct outreach to and supervision of clients. Assertive community treatment also provides ongoing training for clients in communication, coping, and other activities of daily living.

## SELF-AWARENESS ACTIVITY

- What is your first feeling when you see a homeless person?
- What is your first thought when you see a homeless person?
- What is your reaction to reading that nearly 50% of homeless persons are mentally ill?

## QUESTIONS

1. The nurse working in a community mental health center would expect most of his or her clients to be
   a. people with schizophrenia.
   b. people with substance-related mental disorders.
   c. people with chronic mental illness.
   d. people recently released from psychiatric hospitals.
2. Of the following, which is *not* one of the five basic services offered by a community health center?
   a. Inpatient and outpatient treatment
   b. Partial hospitalization
   c. Emergency service
   d. Research
3. Advantages of partial hospitalization programs include
   a. no documentation for health care professionals.
   b. decreased flexibility for clients to work and maintain normal social contacts.
   c. provision of a structured environment that can avert hospitalization.
   d. all of the above.
4. A catchment area is
   a. the 10-square-mile area directly adjacent to a psychiatric hospital.
   b. an area zoned for a community mental health center.
   c. a geographic area with population between 75,000 and 200,000.
   d. an urban area where people with mental disorders tend to meet.

## BIBLIOGRAPHY

Aboleda-Florez, J. (2000). Homeless shelter users in the postdeinstitutionalization era. *Canadian Journal of Psychiatry, 45*(1), 55–62.

Boyd, M., & Nihart, M. (1998). *Psychiatric nursing: Contemporary practice.* Philadelphia: Lippincott Williams & Wilkins.

Malla, A., Norman, R., & Scholten, D. (2000). Predictors of service use and social conditions in patients with psychotic disorders. *Canadian Journal of Psychiatry, 45*(3), 269–273.

Stuart, H., Sadock, B., & Kaplan, H. (1998). *Synopsis of psychiatry: Behavioral sciences/clinical psychiatry.* Philadelphia: Lippincott Williams & Wilkins.

Torrey, W., & Wyzik, P. (2000). The recovery vision as a service improvement guide for community mental health providers. *Community Mental Health Journal, 36*(2), 209–216.

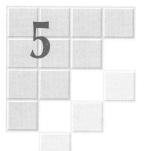

# 5

# Home Care Setting: Client and Family Issues

---

## Behavioral Objectives

*After reading this chapter the student will be able to:*

- Identify the core value of mental health home care.
- List the six holistic health care priorities.
- Describe the importance of nursing assessment in the home care environment.
- List the six reasons why mental health home care is preferable.
- Define intense brief intervention and describe how it is different from traditional home care.

---

## Key Terms

- Collaborative care plan
- Family
- Holistic health care priorities
- Intense brief intervention
- Neuropsychiatric changes
- Social network
- Social system
- Respite care
- Triangle

Home care nursing has seen a nearly threefold increase in size and scope during the last decade. All specialties in nursing, except for intensive and emergency care, have shifted to the home care arena. This shift is a response to the rapidly changing insurance programs of managed medical care, as described in previous chapters. These programs, which are increasingly dictating the health services available to the general public, have mandated a decrease in the cost of all health care. It is interesting to note that the practice arena of nursing has returned to its roots—the home.

## ◆ THE NEW OPTION OF HOME CARE FOR TREATMENT OF MENTAL DISORDERS

### HOME CARE VERSUS HOSPITALIZATION

Traditionally, psychiatric–mental health nursing in the general hospital setting has focused directly on the client. Hospital-based care shifts the client from his or her normal social environment into the unnatural location and experience of the hospital for assessment, treatment, and stabilization.

Table 5-1 compares and contrasts the different perspectives of the medical model, which is practiced in the majority of hospital settings, with the psychosocial rehabilitation model that can be used in home care nursing. In contrast to the medical model of care, the psychosocial model contains components of openness that can support the unique needs and strengths of the client and his or her family in their normal surroundings.

Inpatient admission to the hospital setting is essential in many circumstances. These circumstances include times when the mental symptoms cause

- Risk to the life of the client or others
- The inability of the client and/or family to medicate with appropriately ordered psychotropic medications
- Exhaustion, dysfunction, or any other circumstance that prevents the family or social network from providing the client with a secure environment
- A need for community mental health services when no adequate services are available to meet the individual's needs

In this book, **family** is an inclusive term that means a person's immediate and extended family members who are blood relatives. In addition, the term family is used to designate individuals who are not relatives but reside in the same home and provide significant support for the client. A **social network** comprises all those people whom an individual views as important sources of support. A **social system** is a comprehensive term that includes an individual's family and social network, as well as the general social environment in which he or she lives.

The following section describes the care philosophy and approaches that can contribute to positive outcomes for the client, family or social system, and health care providers.

## ◆ THE PHILOSOPHY OF HOME CARE NURSING

The core value that underlies the philosophy of home care nursing is the ideal of returning the individual to a pre-crisis level of functioning within his or her normal social environment. This ideal also includes

TABLE 5–1. **Comparison of Medical and Psychosocial Rehabilitation Models**

| Medical | Psychosocial Rehabilitation |
|---|---|
| Illness, disease, symptoms | Wellness, health, symptoms deemphasized |
| Person's disability | Person's ability |
| Institutional settings | Normalizing settings |
| Unnatural environments | Natural environments |
| Intrapsychic functioning | Functional behavior |
| Expert to patient | Adult to adult |
| Minimize stress | Take risks |
| Medicate until symptoms are controlled | Minimum amount of medication, symptoms okay |
| Practitioner makes decisions, prescribes treatment | Member and case manager identify strengths and develop a plan for change |
| Dependence and caretaker approach | Self-help, interdependence, support symptoms approach |
| Low expectancy | High expectancy |

Thompson, J., & Strand, K. (1994). Psychiatric nursing in a psychosocial setting. *Journal of Psychosocial Nursing, 32*(2), p. 27. Used with permission.

recognition of the potential for psychosocial adaptation and growth to the highest innate ability of the client and family.

The philosophy of home care nursing is based on the following six **holistic health care priorities,** listed in order of their importance:

1. Life sustenance
2. Security
3. Integrity and balance of the family/social system
4. Integrity of the individual (physical, mental, and spiritual)
5. Discovery of inner strengths and resources to support growth and change
6. Contribution to the betterment of self and others

Assessment of the status of each of these goals can provide the structure for prioritizing decision making at each stage of the nursing process.

These goals are formulated to provide a framework for humane and responsible care of individuals who have mental or physical conditions. They can be generalized to psychosocial nursing care. This home care nursing framework is intended to guide the nurse in maintaining, restoring, or supporting the development of an environment in which the client's holistic sense of well being can potentially occur. Implicit in these goals is the collaborative planning process with nurse, client, and family.

The use of this model in the home care setting recognizes the important role of the family in providing the environment in which rehabilitation and restoration of health and balance can occur. The significance of the assessment phase of the nursing process in the home care environment is emphasized. The nurse's astuteness is essential in recognizing the capabilities and resources within the family to provide the first three of the preceding requirements during an acute phase of mental disorder in a family member.

Also implicit in this model of care planning is the recognition that the client's ability to regain his or her pre-crisis level of functioning depends partly on the family's capacity to provide a stable environment. The assessment of the home environment's capacity to support this provision of adequate care includes the nurse's awareness of the capabilities and current needs of the primary caregiver to provide and maintain the precrisis home environment.

## USING THE MENTAL HEALTH CLINICAL NURSE SPECIALIST TO ASSESS INEFFECTIVE COPING IN THE HOME CARE SETTING

Home health care agencies are increasingly adding the role of mental health clinical nurse specialist to their nursing staffs. The incentives to include this consultant in their home care nursing personnel are related to the aging population and the common incidence of changes in mental state that may accompany physical illness in this population. For example, it is common for different medications customarily used in medically ill elderly persons to create changes in mental state, such as depression and anxiety. Older clients also may experience ineffective coping responses to their physical illnesses. Alternatively, the burden of home care may impose unusual stresses in a family; in such a case, the family will benefit from the recommendations of the mental health clinical specialist.

## IDENTIFYING COMMUNITY SUPPORT SERVICES DURING THE ASSESSMENT PHASE

During this initial phase of assessment, the nurse reviews current and potential gaps in family or caregiver resources that can decrease effective client rehabilitation or exhaust the family's caregiving resources. Recognition of these gaps in resources motivates the nurse to plan collaboratively with the client and primary caregiver for community services to support the home care environment during the time of increased demand on the family.

## IDENTIFYING SOURCES OF SUPPORT WITHIN THE FAMILY OR SOCIAL NETWORK

The nurse also can talk with the client and primary caregiver about calling on the extended family or social network for additional support during times of greater need. It is important to note that, during the initial phase of mental crisis, the primary caregiver is often unable to ascertain his or her personal reserves and the availability of additional family or social supports that may be available to provide respite care.

**Respite care** is possible when extended family or community resources can be called on to provide care for the ill individual in the home to allow rest and recovery for the primary caregiver. Early discussion of the importance of respite care is more likely to ensure the ongoing health of the caregiver and to enhance his or her ability to provide an optimal environment for the client's rehabilitation.

## ◆ BASIC PRINCIPLES OF MENTAL HEALTH REHABILITATION

In 1986, the California Nurses' Association presented an outline of the belief system that is recommended for use as a foundation for mental health and psychosocial rehabilitation. The five basic principles of this belief system are as follows:

1. Each individual has an inherent capacity for change.
2. Ideologies and practices that define the person in terms of mental illness dehumanize the individual.
3. Individual freedom of choice and conscious self-direction are central to change.
4. Interpersonal relationships are essential for bringing about change.
5. Behavior cannot adequately be understood apart from the context in which it occurs.

Table 5-2 reviews the overall values that can contribute to restoring the individual to his or her highest potential. The use of these principles in planning and implementing the mental health nursing care plan enhances the holistic health and integrity of the home care client and family.

## ◆ CRITERIA FOR ASSESSMENT OF SAFE MENTAL HEALTH HOME CARE

When adequate community mental health services are present and the home environment is relatively stable, with a capable caregiver in attendance, home care is preferable for the following reasons:

- Nursing staff are able to assess the status of the client in his or her normal social surroundings and plan individual and home support in a more realistic setting.
- The capacity of the client to perform normal activities of daily living can be observed and specific planning can be recommended more reliably.

**TABLE 5–2. Philosophy of Psychosocial Rehabilitation**

Psychosocial rehabilitation is approached with the following basic values about all people who are engaged in a rehabilitation process:

- The individual contains untapped emotional, physical, and spiritual resources and potentials that can be utilized in the rehabilitation process.
- The individual has a learning and adaptive ability to acquire new coping and vocational skills.
- A holistic approach that recognizes the full capacities of the individual is preferred, rather than one that attends solely to addressing the physical disability.
- The unique capacities and needs of the individual are assessed and supported.
- A collaborative planning process actively involves the client in treatment planning and desired outcomes.
- Care planning involves assessment of the re-entry needs of the client to his or her pre-existing psychosocial environment, including family, social, and vocational arenas.
- The psychosocial assessment of re-entry needs includes communicating with individuals from the home and vocational arenas for reviewing the value systems and reality-based issues that could impact successful re-entry and creating specific approaches to address those needs.
- Care is provided using an integrated care approach by a rehabilitation team with appropriate assessment skills.
- Community and other external resources are utilized in the care planning and delivery of care.

- The normal role in the home of the mentally disordered individual can be more rapidly resumed.
- The client and family are spared the social stigma of psychiatric hospitalization.
- The client and family are saved the financial burden of hospitalization.
- The home health nurse is able to serve as a role model for effective communication with the client and others in the home setting.

Two stages of mental health care are most frequently treated in the home:

1. The acute initial phase of the mental health crisis, when hospitalization can be averted
2. The stabilization phase of the mental health crisis, when discharge from a traditional inpatient setting to an adequately supported home environment may occur

## ◆ HOME CARE SERVICES FOR THE PERSON IN A MENTAL HEALTH CRISIS

Forward-thinking community mental health programs have instituted a new segment of community mental health nursing: home-based mental health crisis intervention. The operating mode and intention of this intervention model are to provide emergency mental assessment and nursing care for individuals using the following general criteria for the assessment of clients at risk:

- The person lives in a predetermined geographic location.
- The person meets specific age criteria (eg, aged 16 to 65).
- The person may be having his or her first mental health crisis or may have a prior psychiatric history.
- There is a stable home environment with adequate community or home support available for the individual to be treated in the home.

The key to success in early intervention community crisis treatment is the presence of a team or teams of mental health nurses who are trained and prepared to intervene in the home when a mental health crisis threatens the well being of a client or others. This type of model uses a rapid assessment team of nurses who respond to a primary caregiver or medical specialist's call for emergency mental health assessment.

These nurses are authorized to arrange direct hospital admission or referral to an acute care mental health home treatment team. According to a 1994 study, 25% of the individuals referred to the service were admitted directly to the hospital, rather than being treated at home.

## ACUTE CARE MENTAL HEALTH HOME TREATMENT TEAM

The purpose of the acute care mental health home treatment team is to provide intensive support in the community to those who are at risk for or are already in a mental health crisis. An essential part of this referral is a planning meeting among the nurses who perform the initial rapid mental and home assessment and nurses on the acute care team who will direct the home care process and provide care.

It is important to note that this form of acute mental health home treatment differs from traditional mental health home care (described in the next section). The character of this early mental health intervention can be described as intense brief intervention. **Intense brief intervention** is a mental health intervention that occurs wherever a client lives. The purpose of the intense brief intervention approach is to rapidly provide acute mental health treatment to an individual who is at risk for hospitalization. This care is provided with the services of a community mental health team, usually consisting of a clinical nurse specialist in psychiatry and mental health as well as other members of the psychiatric care team who assist in lowering the risk of imminent hospitalization.

Mental health providers, clients, and their families describe the acute home treatment model as preferable to hospitalization when inclusion criteria are met. An essential aspect of readiness to provide this type of community care is the immediate availability of a psychiatrist for consultation about treatment setting, medications, and other critical issues that can determine successful intervention outcomes. Research about client outcomes and cost-effectiveness of this type of early-intervention acute mental health care will continue to determine refinements of this approach.

## TRADITIONAL MENTAL HEALTH COMMUNITY AND HOME CARE

The functions of the mental health home care nurse are to provide mental health assessment and nursing care planning and intervention when changes in mental state occur in the following individuals:

- Older adults
- Those with neuropsychiatric changes associated with AIDS. **Neuropsychiatric changes** are caused by the physical deterioration of the anatomy and physiology of the brain, resulting in changes in mental status that produce one or more types of mental disorder.
- Those being treated at home for physical health problems who develop ineffective coping
- Those with chronic mental disorders
- Family members of seriously mentally disturbed children

Another function of the mental health home care nurse is to provide psychosocial support to the primary caregiver and others involved in the care of these clients. The mental health home care nurse may also be called on to consult with the home care nurse generalist in the physical care setting to obtain clinical recommendations for clients or their family members who are coping ineffectively with the strain of physical illness.

## ◆ COLLABORATIVE CARE WITH OTHER HEALTH CARE DISCIPLINES

The nurse who provides psychiatric home care develops collaborative care plans with caregivers from other disciplines. A **collaborative care plan** is one developed by a multidisciplinary mental health team. Communication in home care can be more challenging than in general hospital settings where the client's chart is in a central location and accessible at all times by all care disciplines.

The multidisciplinary home care team can include an occupational therapist, social worker, home care generalist (in the event there is a concurrent physical condition), physical therapist, speech therapist, and home health aide.

## AVOIDANCE OF CONFLICT WITH OTHER CAREGIVERS

Because of the variety of care disciplines in the home care setting, it can be helpful to be aware of the potential for creating conflict when making statements to the client or his or her family. The following scenario illustrates a common example.

While the nurse is with the client, a family member states that the social worker disagreed with a statement the nurse had made the day before. The nurse becomes angry and expresses her anger to the family member. The nurse then returns to her office and tells her clinical supervisor, who makes a call to the social worker's manager to report the incident.

In this scenario, the dynamic of triangulation occurs. A **triangle** is a social dynamic that begins with a conflict between two people. Instead of addressing the problem directly, however, one of the two people describes the conflict to a third person. The third person may then become embroiled in a conflict that he or she never witnessed; such a scenario is called triangulation. The third person may even go on to describe the alleged incident to yet another individual who also may become enmeshed.

Indeed, the family member may have misunderstood the initial event described in the preceding. To reduce the possibility of this type of miscommunication, it is wise not to discuss an alleged statement with anyone other than the individual to whom it has been attributed. Another recommendation is not to discuss it with the family member; the nurse can discuss it later with a clinical supervisor for recommendations about the best course of action to pursue.

## KEY POINTS

- The philosophy of home care nursing has the core value of returning the individual to his or her pre-crisis level of functioning and recognizes the client's and family's potential for psychosocial growth and adaptation.
- Home care nursing recognizes six holistic health care priorities: life sustenance, security, family/social system integrity and balance, integrity, discovery of inner resources to support growth, and contribution to the betterment of self and others.
- Assessment of the home environment includes the client's needs as well as the ability of those in the home environment to provide adequate support, including community support, family or social network, and respite care.
- Home care is preferable because the nursing staff can assess the status of clients in their normal social surroundings, plan individual and home support in a more realistic setting, restore mentally disor-

dered individuals to their normal role in the home, and spare the client and family the stigma and expense of psychiatric hospitalization.

■ The key to success in early intervention community crisis treatment is the presence of a team or teams of mental health nurses who are trained to intervene when a client experiences a mental health crisis.

■ Nurses often must work closely with other disciplines involved in a client's health care. Developing collaborative care plans and avoiding conflict and poor communication practices such as triangulation are essential.

## SELF-AWARENESS ACTIVITY

All families are complex social systems, with rules, secrets, and intricate dynamics that operate between each member of the family and frequently affect each person in the family. The questions in the following are about your family and may also give you an opportunity to understand why home care nursing can be challenging. Illness adds its own level of stress in a family and can activate different types of stress reactions in each member of the family.

- What happens in your family when one person is under more stress than usual?
- Do you begin to see the effects in the family system?
- What are some of the results of this type of stress in your family?
- Is there a peacemaker in your family?
- Is there someone in your family who stirs up trouble or conflict between other family members?

## QUESTIONS

1. The nurse working with clients in the home is aware that one of his or her primary roles is to
   a. teach the family to live with a client's maladaptive behavior.
   b. be a role model for effective communication.
   c. advocate closure of all inpatient facilities.
   d. accept that most mental health clients do not really improve.
2. Which of the following is the highest holistic health care priority?
   a. Security
   b. Life sustenance
   c. Family/social system integrity and balance
   d. Contribution to the betterment of self and others

3. Home care is preferable because
   a. home care can substitute for community care.
   b. nursing staff are able to assess the client's status in his or her normal social surroundings.
   c. home care costs more.
   d. the client does not have to participate in activities of daily living.
4. Successful collaborative care plans include
   a. communicating with other care discipline practitioners, such as social workers or occupational therapists.
   b. using the dynamic of triangulation to resolve conflict.
   c. discussing disagreements with everyone to make sure they are fully informed.
   d. all of the above.

## BIBLIOGRAPHY

Barry, P.D. (1996). *Psychosocial nursing: Care of physically ill patients and their families* (3rd ed.). Philadelphia: Lippincott-Raven.

Boyd, M., & Nihart, M. (1998). *Psychiatric nursing: Contemporary practice.* Philadelphia: Lippincott Williams & Wilkins.

California Nurses' Association. (1986). *The psychiatric-mental health position statement.* San Francisco: California Nurses' Association.

Cnaan, L., & Blankertz, M. (1992). Perceptions of consumers, practitioners, and experts regarding psychosocial rehabilitation principles. *Psychosocial Rehabilitation Journal, 16*(1), 93–119.

Iglesias, G. (1998). Role evolution of the mental health clinical nurse specialist in home care. *Clinical Nurse Specialist, 12*(1), 38–44.

Lefley, H. (1998). Families, culture, and mental illness: Constructing new realities. *Psychiatry, 61*(4), 335–355.

Sadock, B., & Kaplan, H. (1998). *Synopsis of psychiatry: Behavioral sciences/clinical psychiatry.* Philadelphia: Lippincott Williams & Wilkins.

Thompson, J., & Strand, K. (1994). Psychiatric nursing in a psychosocial setting. *Journal of Psychosocial Nursing, 32*(2), 27.

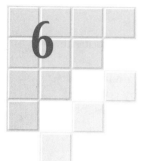

# 6

# Professional, Legal, and Ethical Issues in Mental Health Nursing

---

## Behavioral Objectives

*After reading this chapter the student will be able to:*

- ■ Discuss professional codes for nurses.
- ■ Define socialization, values, and ethics.
- ■ Explain the following legal terms:
  Nurse Practice Act
  Involuntary Commitment
  Competency
- ■ Summarize the rights of a hospitalized person with a mental illness, including:
  The Right to Treatment
  The Right to Informed Consent
  The Right to Confidentiality

---

## Key Terms

- ■ Competency
- ■ Consent
- ■ Ethics
- ■ Habeas corpus
- ■ Involuntary commitment

- ■ Nurse Practice Acts
- ■ Socialization
- ■ Standards
- ■ Statutes
- ■ Value

---

## ◆ THE CODE FOR NURSES

The primary role of nurses is to safeguard the well-being of people entrusted to their care. People receiving nursing services expect nurses to act ethically and professionally. The American Nurses Association (ANA) provides a framework for ethical nursing practice in *The Code for Nurses*, which was revised in 1985. The following are components of this code:

1. The nurse provides services with respect for human dignity and the uniqueness of the client, unrestricted by considerations of social or economic status, personal attributes, or the nature of health problems.
2. The nurse safeguards the client's right to privacy by judiciously protecting information of a confidential nature.
3. The nurse acts to safeguard the client and the public when health care and safety are affected by the incompetent, unethical, or illegal practice of any person.
4. The nurse assumes responsibility and accountability for individual nursing judgments and actions.
5. The nurse maintains competence in nursing.
6. The nurse exercises informed judgment and uses individual competence and qualifications as criteria in seeking consultation, accepting responsibilities, and delegating nursing activities to others.
7. The nurse participates in activities that contribute to the ongoing development of the profession's body of knowledge.
8. The nurse participates in the profession's efforts to implement and improve standards of nursing.
9. The nurse participates in the profession's efforts to establish and maintain conditions of employment conducive to high-quality nursing care.
10. The nurse participates in the profession's effort to protect the public from misinformation and misrepresentation and to maintain the integrity of nursing.
11. The nurse collaborates with members of the health professions and other citizens in promoting community and national efforts to meet the health needs of the public.

The code clarifies the expectations a society has of nurses. Violations of the code may result in the loss of respect for and confidence in the profession of nursing, as well as the individual nurse.

## ◆ THE CODE FOR LICENSED PRACTICAL/VOCATIONAL NURSES

The National Federation of Licensed Practical Nurses (NFLPN) published the *Nursing Practice Standards for the Licensed Practical/Vocational Nurse* in 1996. The NFLPN asserts that upon entering the profession, each LP/VN inherits the responsibility of adhering to the standards of ethical practice and conduct. Each LP/VN is expected to:

1. Know the scope of maximum use of the LP/VN as specified by the nursing practice act of the state in which one is licensed and function within this scope.
2. Safeguard the confidential information acquired from any source about the client.
3. Provide health care to all clients regardless of race, creed, cultural background, disease, or lifestyle.
4. Refuse to give endorsement to the sale and promotion of commercial products or services.
5. Uphold the highest standards in personal appearance, language, dress, and demeanor.
6. Stay informed about issues affecting the practice of nursing and delivery of health care and, where appropriate, participate in government and policy decisions.
7. Accept the responsibility for safe nursing by keeping oneself mentally and physically fit and educationally prepared to practice.
8. Accept responsibility for membership in the National Federation for Licensed Practical Nurses (NFLPN) and participate in its efforts to maintain the established standards of nursing practice and employment policies that lead to quality client care.

## ◆ NURSING PRACTICE STANDARDS FOR THE LICENSED PRACTICAL NURSE

Standards of practice provide descriptions of the essential components of nursing practice. **Standards** provide models for the measurement and evaluation of the quality of nursing care. The NFLPN developed the *Nursing Practice Standards for the Licensed Practical/Vocational Nurse* in 1996. These standards are applicable in any practice setting and include:

### EDUCATION
1. Complete a formal education program in practical nursing approved by the appropriate nursing authority in a state.
2. Successfully pass the National Council Licensure Examination for Practical Nurses.
3. Participate in initial orientation within the employing institution.

### LEGAL/ETHICAL STATUS
1. Hold a current license to practice nursing as an LP/VN in accordance with the law of the state where employed.
2. Know the scope of nursing practice authorized by the nursing practice act in the state where employed.

3. Have a personal commitment to fulfill the legal responsibilities inherent in good nursing practice.
4. Take responsible actions in situations in which there is unprofessional conduct by a peer or other health care provider.
5. Recognize and have a commitment to meet the ethical and moral obligations of the practice of nursing.
6. Do not accept or perform professional responsibilities outside of one's areas of competence.

## PRACTICE

1. Accept assigned responsibilities as an accountable member of the health care team.
2. Function within the limits of educational preparation and experience as related to the assigned duties.
3. Function with other members of the health care team in promoting and maintaining health, preventing disease and disabilities, caring for and rehabilitating individuals who are experiencing an altered health state, and contributing to the ultimate quality of life until death.
4. Know and use the nursing process in:
   a. Planning (assessment of health status, analysis of information gained from the assessment, and identification of health goals)
   b. Implementing (put the nursing care plan into practice to achieve the stated goals)
   c. Evaluating (measure progress toward the stated goals of the nursing care plan)
5. Participate in peer review and other evaluation processes.
6. Participate in the development of policies concerning the health and nursing needs of society and in the roles and functions of the LP/VN.

## CONTINUING EDUCATION

1. Be responsible for maintaining the highest possible level of professional competence at all times.
2. Periodically reassess career goals and select continuing education activities to help achieve these goals.
3. Take advantage of continuing education opportunities that will lead to personal growth and professional development.
4. Seek and participate in continuing education activities that are approved for credit by appropriate organizations, such as the NFLPN.

## SPECIALIZED NURSING PRACTICE

1. Have at least 1 year's experience in nursing at the staff level.

**2.** Present personal qualifications that indicate potential abilities for practice in the chosen specialized nursing area.

**3.** Present evidence of completion of a program or course approved by an appropriate agency to provide the knowledge and skills necessary to effective nursing services in the specialized field.

**4.** Meet all of the standards of practice as set forth in this document.

## ◆ STANDARDS OF PSYCHIATRIC-MENTAL HEALTH CLINICAL NURSING PRACTICE

The ANA further clarified the specialized role of the psychiatric nurse in the *Statement on the Scope and Standards of Psychiatric-Mental Health Clinical Nursing Practice* (1994). The standard and rationale for each are based on the nursing process and are listed below.

### STANDARD 1: ASSESSMENT
The psychiatric-mental health nurse collects client health data.

*Rationale:* The assessment interview (which requires linguistically and culturally effective communication skills, interviewing, behavioral observation, database record review, and comprehensive assessment of the client and relevant systems) enables the psychiatric-mental health nurse to make sound clinical judgments and plan appropriate interventions with the client.

### STANDARD 2: DIAGNOSIS
The psychiatric-mental health nurse analyzes the assessment data in determining diagnosis.

*Rationale:* The basis for providing psychiatric-mental health nursing care is the recognition and identification of patterns of response to actual or potential psychiatric illnesses and mental health problems.

### STANDARD 3: OUTCOME IDENTIFICATION
The psychiatric-mental health nurse identifies expected outcomes individualized to the client.

*Rationale:* Within the context of providing nursing care, the ultimate goal is to influence health outcomes and improve the client's health status.

### STANDARD 4: PLANNING
The psychiatric-mental health nurse develops a plan of care that prescribes interventions to attain expected outcomes.

*Rationale:* A plan of care is used to guide therapeutic intervention systematically and achieve the expected client outcomes.

## STANDARD 5: IMPLEMENTATION

The psychiatric-mental health nurse implements the interventions identified in the plan of care.

*Rationale:* In implementing the plan of care, psychiatric-mental health nurses use a wide range of interventions designed to prevent mental and physical illness and promote, maintain, and restore mental and physical health. Psychiatric-mental health nurses select interventions according to their level of practice. At the basic level, the nurse may select or participate in counseling, milieu therapy, self-care activities, physician-ordered psychobiological interventions, health teaching, case management, health promotion and health maintenance, and a variety of other approaches to meet the mental health needs of clients. In addition, at an advanced level, the certified specialist may provide consultation, engage in psychotherapy, and prescribe pharmacologic agents where permitted by state statutes or regulations.

## STANDARD 6: EVALUATION

The psychiatric-mental health nurse evaluates the client's progress in attaining expected outcomes.

*Rationale:* Nursing care is a dynamic process involving change in the client's health status over time, giving rise to the need for new data, different diagnoses, and modifications in the plan of care. Therefore, evaluation is a continuous process of appraising the effect of nursing interventions and the treatment regimen on the client's health status and expected health outcomes.

The nurse is wise to evaluate his or her practice against NFLPN and ANA standards. Discrepancies would indicate the need for further investigation and re-evaluation of his or her practice, whereas compliance would provide confidence that his or her practice will appropriately meet the needs of clients.

## ◆ LEGAL ASPECTS OF MENTAL HEALTH NURSING

Laws are mandated through federal, state or local authorities. Nurses must function within the guidelines of their state nurse practice act as well as statutory law. **Nurse practice acts** are enacted by each state; each nurse practice act creates a regulatory agency, usually called the board of nursing. The board of nursing has authority for determining the requirements for licensure and practice within its state. Statutory laws, or **statutes**, are laws enacted by legislative bodies such as the United States Congress, state legislatures, and local legislative bodies. Nurse practice acts and statutory law vary from state to state. It is essential that nurses know, understand, and function within the appropriate statutes.

The United States Congress has found that individuals with mental illness are vulnerable to abuse and neglect. Subsequently, United States Code (42 U.S.C.114, 1998) and legal precedents have established rights of individuals with mental illness and provide that states must act to protect these rights. Some of the significant rights of an individual admitted, voluntarily or involuntarily, for the purpose of receiving mental health services include the right to treatment; the right to confidentiality; informed consent and competency; involuntary commitment; habeas corpus; and the right to refuse treatment. They are described in detail below.

## THE RIGHT TO TREATMENT

Appropriate treatment is supportive of personal liberty and individualized to address identified needs. Treatment should occur in the least restrictive environment possible. Treatment is based on a written plan and should include participation by the client, to the extent of his or her capabilities. Treatment plans must be reviewed regularly and revised to reflect changing client needs. Treatment plans will vary from facility to facility; however, all treatment plans guide interactions and interventions by mental health professionals. At a minimum, treatment plans include:

1. A statement of client problems and needs
2. Measurable objectives, with a timetable for implementation
3. Criteria for discharge

## THE RIGHT TO INFORMED CONSENT

Informed **consent** refers to the right of a competent individual to weigh advantages and disadvantages of treatment options and accept or decline treatment. Clients should be given a reasonable explanation of the proposed treatment, as well as the benefits and relative disadvantages and risks of the treatment.

Implied consent is the consent a person gives when allowing himself or herself to undergo routine laboratory work or x-rays, or to take medications administered by a caregiver.

Presumed consent comes into play when an unconscious person is given life-saving treatment in a life-threatening situation. Parents, guardians or conservators give vicarious consent when a person is incapable of deciding for himself or herself.

A health care provider who provides treatment without consent may be held responsible for battery. In an emergency situation, or upon court order, this right may be superseded. It is imperative that the nurse act according to local mental health statutes.

## THE RIGHT TO CONFIDENTIALITY

Confidentiality prevents the nurse from revealing information about the client to anyone who is not directly involved in the client's care, without the consent of the client. Confidentiality protects the nurse–client relationship and fosters therapeutic interactions.

It is important that clients trust the nurse and feel comfortable sharing their thoughts. However, nurses also have a duty to protect the client and others from harm. When clients report suicidal or homicidal ideations or when they discuss plans that may produce significant harm, nurses must report this to the appropriate supervisor or authority.

It is unwise for a nurse to agree to a client request that the nurse "not tell anyone else" about a conversation. Because the nurse is a member of a treatment team, such information should be shared verbally with the director of the team, whose clinical judgment forms the basis of the decision about whether and how this information should be shared with the team.

Inexperienced students or nurses sometimes may want to maintain this requested confidentiality, but it can sometimes have tragic consequences if the information would have averted danger to the client or others. In addition, a request for confidentiality is often an attempt by the client, consciously or otherwise, to split the members of the health care team.

It is also important to remember that a client's chart can be used at any time in a legal proceeding. The client's chart should contain accurate documentation using the guidelines established by the institution where the nurse is employed. Guidelines may vary from institution to institution. When clients share information that may be sensitive or potentially damaging, the nurse should follow institution policies. If the nurse is in doubt about how to document a conversation or incident, the nurse should discuss his or her concerns with a supervisor.

Many people with mental illness may voluntarily seek assistance from mental health professionals and readily accept hospitalization when it is recommended. Others, whose judgment and sense of reality are altered, may reject assistance or hospitalization.

States, in order to protect all its citizens, have the authority to hospitalize a person with mental illness against his or her will. This process is known as **involuntary commitment**. Involuntary commitment is based on an assessment of the clients' danger to self or others. In order to be involuntarily committed, the client must generally exhibit behaviors or conditions that, if left untreated, would lead to serious bodily harm to the client or others. If these conditions are met, based on the expert opinion of qualified mental health professionals, an emergency placement may be made. After an emergency placement is made, a civil court judge reviews the case, and judicial orders for hospitalization or release are made. Clients are generally committed to the least restrictive environment that can provide treatment, which may include acute, long-term, or community agencies.

A clients who is held in a hospital against his or her will may apply for a writ of **habeas corpus**. A writ of habeas corpus compels the court to have an immediate hearing to determine a person's sanity. If the person is declared sane, then he or she must be released from the institution immediately.

**Competency** is a legal determination and relates to a person's ability to make sound decisions and manage his or her own life circumstances. Decisions to obtain a court decision on mental competency are usually made when family members or caregivers are concerned about a person's ability to make life decisions.

During court proceedings, sufficient evidence must be presented for the judge to order that the client is not competent and then appoint a guardian, conservator, or committee to safeguard the client's well-being. A diagnosis of a mental illness, without evidence of severely impaired function, is not sufficient for a determination of incompetence.

As discussed earlier in the chapter, any competent individual has the right to decline or refuse treatment. Unless found incompetent, a person with a diagnosed mental illness maintains the right to decline or refuse treatment. However, there are legal precedents for the administration of medications and some biologic treatments against the will of a person with a mental illness, in certain situations.

Legal issues surrounding mental health nursing practice are dynamic and complex. Nurses are advocates for their clients and must work to protect the rights of the mentally ill client in their care. Additionally, nurses are responsible for maintaining legal practice under the nurse practice acts and statutes where they are employed.

## ◆ THE ETHICS OF NURSING PRACTICE

Standards, laws, and rules are generally based upon ethical determinations by members of professional groups and society. **Ethics** is defined as the knowledge of the principles of good and evil. Sensitivity to ethical issues should be prerequisite for any profession that holds a public trust. Nursing holds a public trust and must, therefore, be aware of ethical concerns when dealing with clients. The study of ethical principles assists the nurse in determining the answer to the question "What should I do?" in a given situation. An ethical dilemma exists when it is difficult to know or decide what is right or wrong. When there is an ethical dilemma, more than one thing may be right or wrong.

When the ethics of a particular field or discipline are discussed, it is expected that the individual within that field possesses a basic set of ethical values about his or her conduct individually and in interpersonal relationships. Professional ethics are then built on the foundation of personal ethics. The *ANA Code for Nurses* describes ethical principles, such as respect for human dignity, confidentiality, and acting to safeguard the client, that are essential to nursing.

Personal ethics are formed as a person is socialized. **Socialization** is a developmental process during which the young child gains acceptance from his or her parents and other authority figures by conforming to their rules. These rules are the "do's and don'ts" that are gradually internalized to form the child's value system. A **value** is a basic internal guideline that causes an emotional response in a person.

These values or personal guides develop and evolve throughout one's lifetime. They form the basis, either consciously or unconsciously, of a person's decisions and actions. Values, which are at the core of a person's selfhood, do not change easily or quickly. Ideally, they are dynamic and are subject to modification and change as a person matures and acquires more wisdom and knowledge about himself or herself and others.

Clients with mental illness pose unique nursing practice opportunities. Nurses who work in psychiatric-mental health settings are continually challenged to evaluate and clarify their values. The nurse must be aware of his or her personal values, professional standards, and expectations, as well as legal constraints, to provide the best care possible.

## KEY POINTS

- Codes of nursing describe how nurses should carry out their role of safeguarding the well-being of people in their care.
- Standards of nursing practice provide guidelines for measuring and evaluating nursing care.
- Clients with a mental illness have the right to:
  —Treatment
  —Informed Consent
  —Confidentiality
  —Determination of Competency (habeas corpus)
  —Refuse Treatment
- In cases where a mentally disordered client is a danger to self or others, the client can be committed involuntarily.
- Legal statutes vary from state to state. Nurses are responsible for knowing and following mental health statutes and their nurse practice act.

■ Ethics is the knowledge of principles of good and evil and helps nurses determine what they should do in a given situation.

### SELF-AWARENESS ACTIVITY

- Do you believe a person with a mental illness can make informed decisions? Why or why not?
- In what situation would you, personally, be able to justify breaking confidentiality? What would be the impact on your licensure?
- What would you do if your client refused to take a medication "because it has arsenic in it"?

## QUESTIONS

1. Nurses must be aware of the ethics of treating clients with mental illness because:
   a. each treatment plan contains an "ethics" section that must be completed.
   b. otherwise clients cannot become socialized.
   c. the *Code for Nurses* requires it.
   d. mental health nursing involves working with people who have varying degrees of mental competence or judgment.
2. Vicarious consent is given:
   a. by the client at least 6 months before hospitalization occurs.
   b. when the client is competent but not able to decide for himself or herself.
   c. by parents, guardians, or conservators when the client cannot decide for himself or herself.
   d. only in cases of outpatient treatment.
3. If a person held in a hospital applies for a writ of habeas corpus, what must happen?
   a. The person must be immediately released from the hospital.
   b. The person must sign a document declaring that he or she is mentally disordered.
   c. The person must undergo blood tests to check for substance abuse.
   d. The person immediately receives a court hearing to determine his or her sanity.
4. When a nurse is unsure of a client's wishes concerning treatment, the nurse should:
   a. do whatever, in the nurse's opinion, is best for the client.

b. let the doctor decide what should be done.
c. take it to the ethics committee for a decision.
d. clarify the client's wishes with the client.

## BIBLIOGRAPHY

American Nurses Association (1985). *Code for nurses with interpretive statements.* Washington, D.C.: American Nurses Association.

American Nurses Association (1994). *Statement on the scope and standards of psychiatric-mental health clinical nursing practice.* Washington, D.C.: American Nurses Association.

Bandman, E.L. & Bandman, B. (1995). *Nursing ethics across the life span* (3rd ed.). Norwalk, CT; Appleton & Lange.

Brent, N.J. (1997). *Nurses and the law: A guide to principles and applications.* Philadelphia: W.B. Saunders Company.

Fiesta, J. (1998). Psychiatric liability: Part 2. *Nursing Management, 29*(8), 18–19.

Isaacs, A. (2000). *Lippincott's review series: Mental health and psychiatric nursing* (3rd ed.). Philadelphia: Lippincott Williams & Wilkins.

Lego, S. (1996). *Psychiatric nursing: a comprehensive reference* (2nd ed.). Philadelphia: Lippincott-Raven.

Ludwick, R. (1999). Ethical thoughtfulness and nursing competency. *Online Journal of Issues in Nursing* (http://www.nursingworld.org/ojin/ethicol/ehtich_2.htm )

National Federation of Licensed Practical Nurses. (1996). *Nursing practice standards for the licensed practical/vocational nurse.* Garner, NC: National Federation of Licensed Practical Nurses.

Offer, P.A. (1994). Nursing and patient rights: Can both be protected? *Journal of Psychosocial Nursing and Mental Health Services, 32*(12), 48.

Trandel-Korenchuk, D. M. & Trandel-Korenchuk, K. M. (1997). *Nursing and the law* (5th ed.). Gaithersburg, MD: Aspen Publishers.

United States Code. (1998). *The public health and welfare: Protection and advocacy for mentally ill individuals.* 42 USC, Chapter 114.

## DEVELOPING CRITICAL THINKING SKILLS THROUGH CLASS DISCUSSION

### UNIT 1 Case Study
# Patterns of Mental Health Care

Mike is a 32-year-old male who was diagnosed with schizophrenia, a chronic mental illness, when he was 22 years old. He is the son of a prominent businessman in a small community. Mike has been hospitalized several times for treatment of his mental illness. He was recently discharged from a state institution and is now living at a community residential treatment facility. Mike has a small apartment at the facility. Meals are provided for the clients and medications are supervised. He attends groups during the week, including social skills, medication, and current events. He has individual therapy with a social worker once a week and meets with a psychiatrist every 2 weeks. Mike has been at the facility for 1 month.

Karen is an LPN working at the residential treatment facility. She is responsible for helping Mike manage and understand his medications. To help Mike be more responsible in managing his illness, she takes him to the pharmacy to have his prescriptions filled. The day after taking Mike to the pharmacy, Karen sees the pharmacy clerk at the grocery store. The clerk says to Karen, "I had no idea Mike was so ill, his medications are really strong. His parents sure have hidden his illness well."

## DISCUSSION QUESTIONS

1. What are the benefits of Mike being treated at a community residential facility?
2. What should be done to facilitate coordination of treatment between the inpatient and residential facilities?
3. What is the role of the practical/vocational nurse at a residential facility?
4. Will Mike be able to function independently? What more could the nurse do to facilitate Mike's independence?
5. What other members of a treatment team should be involved in Mike's care? How could they facilitate Mike's treatment?
6. How should Karen respond to the clerk's statement? Why?

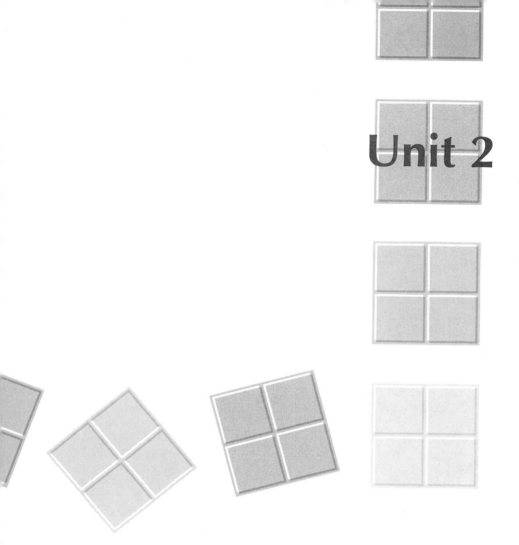

# Unit 2

# FOUNDATIONS OF THE THERAPEUTIC RELATIONSHIP

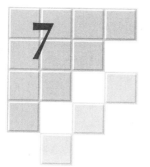

# Communicating in the Therapeutic Relationship

---

## Behavioral Objectives

*After reading this chapter the student will be able to:*

- Define empathic care.
- Explain the concept of acceptance and describe why it is an important part of the therapeutic relationship.
- Describe why explanations are important to the mentally ill person.
- Explain the difference between empathy and sympathy and give an example of each.
- Describe why limit setting is important in the treatment of the mentally ill person.
- Explain five functions of the ego.
- Name the important personal qualities in a therapeutic relationship.
- Discuss the differences between open-ended and closed-ended questioning.
- Explain the importance of contracting and terminating of the counseling relationship.

---

## Key Terms

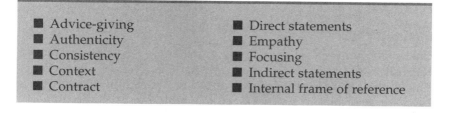

- Advice-giving
- Authenticity
- Consistency
- Context
- Contract

- Direct statements
- Empathy
- Focusing
- Indirect statements
- Internal frame of reference

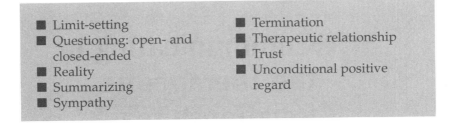

- Limit-setting
- Questioning: open- and closed-ended
- Reality
- Summarizing
- Sympathy
- Termination
- Therapeutic relationship
- Trust
- Unconditional positive regard

This chapter presents general concepts that form the basis of beginning a therapeutic relationship. It also describes the various counseling techniques that promote a therapeutic relationship. A **therapeutic relationship** is a unique type of relationship in which nursing care is provided to clients and families. A therapeutic relationship uses professional knowledge and skill in a manner that is constructive to the well being and adaptation of the client. The information presented here will enhance your comfort as well as that of your clients while you are working in mental health as well as all practice settings. Table 7-1 describes the principles of therapeutic communication.

### ◆ IMPORTANT ELEMENTS IN A THERAPEUTIC RELATIONSHIP

#### EMPATHY AND SYMPATHY
One of the important qualities in a helping relationship is **empathy.** Empathy is the ability to hear what another person is saying and be able to borrow the other person's feelings temporarily but still maintain one's own. When with a client, it is important to maintain one's own objectivity in order to assess accurately the client's mental functioning. **Sympathy** occurs when the caregiver adopts the same feelings as the client and loses objectivity.

The following scenario illustrates the difference between empathy and sympathy. You are in a boat with someone who falls overboard. Choosing to throw him a line and pull him to safety is comparable to an empathic therapeutic intervention. Jumping into the water with him, even if you do not know how to swim, is comparable to sympathy.

#### CARING
There are many qualities that support therapeutic nursing practice. Regardless of the pattern of behavior that may characterize a client's illness, certain general principles apply to the care of all who show behavior disorders. Everyone has certain basic and psychosocial needs that must be met, no matter how different the surface behavior may be. Caring is a distinguishing characteristic of nursing practice. Patricia

## TABLE 7–1. **Principles of Therapeutic Communication**

1. The patient should be the primary focus of the interaction.
2. A professional attitude sets the tone of the therapeutic relationship.
3. Self-disclosure should be used cautiously and only when the disclosure has a therapeutic purpose.
4. Social relationships with patients should be avoided.
5. Patient confidentiality should be maintained.
6. Intellectual competence should be assessed to determine the level of understanding.
7. Implement interventions from a theoretical base.
8. Maintain a nonjudgmental interaction. Avoid making judgments about patient's behavior and giving advice. By the time the patient sees the nurse, he or she has had plenty of advice.
9. Guide the patient to reinterpret his or her experiences rationally.
10. Track the patient's verbal interaction through the use of clarifying statements. Avoid changing the subject unless the content change is in the best interest of the client.

From Boyd, M., & Nihart, M. (1998). *Psychiatric nursing: Contemporary practice.* Philadelphia: Lippincott Williams & Wilkins.

Benner studied this characteristic of nursing practice and nurses. Benner says that nurses have the potential to provide skilled, empathic, and effective care. She describes the heart of caring as the ability to be empathic. Other abilities that expand one's empathy are "being there" and understanding the meaning of illness to the client; touching; listening; communicating verbally and nonverbally so that the client feels that he or she is understood; and demonstrating technical competence.

## ACCEPTANCE

The client needs to be accepted exactly as he or she is, as a person of worth and dignity. Each of us has certain standards of conduct that we strive to maintain. When others fail to meet our standards, we tend to pass judgment on them and punish them in one way or another for their transgressions. This is acceptable behavior for normal individuals, but an emotionally ill person needs a reasonable and reliable social environment in order to learn to function in an adaptive manner again with others.

Acceptance does not mean that we sanction or approve of a client's behavior, but neither do we judge or punish him or her for it. Do not call attention to defects, or show disapproval by word, action, attitude, or expression. It is important to show interest in a client as a human being—as an individual possessed of dignity and worth.

Acceptance often starts out as one-sided. Frequently, the client wants no part of you or other staff members, or your help. He or she may be fearful of any closeness and be suspicious of your intentions. If previous interpersonal experiences have convinced the client that he or she is not acceptable to others, it may be difficult to change this self-concept. However, you must convey to the client that he or she is a worthwhile person, and that even though some behavior may be unacceptable, he or she—as a person—is acceptable. If you set limits on behavior in order to help the client behave more appropriately, but demonstrate warmth and support while doing so, he or she will slowly begin to feel accepted and viewed as a worthwhile person.

The mentally ill person may need to test the sincerity of the therapeutic relationship over and over again before fears and doubts are swept away. Acceptance is a way of expressing belief in the fundamental worth of another person. We all have a need for acceptance; the mentally ill have a very great need for it.

## EXPLANATIONS

Routines and procedures should always be explained at the client's level of understanding. Most of us like to be informed about what to expect in any given situation. Mentally ill clients are no exception. Always explain what is being done and why it is being done in such a way that full allowance is made for the client's symptom-imposed limitations. A client with a limited attention span needs a brief, clear, pointed explanation. An apprehensive client needs a firm explanation that assumes he or she will accept the procedure. An indecisive client needs us to make decisions for him or her and to outline procedures to minimize the necessity of deciding. The purpose behind an explanation is to reduce anxiety whenever possible by preparing the client for what is to come.

## EXPRESSION OF FEELINGS

The client needs to be able to ventilate feelings without fear of retaliation. Encouraging the client to express feelings helps lower his or her frustration level and assists you in assessing real feelings and the motivation for behavior. Talk and *actively listen* to the client. Conversation should center on the client—on his or her needs, wants, and interests—not on those of the listener. Allow the client to express emotions such as anxiety, fear, hostility, hatred, and anger.

A client's ability to express a negative emotion can be a healthy sign because strong emotions, when bottled up, are potentially explosive and dangerous. Strange as it may seem, we can frequently be more help to a psychiatric client if we are the objects of his or her hostility rather than if the client likes us. Our quiet acceptance of hostility permits him or her to discharge emotion without retaliation. One of the real dangers of hatred and hostility to the person who feels these emotions is the fear of retribution they carry; therefore, the client needs an atmosphere in which his or her behavior is calmly accepted.

## CONSISTENCY

**Consistency** is the experience of a reliable environment, one in which the client understands what the rules and expectations are and they remain reliable, not changing frequently without explanation. Consistency is a measure that contributes much to client security. All mentally ill clients are insecure and uncertain. Not knowing what to expect produces anxiety. Consistency in all areas of experience is valuable to the psychiatric client, because it builds something to depend on into his or her environment.

A consistent hospital routine with firm limit-setting is very important to the client. It reduces the number of decisions that must be made daily, and he or she learns what to expect from the environment. The attitude of the entire hospital staff toward the client, likewise, must be consistent; this consistency in attitude should extend from person to person and from shift to shift. Continuous exposure to an atmosphere of quiet understanding causes the client's anxiety to lessen, and he or she becomes increasingly aware of the acceptance of the staff.

## MUTUAL TRUST

Like the need for acceptance, the need for mutual trust is vital to a therapeutic relationship. **Trust** is the ability of one person to rely on another, to experience consistent and reliable interactions, and to expect to be treated with dignity. If we find our world a friendly and trustworthy place to live in, we bring this ability to trust to our work. If a series of experiences have convinced the client that he or she cannot trust others, we must start at the beginning to establish a basis for trust, building slowly and carefully. Honesty, integrity, and consistency are all building blocks in laying such a foundation.

Explain in clear, simple language what you intend to do with and for your client and let nothing interfere with carrying out your contract or pact. If you promise to visit a client daily, then arrive at the appointed time, stay the length of time promised, and leave when the time is up. Should something unavoidably cause a delay or prevent a visit, notify the client. This is the way to build trust.

If you tell a client that he or she may discuss problems, it is important to sit quietly and listen openly. Afterward in this chapter, counseling techniques are presented that are helpful in this communication. If the client's behavior becomes unacceptable, it is important to set reasonable limits so he or she can express emotions constructively, not destructively.

## UNDERSTANDING

When we as staff members increase our own self-understanding, we are better able to understand client behavior. We each need to analyze our own feelings and motivations and usually need some help in developing skills in interpersonal relationships. Group discussions on emotions and their effects are very valuable in deepening self-awareness. We can become comfortable in our relationships with clients only when we feel secure about our ability to respond appropriately to client behavior.

When we are able to understand a client's behavior and find the underlying motivation, then and only then can we organize these findings into a truly therapeutic care plan designed to meet his or her needs. We must then constantly evaluate the client's behavior to see if those needs are being effectively met. Place yourself in the client's position to understand whatever he or she is experiencing. At the same time, make efforts to establish and improve communication, especially in the field of active listening.

## LIMIT-SETTING

We have been stressing the acceptance of clients' behavior and the value of a permissive, therapeutic atmosphere; however, permissiveness must have a limit. **Limit-setting** is the communication to the client of which behaviors are acceptable and which are not. If a client engages in unacceptable behaviors, pre-established consequences must be put into action. Clients cannot be allowed to do only as they please—they must conform to the expected rules of the unit. The entire team to whom they are assigned should determine the actual limitations on clients' behavior. Everyone who comes in contact with them should consistently enforce those limitations.

If, for example, a client is overactive, do not allow him or her to become exhausted. We accept the fact that the client has a right to feel the way he or she feels, but limitations must be drawn and behavior kept within these limits. If limit-setting is enforced in a consistent, quiet, matter-of-fact way by the staff, then these rules contribute to the client's security.

Avoid physical and verbal force. None of us likes being forced to comply with the wishes of others; however, in spite of every precaution, occasions may arise in which the use of force cannot be avoided. When force must be used, adequate help should be secured and the action carried out quickly and efficiently. When employing force, never show annoyance or anger toward the client. Self-control in this situation is very important. The rules for forceful restraint are described in the policy manual of all hospitals and must be followed carefully in order to ensure the safety of both clients and staff.

## REALITY

The mind may use defense mechanisms that alter a person's perception of what is really happening in an attempt to protect itself from internal or environmental awareness that is potentially anxiety provoking.

**Reality** is a person's accurate perception of what is really happening within his own experience or environment. Reality testing is the experience of a person whose mental perceptions may be inaccurate because of mental disorder or medication—the experience of a person who is trying to determine what is real and what is not.

The ability to differentiate between reality and unreality often is seriously affected in a mentally ill person. What he or she observes and hears may be very distorted. If a client is hallucinating, what the client hears and sees may cause him or her to respond to his or her own unconscious motivation. The client may interpret and respond to the behavior of others in a very inappropriate way because of this faulty perception. If you can gain the trust and acceptance of such a client, you will be in a position to help validate his or her concepts of reality and bring him or her back gently and slowly into the real world. While making the assessment, always try to establish the approximate degree of the client's distortion and ability to respond to reality.

## REASSURANCE
All of us need reassurance occasionally; the psychiatric client needs it constantly. Make every effort to see a situation as the client sees it. Reassurance is effective only if it does not contradict a false concept that the client holds (ie, a concept or defense mechanism to protect his or her own belief system). The best way to reassure a client, in addition to well-placed verbal assurance, is by giving attention to matters that are important to him or her and by doing things for and with the client without asking anything in return, such as showing appreciation for an improvement in his or her behavior.

We do not change a client's behavior by reasoning with him or her. Simply telling a client why he or she ought to do something is not an effective way of getting cooperation, especially when he or she has emotional difficulties. The client has developed a pattern of behavior that functions as a defense against anxiety-producing stress, and the client uses what reason he or she is capable of to bolster defensive patterns of thinking. If a false belief is based on strong emotional needs, the more we challenge it, the more the client will defend it. Work at helping to develop the client's emotional security. With an improvement in this area, the client will slowly tend to develop some insight into his or her behavior and the forces behind it. However, insight can be a threat as well as a help to the emotionally disturbed client. Thus, behavior should only be interpreted when the client is ready for it, secure enough to tolerate it, and able to apply it to alter his or her behavior. This help is best left in the hands of the psychiatrist.

It is important not to meet your own emotional needs through your clients. Be trained and prepared to understand their needs and meet them, with no expectations for benefit to yourself other than to see your clients recover. Whenever we find ourselves evaluating a client's behavior in terms of right or wrong, or criticizing a client or defending or justifying ourselves, we are in danger of letting our own emotional needs take precedence over those of the client.

## ◆ IMPORTANT PERSONAL QUALITIES IN A THERAPEUTIC RELATIONSHIP

In addition to supporting the concepts described in the preceding, there are additional personal qualities in the nurse that help to establish a helping, trusting relationship with a client. They are described by Carl Rogers:

1. *Unconditional positive regard.* Accept the client without negative judgment of his or her basic worth.
2. *Empathic understanding of the client's internal frame of reference.* A person's **internal frame of reference** is the unique perspective and meaning that one has about his or her own personal circumstances and life experiences. It is helpful for the nurse in the mental health setting to be aware of and have the capacity to empathize with the client's personal life situation and the various dynamics that are contributing to it. As described, empathy is the capacity of one person to hear the emotional circumstances of another's life or personal circumstances and maintain caring—a clear sense of boundary between the client and the one who is listening and emotional perspective. Another word for the circumstances that contribute to the client's current difficulty is **context.**
3. *Authenticity.* Allow yourself to be known to others (also called genuineness).

## ◆ COMMUNICATION PATTERNS IN THE COUNSELING RELATIONSHIP

The following section discusses specific counseling approaches that can ease conversations with a client and contribute toward a therapeutic outcome.

### NONVERBAL COMMUNICATION IN THE COUNSELING SETTING

The essence of a helping relationship is the communication or message that is relayed from the helper to the client *and* from the client to the helper. There are two types of messages: verbal and nonverbal. In the field of psychiatry, the way that we communicate nonverbally is very important. Psychiatric clients are particularly sensitive to the many nonverbal messages they receive from caregivers. They know whether they are liked, respected, distrusted, or considered a nuisance. We give off messages, usually without being aware of them. Clients give the same messages to us.

The means with which we tell clients how we are feeling about them are our eyes, posture, and gestures. The ability to maintain consistent eye contact is a strong indicator of relationship potential. When a person frequently looks away or keeps his or her eyes in a downcast position, we know that he or she is not comfortable. Posture is another indication of what a person's true feelings are about a given situation. A person who is standing or sitting erect is usually interested in what he or she is doing or the person he or she is with. Conversely, one who is slouched and half turned away is saying "I really don't want to be here." Finally, gestures that we unconsciously make can be important nonverbal signs. For example, a quick movement by a caregiver in the presence of a markedly paranoid client can trigger a defensive reaction. A depressed client would meet the same movement with hardly a glance.

## VERBAL COMMUNICATION IN THE
## COUNSELING SETTING

When we are talking with a client we are essentially inviting him or her to join in verbal communication. The words we speak may prompt him or her to engage in a discussion or to "shut down" and not respond. The various methods of leading the client into discussion are as follows:

Indirect statements
Direct statements
Focusing
Questioning: open-ended and closed-ended
Advice-giving
Summarizing

An **indirect leading statement** is intentionally general and nonspecific, such as "Tell me about your childhood." A **direct leading statement** is more specific: "You said your mother died when you were 6 years old." **Focusing** is a helpful technique when you have explored a broad range of subjects and have a general idea about the client's circumstances. When you focus, you pay particular attention to a topic that seems especially sensitive for him or her. For example, you might ask, "Do you remember how you felt when your mother died?"

**Questioning,** particularly when open-ended questions are used, is a helpful way to encourage the client's insights into his or her difficulties. An **open-ended question** invites the client to give as much information as he or she wants. For example, you could ask, "You told me earlier you went to live with your aunt when your mother died. How was it for you to live with her?" In contrast, a **closed-ended question** is one that frequently requires a one-word answer that ultimately closes off further discussion. You might say, "John, are you sad today?" If John answers "no," it shuts off further therapeutic discussion. Instead say, "John, how are you feeling today?" His answer to this will make it easier to explore how he is feeling.

**Advice-giving** is a counseling technique that *rarely* should be used in the counseling or psychiatric setting. Advice is actually "the easy way out" that can encourage the client's dependence and delay his or her rehabilitation. When a client asks for advice, gently turn the question back to him or her. The response, "John, what would you like to do?" for example, allows him to explore his options out loud with a caring but impartial person. Often, clients learn to form their own conclusions and trust their own judgments when this process is implemented.

If the client is in crisis or experiencing severe anxiety, turning the question back to him or her is not helpful. Before responding to such a client, check with the client's primary nurse, who knows him or her well and may be able to recommend alternative approaches.

**Summarizing** is a skilled form of verbal communication that occurs at the end of a session in which the nurse and client have explored a number of issues. The nurse briefly describes the affective and intellectual experiences that occurred during their time together. The use of summarizing leaves the client with the feeling that he or she accomplished something during the interview.

## ◆ OTHER ASPECTS OF THE THERAPEUTIC RELATIONSHIP

### CONTRACT

Whenever we tell someone that we will do something, we are entering into a contract. In a therapeutic relationship, a **contract** is an agreement, direct or indirect, with another person. A **direct contract** is one that involves setting formal appointment times with a client or entering a primary nurse–client type of commitment. An **indirect contract** is less formal. Here you can commit to see a client at some time during a working shift—but remember, clients will come to depend on you. It promotes their trust in you and their sense of security, both important aspects of returning to good mental health. For example, if you will be off the next day or working a different shift, let your clients know when they can expect to see you next. Keep clients informed of your schedule; this indicates your respect for them and your regard for their needs and feelings.

## TERMINATION OF RELATIONSHIP

The therapeutic relationship is a very close, delicate, and intimate relationship between two people. During the course of interaction, if the client fully accepts the nurse or health care professional and cooperates toward an improved mental health goal, he or she tends to become quite dependent on and emotionally attached to the nurse. It is not easy to **terminate** an emotional dependency. It is usually quite traumatic for the client, and it may also be hard for us as staff members. If we give deeply of our professional skills, we will terminate those relationships with genuine regret and loss.

It is not easy to determine, at the start of a therapeutic relationship, just how long it may take to help a client gain enough insight to be able to manage his or her feelings and behavior in an acceptable way. Ideally, you can indicate, both at the initiation of the relationship and at intervals during it, that hopefully the day will arrive when the client will no longer need specific help, when he or she will reach a plateau of emotional stability that will enable him or her to handle problems without your intervention.

The client is often fearful of his or her ability to make decisions and act responsibly. He or she may fear the approaching time of return to family and job, and be concerned about not being well enough yet to carry on work and family responsibilities. He or she may fear acceptance by family and friends or may wonder whom to call on for help. The client may feel quite threatened by the withdrawal of your help—you have earned his or her trust and helped him or her face personal needs and adjust behavior to an acceptable level.

Discuss these fears long before the relationship is terminated. Find ways to handle them. Slowly include other members of the treatment team to prepare the client for discharge or for further therapy in or out of the hospital, as his or her needs may indicate. As you slowly withdraw from the relationship, include other clients on the ward in an enlarging circle to help promote the client's ability to socialize with others.

To make termination easier, assure the client that you would like to hear from him or her to know how he or she is. Encourage the client to come back to visit you in the hospital from time to time. The invitation to maintain contact is rarely abused by clients. Instead, such assurances, during the period before discharge when the client's anxiety about independence is high, will enhance his or her sense of security. In addition, during the immediate postdischarge period, the knowledge that he or she can call you often provides security without his or her ever actually placing a telephone call.

## KEY POINTS

- Mentally disordered individuals need the following:
  - —Acceptance: Acknowledge the client's basic worth and dignity.
  - —Explanations: Explain routines and procedures at the client's level of understanding.
  - —Safety to express feelings: Allow the client to vent feelings without fear of retaliation.
  - —Trust: Develop trust by honesty, integrity, and consistency in dealings with client.
  - —Consistency: Consistency reduces client's anxiety about not knowing what to expect.
  - —Reassurance: Reassurance helps the client feel secure and develop insight about his or her behavior.
- It is important for nurses to understand client behavior and its underlying motives in order to create an effective therapeutic care plan.
- Empathy means that the nurse temporarily borrows the client's feelings to gain insight but maintains his or her own feelings and boundaries.
- Sympathy means adopting the same feelings as the client, which is not effective for assessing a client's status or needs.
- Psychosocial adaptation is a person's ability to perceive reality and respond to it in a way that supports emotional and physical well being. Psychosocial maladaptation is the result of ineffective coping.
- Caregiver qualities that help a client establish trust are:
  - —Unconditional positive regard
  - —Empathic understanding of the client's internal frame of reference
  - —Genuineness or authenticity
- Effective verbal communication techniques include indirect and direct leading statements; focusing; open-ended questioning; and summarizing.
- Nonverbal communication includes posture, gesture, and eye contact.
- In a therapeutic relationship, a contract is an agreement with another person. A caregiver's contract with a client may be direct (formal) or indirect (informal).
- Termination of the therapeutic relationship can be difficult for both clients and caregivers. It is important to discuss client fears about the end of the relationship well before termination.

## SELF-AWARENESS ACTIVITY

Imagine yourself with a client who has a mental disorder. Imagine that this person has a high level of anxiety.

- How do you feel?
- What are your fears?
- Do you wonder what to say?
- Are you afraid that you will say the wrong thing?

When you are with such a person, one of the most important things you can do is just sit with him or her. Every person who has ever worked in a mental health care setting has had the same fear.

- You do not have to find the "perfect" thing to say.
- Your caring is the most important therapeutic intervention you can bring to this person.
- Ask the person, "How are you?"
- Then, whatever the person says, ask a question about whatever he or she says.
- After the person answers, ask another question about the most recent answer, and so on.
- This is one of the most caring ways you can communicate therapeutically with this person.

## QUESTIONS

1. Which of the following is true?
   a. Reality is a person's accurate perception of what is happening.
   b. A mentally disordered client often cannot distinguish between reality and unreality.
   c. Nurses who gain a client's trust can help the client move back into the real world.
   d. All of the above.
2. When working with a mentally ill client, the nurse may enter into a direct contract with him or her. The best way for the nurse to implement this contract is to
   a. ask questions that require the client to respond with more than a "yes" or "no" answer.
   b. explain all procedures in a detailed and consistent manner.
   c. be on time for all scheduled appointments.
   d. review the results of each session with the client.

3. Setting limits when working with the mentally ill is
   a. not recommended, because it may discourage expression of feelings.
   b. essential, because it establishes acceptable and unacceptable behaviors.
   c. only the responsibility of the nurse on duty.
   d. important, but always negotiable.
4. Which of the following responses *best* exemplifies an empathic response?
   a. "Given all you've been through, I can understand why that situation was difficult."
   b. "You've been through a lot with your mother, I certainly don't blame you for not wanting to speak with her."
   c. "You have a right to whatever you're feeling right now."
   d. "Tell me how you feel after receiving that phone call."

## BIBLIOGRAPHY

Barry, P. (1996). *Psychosocial nursing: Care of physically ill patients and their families* (3rd ed.). Philadelphia: Lippincott-Raven.

Benner, P. (2001). *From novice to expert: Excellence and power in clinical nursing practice.* Upper Saddle River, NJ: Prentice-Hall.

Boyd, M., & Nihart, M. (1998). *Psychiatric nursing: Contemporary practice.* Philadelphia: Lippincott Williams & Wilkins.

Cleary, M., Edwards, C., & Meehan, T. (1999). Factors influencing nurse–patient interaction in the acute psychiatric setting: An exploratory investigation. *Australian New Zealand Journal of Mental Health Nursing, 8*(3), 109–116.

Delaney, K. (1999). Time-out: An overused and misused milieu intervention. *Journal of Child and Adolescent Psychiatric Nursing, 12*(2), 53–60.

Hirose, H. (1999). Classifying the empathic understanding of the nurse psychotherapist. *Cancer Nursing, 22*(3), 204–211.

Litwack, L., & Lewis, M. (1997). *Community counseling* (2nd ed.). Pacific Grove, CA: Brooks-Cole.

Peplau, H. (1999). Psychotherapeutic strategies. Perspectives in psychiatric care. *The Journal for Nurse Psychotherapists, 35*(3), 14–19.

Sadock, B., & Kaplan, H. (1998). *Synopsis of psychiatry: Behavioral sciences/clinical psychiatry.* Philadelphia: Lippincott Williams & Wilkins.

Walsh, K. (1999). Shared humanity and the psychiatric nurse encounter. *Australian New Zealand Journal of Mental Health Nursing, 8*(1), 2–8.

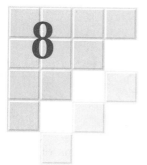

# 8

# Theories and Stages of Personality Development

## Key Terms

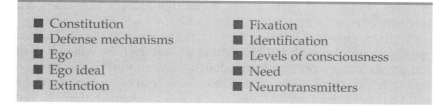

- Constitution
- Defense mechanisms
- Ego
- Ego ideal
- Extinction
- Fixation
- Identification
- Levels of consciousness
- Need
- Neurotransmitters

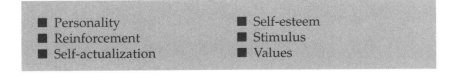

- Personality
- Reinforcement
- Self-actualization
- Self-esteem
- Stimulus
- Values

The formation of personality is one of the most profound forms of development in the human experience. Personality development is shaped by a multitude of factors. The fundamental core of personality is endowed by genetics. Using the analogy of the computer with its hard drive or "hard wiring" already in place, genetics sets out the basic foundation of the personality that evolves. Genetics also determines the basic constitution of the child. The **constitution** is the basic temperament or disposition inherited by the child. For example, some children are born with even, easygoing dispositions. Regardless of what happens, such children adapt easily to new or unexpected events. Other children are more prone to anxiety or anger. As new events occur, their responses are colored by their anxious or anger-prone constitutions.

## ◆ HEREDITY

When a sperm and an ovum unite to form a new life, each germ cell contributes 23 chromosomes on which a vast number of genes or genetic factors are arranged. These genes determine the type of body build the child will have, his or her skin and hair texture, eye color, general intellectual capacity and abilities, talents, and many other physical and mental characteristics. In short, they constitute the child's heredity. Heredity can also be described as genetic endowment.

Part of an infant's heredity includes the makeup of his or her neurologic system. **Neurotransmitters** are the biochemical substances that send messages to and from the central nervous system and all body tissues and organ systems. These substances include adrenaline (epinephrine), noradrenaline (norepinephrine), and serotonin, to name a few of the many that are present in the body. Theorists believe these neurotransmitters strongly influence the human drives for sleep, nourishment, and sexual gratification. Neurotransmitters also affect the intensity of emotions and stress tolerance.

After 9 months of sheltered prenatal life, when every need of the growing fetus is supplied by the mother's body, the baby emerges from the uterus into a world that immediately begins to make demands on him or her and will continue to do so throughout his or her life. If the child has developed normally, he or she is well designed to live in and adapt to this world.

Babies come into the world with basic temperaments or personality dispositions. For example, some infants are more placid than others. In addition, the temperaments of the baby's parents can be similar to or quite unlike that of their newborn. Depending on the compatibility of the baby's inborn disposition and those of his or her parents, the environment may hold varying degrees of conflict for the developing child.

Dr. T. Berry Brazelton, a pediatrician who researches the development of newborns, has identified certain inborn personality characteristics. These personality characteristics include 26 behaviors and 20 reflexes that can be observed and rated. The most easily observable of these appear in the following list:

Alertness
General physical tone
Cuddliness
Motor maturity
Tremulousness
Activity
Irritability
Startle reflex during examination
Lability of skin color
Lability of states
Self-quieting activity
Hand-to-mouth facility
Smiles
Response to light
Response to rattle
Response to bell
Response to pinprick
Orientation to various auditory and visual stimuli
Defensive movements
Consolability with intervention
Peak of excitement
Buildup of excitement
Pull to sit
Environment

The child's environment is a limited world—one reflected by his or her parents and their home—and it causes him or her to react to a multitude of new situations and to other human beings. The child's personality forms as the result of interaction between environment and heredity.

One important effect of environmental influences is the child's acquisition of values. **Values** are deeply held beliefs the child acquires during the formative years as the result of exposure to people who are important to him or her. In the desire to be accepted and avoid disapproval, the child gradually takes on their values and beliefs. Conversely, the child also develops a value system based on exposure to individuals who displease him or her, forming values unlike theirs in order to be different from them. Values are the basis of much of adult behavior and decision making.

## ◆ DEVELOPMENTAL STAGES

Just as bodies go through successive stages of physical development until they reach adulthood, so too personalities normally undergo developmental stages until they reach maturity. Harmful influences may interfere with the normal physical growth and functioning of a tissue, an organ, or the entire body. Similarly, disturbing early experiences and unsatisfied emotional needs may lead to an arrest or **fixation** of the normal growth pattern of the personality and can result in personality distortions and immaturities.

Psychologists consider a wholesome mother–child relationship to be essential for the normal growth and personality development of the child. The child must feel wanted, loved, and enjoyed by his or her parents, and especially by his or her mother or the mother-figure.

If the child feels loved and cared for, then a desirable sense of security follows. If, on the other hand, the child experiences rejection, harshness, and frustration, then his or her personality is often characterized by anxiety, insecurity, and depression. He or she may develop hostile and aggressive tendencies. The emotional experiences of early years leave permanent imprints on the personality, although they may no longer be a part of the individual's consciousness.

One of the most important processes in influencing personality development is called **identification.** Through this process, the child, because of his or her love for and wish to be like the parent, particularly the parent of the same sex, molds himself or herself after that parent and adopts the parent's characteristics and attitudes. This is not a conscious imitation; it is automatic. If the parent is emotionally mature and well adjusted, this process of identification can greatly contribute to the development of similar characteristics in the child's personality.

As the personality continues to grow, it is influenced and molded by many factors. Some of the child's experiences stimulate personality growth; others block or distort its development. If the child experiences difficulties with the issues of security, love, aggression, and dependence, he or she may develop emotional problems. As the child begins to strive for independence, he or she finds it difficult to meet the new responsibilities that independence entails. Growth brings new problems and contradictory urges. Such challenges sometimes may result in emotional turmoil and sometimes in healthy, adaptive behavior.

Emotional development often progresses on an uneven course, but if early identifications have been healthy and if most conflicts have been successfully resolved, eventually a mature, adult personality should emerge. A person with a mature personality has achieved a harmonious adjustment to his or her environment and can meet life's inevitable stresses realistically and effectively.

In order to understand deviant personality, it is important to understand how a normal personality develops. For our purposes, personality does not mean personal charm and distinction; rather, **personality** is the total of all individual tendencies—including strengths and weaknesses, attributes, aspirations, and drives—that determine a person's adjustments to his or her material and social environment. Personality has been referred to as the internal psychophysiologic organization of an individual as he or she interacts with the external organization of the environment.

Personality is always in a state of flux. It is always in the process of becoming something else, yet ordinarily it retains an identifiable continuity from situation to situation, from year to year, and from birth to death.

Although definitions of personality vary greatly, most theorists agree on the following six points:

1. Personality is a relatively enduring organization of patterns of behavior characteristic of the individual.
2. Personality results from the complex interactions of heredity and environment. (Theorists do not agree whether biological forces or psychosocial factors are more important.)
3. Dynamic forces, including psychobiological drives produced by neurotransmitters, cause behavior.
4. Some of these dynamic forces are unknown to the individual; that is, unconscious causes of behavior do exist.
5. Childhood is an important time for forming and organizing relatively enduring patterns of behavioral characteristics of an individual.
6. Behavior, both in its outward and inward manifestations, is a function or expression of personality.

## ◈ DEVELOPMENT OF NEEDS

The newborn shows a generalized response to all stimuli. Emotions develop as the baby reacts to his or her environment. For the infant, life is first of all a biological fact. All infants have basic needs that must be met. A **need** is a necessity, a fundamental requirement for something or someone. The infant responds physiologically to the unpleasantness of hunger and cold and to the need to move his or her muscles. It soon becomes necessary for the infant to react to a multitude of new situations and to other human beings.

One ability the infant possesses is highly significant—the inexplicable power to communicate emotional feeling tones. The baby is able to sense and respond to feelings of approval and disapproval from the mother or mother-figure. Feelings of approval increase the newborn's sense of well being, and the opposite feelings cause discomfort. This happens long before the baby is capable of understanding the meaning of either feeling.

Although all experiences are planted forever in the mind, at this time the infant only vaguely associates them with the mother-figure. Satisfactions are achieved with the first magic tool, crying, and comfort and discomfort are known but not understood. The baby's responses to comfort and discomfort begin to form a patterned behavior.

Experiences in childhood that are particularly important in future development are as follows:

- Availability of a consistent, concerned caregiver
- The feeding situation in early infancy (including weaning)
- Toilet and cleanliness training
- Early training about sexuality
- Training for control of anger and aggression

Adjusting to these situations can be quite upsetting to the child, and it takes patience and understanding on the part of the parents to help him or her accept social rules and regulations. If the parents approve of the child as a person, even when they may disapprove of his or her actions, the child usually accepts their rules and values as his or her own and builds them into a growing personality.

## ◆ HIERARCHY OF HUMAN NEEDS

Abraham Maslow, a psychologist, was one of the founders of the field of humanistic psychology. He believed that humans have levels of needs that must be met before each can develop into a psychologically mature person. Maslow called these the hierarchy of human needs:

1. Physiologic needs
2. Safety needs
3. Love and belonging needs
4. Esteem needs
5. Self-actualization needs

According to Maslow, it is impossible to progress from one stage of psychological development to the next higher stage until the needs at the lower level are met. For example, until a person has obtained the basic physiologic needs of the first level, it is impossible for him or her to move to the level of feeling safe and secure. Accordingly, until a person has a safe and secure environment, he or she is unable to continue the process of feeling loved and accepted in that social environment.

## PHYSIOLOGIC NEEDS

The growing child has many needs; some are physiologic and some are psychosocial. The physiologic needs are often called basic or primary needs because they are basic to physical survival. Six basic requirements are oxygen, food, water, sleep, protection from temperature extremes (clothing and shelter), and excretion. Extreme deprivation of any one results in a person's death.

To these six should be added a seventh—sexual activity—not because deprivation of this activity would result in death, but because, without it, the human race would become extinct. If these physiologic or biologic needs were humans' only concern, they would live on a very primitive level indeed. Brute force would determine survival.

## SAFETY NEEDS

It is important that a person feel safe and secure from harm in order to develop in a psychologically healthy way. This requires a predictable social and physical environment. Without feelings of safety, humans of any age, from infants to elderly adults, live with a chronic sense of fear that inhibits personal growth and fulfillment.

It is important to note that, in a psychiatric inpatient setting, the client's need for feeling safe and secure is crucial. These safety requirements and the nursing care measures needed to provide them are discussed in the chapters covering specific mental disorders and appear elsewhere in this book. Clients whose needs for safety in the inpatient setting are not met are not able to progress to higher levels in the hierarchy.

## LOVE AND BELONGING NEEDS

Probably the deepest psychosocial need most of us have is the need for love or emotional security. Love is a complex feeling of trust, warmth, and understanding—of closeness, intimacy, and emotional give-and-take. Humans need to feel accepted from infancy. All babies need a sense of emotional security; they need to be "mothered" regularly—held against the mother's body, stroked, caressed, cuddled, spoken and sung to, and rocked. This need is so deep that some psychologists place it with the seven basic needs. Humans do not outgrow the need to love and be loved. They merely shift where they look for the need to be filled—from the parental figure to peers (those of one's own age).

## ESTEEM NEEDS

A person must feel accepted and loved by others in order to love and accept himself or herself. The young child's sense of self-worth or self-esteem forms the basis of his or her supply of self-esteem in adulthood. **Self-esteem** is a feeling of self-acceptance and positive self-image. Esteem needs have two main parts: a sense of competence about oneself and the need for recognition and a good reputation. If these needs are not fully met, a person lacks the feelings of confidence and competence necessary to move to the next and highest level of human needs.

Within the esteem level of human needs is the need for status and recognition. Status is a person's particular place in society; this place is allotted to him or her by virtue of age, sex, abilities, vocation or profession, his or her parents' status, and his or her socioeconomic standing. Recognition is the approval or acceptance given the individual by society as he or she performs in keeping with the role society has accorded. The esteem of others nourishes and supports an individual's self-esteem.

Although in the United States we have a so-called classless society—that is, one without aristocratic titles—we do have criteria, such as success and money, that substitute for aristocracy and help to determine status. The pressure to succeed, achieve, and excel begins very early in our lives. Power and possessions are two very important symbols of success. The need for status and recognition is probably related directly to our need to belong—the need for approval and acceptance—first within the family, and then within the group.

## SELF-ACTUALIZATION NEEDS

Finally, there is the need to achieve—the need to accomplish and do. Maslow believed that **self-actualization** is the inborn need of all people to fully develop their potential. He theorized that the need for self-actualization is a constant driving force in all people, regardless of age. When adults feel vague discontent with their lives, it is often because they have not fully developed their potential. This usually occurs because a person is limiting his or her own capacity for further development, personally, educationally, or professionally. It also can happen when another person, financial circumstances, or other environmental factors thwart a person's attempts at full personal development. Full actualization requires that these self- or other-created obstacles be overcome.

If the child's struggle to crawl, stand, walk, talk, and master the environment is rewarded by the approval of the significant figures in his or her life, the child will learn the satisfaction of accomplishment and build a healthy concept of himself or herself as a "doer of deeds," a success. If the child fails to earn the approval of those around him or her, if small achievements are ignored, or worse yet, criticized severely, the child will build a picture of himself or herself as "one who fails." The child whose pride is diminished may lose the ambition or drive to develop his or her potential in adulthood. The child's rights and limits should be clearly defined and respected by the family. Accordingly, the child will grow to respect his or her own rights as well as the rights of others.

Self-development in the child is vital. The child must gradually acquire a concept of *who* he or she is, *what* he or she is, and *what he or she can do*. By the time the child is 4 or 5 years old, he or she tends to have an exaggerated self-concept and feels able to do anything. The lessons slowly learned from the environment, however, level off this concept to a more realistic one. Some self-idealization continues in most adults. They have a strong tendency to see themselves as much closer to perfection than they really are.

## ◆ PERSONALITY DEVELOPMENT AND LEARNING

Few subjects have been as fully studied as the field of animal and human learning. Yet much remains to be understood about how learning occurs. Psychologists studying the process of learning have organized it into four steps:

1. First a person must want something (the drive, the **need,** or motivation).
2. The person must then notice something that will satisfy his or her need (the **stimulus,** or cue).
3. The person must then act on the stimulation (the **response**).
4. He or she must then get something (the reward, the **reinforcement,** or need reduction).

These four steps of learning, of course, are very oversimplified. Learning is a process; each step can be infinitely elaborated. For example: A newborn baby becomes hungry and needs impel him or her to restless activity. The mother offers food, the baby sucks, and the hunger pangs subside. The baby becomes comfortable and drowsy. Here are all the ingredients of a learning situation—a need (hunger), a stimulus (the feel of a nipple in the baby's mouth), a response (sucking), and reinforcement (relief from hunger). Accordingly, learning takes place.

At birth, a baby actively seeks the nipple, turning his or her head from side to side and making sucking responses if his or her cheek is stroked when he or she is hungry. The baby then learns that food (nipple plus sucking) brings relief. After a few weeks, the learning extends to include other elements of this sequence. Now the baby may stop crying from hunger when he or she is picked up. New cues have been tied in or associated with the food-brings-comfort pattern. Soon baby will smile when mother bends over him or her, even when he or she is not hungry, which indicates that the original food-brings-comfort learning has been elaborated into "mother is something good." The baby may learn to associate the feel of his or her mother's body with nursing, and he or she will wiggle with anticipation.

**Reinforcement** is the process by which behavior is learned. A reinforcer is anything that causes behavior to be repeated. The greater the reinforcement, the stronger the learning. The reinforcement may have to come in succeeding episodes, or, if strong enough, a single reinforcement may result in fixing the pattern of learning. For instance, toilet training or learning to eat with the fingers and later a spoon becomes effective only after repeated efforts followed by the reinforcement. Reinforcement of eating behavior can be the pleasant feeling of satiety, a smile from mother, or the feeling of accomplishment from feeding oneself.

On the other hand, a single experience that is very painful or surprising, such as a burnt finger or tumbling down several stairs, usually results in a clearly remembered learning experience. The baby will avoid the hot object and refuse, even when coaxed, to try the stairs again until his or her coordination is much better.

When the pattern of learning no longer serves the need, reinforcement ceases to operate. When this happens, the learning process progressively decreases and finally ceases altogether. This is called **extinction,** or, in ordinary language, forgetting. Although lack of reinforcement is just one cause of forgetting, it is the chief one. Many things that are important to a child lose importance as the child matures, and lack of reinforcement causes a progressive decrease in the sharpness of the mental image, until memory finally ceases.

Nonetheless, something well learned once is never fully forgotten. We store it in our subconscious mind, and it can be brought back to immediate awareness. Sometimes remembrance is immediate; sometimes we must concentrate quite a bit before a dim memory emerges clearly into view. Learning of many activities, such as playing the piano, typing, or tying an intricate knot, improves with reinforcement but fades away or becomes extinct if the activity is not used. On the other hand, relearning a once-acquired skill is usually accomplished with a little practice.

## ◆ THE EGO

The **ego** is the part of the self that is most closely in touch with reality. The primary role of the ego is to balance a person's biological urges with one's own conscience or the expectations of the environment and to satisfy both in a way that coincides with physical and social reality. The **conscience** is one's inner voice that judges whether thoughts and actions are good or bad. The ego is equivalent to the terms "conscious awareness" or "the self." As it develops, the ego overrules or operates in concert with one's biological urges in guiding behavior.

By the age of 3, the average child has learned that there are many things he or she may not do and other things that he or she must do. The child is also learning to defer immediate satisfactions for anticipated or delayed satisfactions. For example, the child will stop doing something that feels good in order to obtain his or her mother's approval. During this time, the child has learned to accept the attributes and standards of his or her parents as his or her own. The child is not yet able to understand the reasons behind behavior, but readily accepts his or her parents' judgment about what is right or wrong to do or say.

The child tends to idealize and view himself or herself as close to perfection. Thus, his or her ego ideal is formed. The **ego ideal** is a high standard within the ego that motivates the individual to continued growth and self-actualization.

The ego encompasses a large variety of functions that are essential to mental and physical well being. They include the following:

Consciousness
Mastery of motor skills
Mobility
Perception
Judgment
Sense of reality
Regulation and control of emotions and impulses
Object relations
Memory
Thinking
Defense mechanisms

The id, ego, and superego are involved in constant conflicts. These conflicts and frustrations give rise to our behavior and result in emotional growth. Without conflict and frustration, there would be no personality growth. Some conflicts are apparent to us; we are aware of some, consciously involved in many, but unaware of other conflicts. Because the conflicts that are unknown to us function at a deeper level, we cannot resolve them. Nevertheless, they act as strong motivators of our behavior.

## ◆ LEVELS OF CONSCIOUSNESS

Many view Sigmund Freud as the father of the field of personality theory. One of Freud's greatest contributions to the understanding of human behavior was his concept concerning **levels of consciousness**. He saw the mind as consisting of three levels of consciousness. These he labeled, from the one we are most aware of to the one we are least aware of, the conscious mind, the subconscious mind, and the unconscious mind, likening them to parts of an iceberg.

The **conscious mind** refers to that part of the mind that is focused in a here-and-now awareness (the part of the iceberg that is above the water level, freely visible).

The **subconscious mind** refers to that part of the mind just below immediate awareness—the storehouse for memories. These memories are either those that have ceased to be important to us or those that we suppressed because they are mildly uncomfortable. They can be brought back into awareness at will. (This is the part of the iceberg below the water level that can be seen by peering down into the water.)

The **unconscious mind** refers to that part of the mind that is closed to immediate awareness. It is a vast reservoir of memories, experiences, and emotions that cannot be recalled. (This is the part of the iceberg that cannot be seen at all and may extend a great distance down into the water, completely unknown to the observers above it.)

## ◆ CONFLICT

Conflicts among the three parts of the personality may result in behavior that is wholly conscious, partly conscious, wholly subconscious, or wholly unconscious. *The important aspect of behavior is that it usually resolves conflict.* Faced with an upsetting situation, people ordinarily do one of three things: (1) they become aggressive and oppose the situation, (2) they flee from it, or (3) they compromise with it. This last way of handling a situation seems to be the most realistic and the one most likely to resolve the conflict or anxiety.

Conflicts are resolved through the use of certain methods of thinking and acting that either eliminate the conflict or reduce its severity. These methods, commonly called **defense mechanisms** or **mental mechanisms,** are not always clear-cut; in fact, they often overlap or may be used simultaneously. Many defense mechanisms have been identified; they are described in Chapter 13, Stress: Ineffective Coping and Defense Mechanisms.

Why do people seem so different? Why is one person angry, aggressive, and ready to fight at the slightest provocation, whereas another is passive and gentle, always willing to compromise and bend in order to seek a peaceful solution?

The differences in basic personality style and energy level are apparent in any newborn nursery. One-day-old infants vary greatly in their amount of movement, crying vigor, sucking strength, and tolerance for discomfort. Any mother with more than one child will readily admit that each child exhibited definite differences throughout the neonatal period and infancy. One child was weaned more easily, another was more difficult to toilet train, and so forth.

## ◆ FACTORS IN PERSONALITY DEVELOPMENT

One can observe that even with the same parents, the genetic makeup of each sibling is different. One may "take after" his or her mother and the other "lean to the father's side of the family." One child may be significantly brighter than another. Literature is full of references to "the beautiful sister" and "the ugly sister," to the son who is "the dreamer" and the son who is "the doer."

The order of birth also plays a role in personality development. The first child is born into a home where childbearing is a new experience for the parents. Not only is the infant new at the job of being an infant, but also the parents are new at the job of being parents. The second child is born into a different situation. His or her parents have had some experience at being parents. They may be practiced at limit-setting. They have, perhaps, made the house more childproof so that the second child is less likely to break valuable possessions or stray into situations of physical danger.

The first child is an only child until his or her brother or sister is born. He or she has the parents' full attention until suddenly the parents have a new baby, and he or she is an only child no longer. The second child is never an only child.

Although they often deny it, parents have preferences among their children. The father may like boys or more aggressive children, whereas the mother may prefer girls or quiet, obedient children. Often the reverse is true, the mother favoring her sons and the father favoring his daughters.

With all of these variables, it is little wonder that a great number of theories or belief systems have evolved regarding the issue of how personality development occurs. That genetic factors play a part is virtually beyond dispute. The most universally accepted belief about heredity is that it is the background, the set, on which environmental factors play to form the personality.

For example, it is believed by some, although by no means proved, that an infant with a genetic predisposition to schizophrenia may develop into a quiet, sensitive, artistic youth in one family and into a person with schizophrenia in another family (see Chapter 18, Schizophrenia and Other Psychotic Disorders). On the other hand, studies on identical twins, who have identical genetic structures, show that there is a very high likelihood of each twin developing the same mental disorder even when they are separated at birth and reared in different families.

Related to the heredity-as-cause belief system, but containing some of its own special concepts, is the biochemical (or neurotransmitter) theory. There are subtle, but distinct, biochemical differences between people with no mental disorder and people with major mental illnesses. Which comes first—the biochemical disorder or the mental disorder—is still under dispute, but this area of investigation is among the most promising in psychiatric research today.

## ◆ THEORIES OF PERSONALITY DEVELOPMENT

Most belief systems, however, have little to do with heredity or biochemistry. They are concerned with one or another facet of the individual person's development from birth onward. They focus on the various forces that impinge on the child, such as the father, mother, siblings, family, or society; or the intrinsic developmental forces, such as the child's initial dependence and growth toward independence, the development of language, the development of motor skills, and bowel and bladder control.

It should be well understood by the student at the outset that no theory is entirely and absolutely correct. At the same time, there is no place for a negative attitude that says, "since nobody knows, there's no reason for listening to anybody." Each theory contains plausible elements that assist in understanding the formation of personality.

Carl Jung emphasized concepts of the collective unconscious, individuation (becoming an individual), and introversion and extroversion.

Sigmund Freud was a Viennese physician who made important contributions to our understanding of personality development. These theories are a part of the system of psychology he named psychoanalysis. The word is obtained from the term *psyche*, or mind.

Harry Stack Sullivan believed that the individual could be studied only in relation to his or her social interactions with others. Sullivan developed four basic postulates that underlie his theories:

1. The *biological postulate*, which states that man (as an animal) differs from all other animals in his cultural interdependence.
2. *Man's essentially human mode of functioning*, which refers to those characteristics that distinguish humans from all other animal life.
3. *Significance of anxiety*, which refers to the central role of anxiety in human development.
4. The *tenderness postulate*, in which Sullivan states that "the activity of an infant which arises from the tension of his needs produces tension in the mothering one which is felt by her as tenderness." Man has a growing capacity for tenderness.

Gertrude Mahler described the important psychological development that occurs in children during the first 2½ years of life. She believes that the availability of a consistent, loving caregiver, ideally the mother, is essential if the child is to avoid feeling abandoned and insecure during later life.

Erich Fromm's theories reflect the orientation of the social scientist. He emphasizes the role of society in mental disorders rather than the role of the individual, which is the classic psychoanalyst's concern. Fromm believes that "self-love" is really self-affirmation, which is the basis of the capacity to love others.

Alfred Adler influenced child psychiatry a great deal with his early considerations of organ inferiority and nervous character. He later became preoccupied with educational, social, and political issues as the causes of mental illness.

Karen Horney believed that specific cultural values and beliefs cause disturbances in human relationships leading to neuroses.

Jean Baker Miller describes the psychological development of women as a process in which they learn the value of being subordinate in order to gain acceptance from the larger social system, which includes men and authority figures. She also identifies several important traditional roles of women: the giver of care; the mediator, who avoids and mediates conflicts; and the avoider of power. She believes that these roles undermine women's ability to develop their full potential as human beings.

Wilhelm Reich made a valuable contribution to the understanding of how the character or personality style evident in adulthood is developed.

Otto Rank was primarily concerned with the application of psychoanalysis to mythology and literature.

Eugen Bleuler published a comprehensive study of schizophrenia (a term he coined).

Hermann Rorschach, who developed the ink blot test, was a pioneer in the elaboration of projective psychological testing.

Carl Rogers' theory of personality states that the values of a society and of a person living within that society may differ. If a person replaces his or her own values and choices regarding self-actualization with those of the social environment in order to gain acceptance and approval, conflict occurs in the form of anxiety.

## ◆ ERIKSON'S CONCEPT OF PERSONALITY DEVELOPMENT

Erik Erikson's concept of personality development compares the evolution of the personality to the evolution of tissues in the early stages of embryonic development. He believes that there is a timetable inherent in the development of various specialized tissues, organs, and systems tasks to be accomplished. In his view, a developmental task not only contributes some vital attribute in the physical body but also lays the groundwork for the next task. The stages of psychosocial development identified by Erikson and the developmental challenges of each stage are listed in the following:

1. Early infancy (birth to 1 year): trust versus mistrust
2. Later infancy (1 to 3 years): autonomy versus shame and doubt
3. Early childhood (4 to 5 years): initiative versus guilt
4. Later childhood (6 to 11 years): industry versus inferiority
5. Puberty and adolescence (12 to 20 years): ego identity versus role confusion
6. Early adulthood (20 to 40 years): intimacy versus isolation
7. Middle adulthood (40 to 60 years): generativity versus stagnation
8. Late adulthood (60 years and older): ego integrity versus despair

He builds the theory upon this concept that a whole or partial failure at one step means that the personality will be deficient in the trait that should have arisen at that particular time. If succeeding stages are developed on too weak a foundation, the total personality may suffer as a result. Erikson points out that these successive stages of personality development should not be thought of as arising at exact time periods but, rather, at approximate age levels, with considerable individual variation, and that the developmental tasks of each stage overlap. According to Erikson, if a developmental task is not fully mastered during a particular stage of development, it is possible for the unresolved issues of that stage to be worked through during later stages. Following is a brief description of Erikson's stages of psychosocial development.

## EARLY INFANCY

This period is characterized by *basic trust*. An infant is completely helpless and at the mercy of adults. The baby who is warmly accepted, wanted, and loved comes to know the world as a nice place and the people in it as friendly and helpful. He or she develops a cheerful confidence that his or her needs will be met. On the other hand, the baby who feels unloved and unaccepted develops a diffuse anxiety, a distrust of his or her small world. The baby may become preoccupied with his or her own needs as a result of uncertainty over whether they will be met. Because the baby is given so little opportunity to respond positively to others, he or she is likely to become demanding, fearful, hostile, or simply cold and withdrawn.

Basic trust is the necessary foundation for the capacity to love. The histories of people with schizophrenia, the largest group of mentally ill individuals, all have a remarkable sameness; they felt unloved and unwanted in childhood, so unloved that they failed to develop the basic trust that enables them to build binding ties with other human beings. The schizophrenic is afraid to love, afraid to invest affection in others. Thus, he or she lives in a world of isolation.

## LATER INFANCY

This period is characterized by *autonomy*. Between the ages of 2 and 4 years, the young child comes into contact with increasing restrictions. He or she must adapt to the family and its practices and learn to adjust to social and moral norms. The child becomes fiercely rebellious at all these restrictions and impatient with routines and regulations. His or her favorite word is "no." Because the child is still dependent on the very adults he or she defies, however, and because he or she desires their love and approval, the child usually builds a fine but precarious balance between independence and conformity.

## EARLY CHILDHOOD

This period is characterized by *initiative* and occurs during the fourth and fifth years. As trust represents the first phase and independence the second, so the third is characterized by an outstanding attribute of personality—initiative. Early childhood is the period during which the child expands his or her imagination. He or she starts trying on, or identifying with, the role of the same-sex parent. The boy unconsciously adopts the mannerisms and attitudes of his father, whereas the girl adopts those of her mother. The underlying dynamic in the child who attempts new situations is positive self-esteem. Positive self-esteem is the internalization of the acceptance and approval the child received from his or her parents during the first years of life.

## LATER CHILDHOOD

This period is characterized by *industry* and *accomplishment*. Children between 6 and 11 years of age have much energy that needs channeling into constructive accomplishments. The child is in school, and he or she learns to compete with peers in many areas. Pride in achievement develops as a result of praise and attention to his or her efforts. Group projects become absorbing; interests develop into hobbies. These are the joyous, exciting years of childhood, when the child learns to work beside and with others, when he or she begins to learn the skills, both intellectual and mechanical, necessary for a future role as a citizen in a complex society. It is the lull before the turbulent years of adolescence. Parents can assist the child's transition during latency by being actively involved in his or her activities and supporting his or her self-esteem.

## PUBERTY AND ADOLESCENCE

This period can be a stormy one, characterized by a *search for identity*. The young boy or girl is usually ill-prepared for the great physiologic changes that must occur before the body becomes ready for reproduction. During the same period, emotions must stabilize in preparation for assuming the responsibility of a family. An adolescent's new surge of sexual feelings, striving for independence from family restrictions, self-doubt about his or her abilities, and a strong sense of ambivalence can cause confusion.

The teenager needs to choose a vocation or career but often has qualms about the selection of a life's work. He or she may be bewildered by the vast array of possibilities and uncertain about what course he or she really wishes to follow. Sympathetic and understanding parents and teachers can do much to lighten the emotional burdens of the adolescent. They must understand the adolescent's need to reject their standards and ideals temporarily and find security in identifying with the mannerisms, dress, speech, and activities of peers. If the teenager feels loved and knows that his or her parents stand as safe ports in a storm who will provide temporary shelter when the going gets too rough, he or she will emerge from the turmoil with a renewed sense of identity and with good, fundamental human values intact. The teenager's redefined identity is founded on inner integrity—a conviction that he or she is truly a person worthy of respect in the adult world.

## EARLY ADULTHOOD

The developmental challenge of the young adult between 20 and 40 years of age is to be capable of intimacy. *Intimacy* is the capacity to trust oneself and another in a deep and committed relationship. The challenge is to know and be known by another. This includes accepting one's own foibles, as well as those of another. Intimacy in a long-term sexual relationship is marked by love, concern, compassion, and commitment to the well being of the other. A capacity for intimacy is also an essential characteristic of long-lasting, deep friendships. When a person is incapable of intimacy, he or she is aloof and isolated, shunning closeness with others.

## MIDDLE ADULTHOOD

The middle-aged adult between 40 and 60 years is engaged in developing and guiding the next generation—children, grandchildren, coworkers, or young people in various types of social groups. The psychologically mature adult is productive rather than stagnant. The person who does not master this developmental hurdle is preoccupied with himself or herself to the exclusion of others' needs. The immature adult also exhibits a tendency toward hypochondriacal sickness and general dissatisfaction with life. Hypochondriasis is the belief that one is ill when there are no identifiable symptoms of illness.

## LATE ADULTHOOD
This period is characterized by integrity. To Erikson, *integrity* is the ability to live out the later portion of life with dignity and an assured sense of order and meaning in the total scheme of life. The facets of integrity are serenity, continual joy in living, a sense of accomplishment, and anticipation of worthwhile endeavors yet to be accomplished. These traits contrast with the despair that eventually develops in elderly adults who are unable to resolve the losses of later life or master this last stage of psychosocial development.

## K E Y   P O I N T S

- A child's heredity, also known as genetic endowment, includes genetic traits such as constitution or temperament, eye and skin color, general intellectual capacity, talents, and the makeup of his or her neurologic system.
- Just as a child's body goes through successive stages of physical development, the child's personality undergoes developmental stages. Disturbing early experiences or unsatisfied emotional needs may lead to an arrest of normal development.
- Most theorists agree that:
    —Personality results from complex interactions between heredity and environment.
    —Dynamic forces cause behavior.
    —Some of these dynamic forces are unconscious or unknown to the individual.
    —Childhood is an important time for forming enduring behavior patterns.
    —Behavior is a function or expression of personality.
- Learning consists of four steps: need, stimulus, response, and reinforcement. Extinction (forgetting) occurs when reinforcement ceases.
- Certain experiences are crucial in a child's development:
    —Availability of a consistent, concerned caregiver
    —Feeding situation (including weaning) in early infancy
    —Toilet and cleanliness training
    —Early sex training
    —Training for control of anger and aggression

■ According to Abraham Maslow's theory, a hierarchy of needs must be met for people to develop psychological maturity. These needs, from lowest to highest, are physiologic, safety, love and belonging, esteem, and self-actualization.

■ The conflicts that arise among these parts of the personality give rise to behavior. Satisfactory resolution of the conflicts, usually through defense or mental mechanisms, results in emotional growth.

■ According to Freud, the human mind consists of the conscious, the subconscious, and the unconscious.

■ The major factors in personality development are genetic makeup and environmental impacts and influences.

■ Most personality theories focus on the various forces that affect the child, such as heredity, family structure, societal expectations, and other developmental forces.

■ A number of theories of personality exist, although no one theory is completely correct or incorrect.

■ Erik Erikson's concept of personality proposes eight stages of development, from infancy to old age, each of which has a developmental task to accomplish. The stages and tasks are as follows:
1. Early infancy—trust versus mistrust
2. Later infancy—autonomy versus shame and doubt
3. Early childhood—initiative versus guilt
4. Later childhood—industry versus inferiority
5. Puberty and adolescence—ego identity versus role confusion
6. Early adulthood—intimacy versus isolation
7. Middle adulthood—generativity versus stagnation
8. Late adulthood—ego integrity versus despair

### SELF-AWARENESS ACTIVITY

This chapter provides many types of information about the complexity of human development.

• As you were reading about the formation of personality, what thoughts came to your mind about your own development?

• Can you name three different factors that have most strongly contributed to your own personality characteristics?

• Is there someone in your family who you resemble physically?

• Do you have similar personality characteristics to this person? If not, is there someone in your family with whom you share similar personality characteristics?

• If you would like to have a child some day or currently have one or more children, name three of your most important beliefs about providing an environment that is most nurturing for a child.

- As you review the information about Maslow's hierarchy of human needs, where do you place yourself on the hierarchy? Why?

## QUESTIONS

1. Identification is important in personality development because:
   a. children can identify their parents' outdated ideas and attitudes and avoid them.
   b. it indicates a child's intelligence.
   c. healthy identifications can help people develop mature adult personalities.
   d. it means the child's personality is never in a state of flux.
2. Which of Maslow's needs would have the highest nursing *priority?*
   a. Esteem
   b. Self-actualization
   c. Love and belonging
   d. Physiologic
3. When working with an 8-year-old child the nurse should be aware that, according to Erikson, it is *most* important to
   a. provide praise and attention for accomplishments.
   b. encourage the child's imagination.
   c. openly discuss the child's emerging sexuality.
   d. reinforce social norms.
4. The four steps involved in the process of learning are
   a. need, stimulus, reinforcement, and repetition.
   b. desire, stimulus, reinforcement, and repetition.
   c. need, stimulus, response, and reinforcement.
   d. desire, stimulus, response, and reinforcement.

## BIBLIOGRAPHY

Boyd, M., & Nihart, M. (1998). *Psychiatric nursing: Contemporary practice.* Philadelphia: Lippincott Williams & Wilkins.

Brazelton, T. (1991). What we can learn from the status of the newborn. *NIDA Research Monograph, 114,* 93–105.

Gerow, J., & Bordens, K. (2000). *Psychology: An introduction.* Carrollton, TX: Alliance Press.

Ginsburg, H. (1992). Childhood injuries and Erikson's psychosocial stages. *Social Behavior and Personality, 20,* 95–114.

Kaplan, H., & Sadock, B. (1998). *Comprehensive textbook of psychiatry* (6th ed.). Baltimore: Williams & Wilkins.

Maslow, A. (1970). *Motivation and personality.* New York: Harper & Row.

Ogden, J. (2000). *Health psychology: A textbook.* Buckingham: Open University Press.

Rathus, S. *Psychology: The core.* Fort Worth, TX: Harcourt College Publishers.

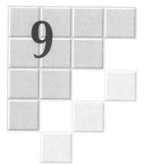

# 9

# Influences of Family and Social Environment on the Individual

---

## B e h a v i o r a l    O b j e c t i v e s

*After reading*
*this chapter*
*the student*
*will be able to:*

■ Describe the concept of personality disposition.

■ Explain the concepts of system, subsystem, and supersystem.

■ Define the term dynamic and explain the dynamics in a closed versus open family.

■ Explain how the dynamics of a family are altered when one of its members is treated for mental illness.

■ Explain why sibling position in a family can have an effect on personality development.

■ Describe homeostasis in the family.

---

## K e y    T e r m s

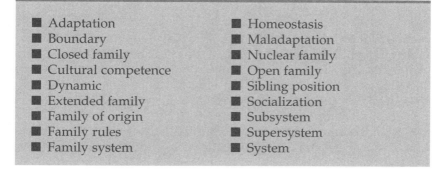

■ Adaptation
■ Boundary
■ Closed family
■ Cultural competence
■ Dynamic
■ Extended family
■ Family of origin
■ Family rules
■ Family system

■ Homeostasis
■ Maladaptation
■ Nuclear family
■ Open family
■ Sibling position
■ Socialization
■ Subsystem
■ Supersystem
■ System

The family is the first social group experienced by a developing infant. The comfort of an individual with any social group during childhood and adulthood is shaped by his or her relationships with mother, father, siblings, and the extended family. The **extended family** includes grandparents, aunts, uncles, and cousins. Because of today's mobile society, some of the important roles usually performed by family members may be filled by friends, neighbors, teachers, ministers, and so on.

As described in Chapter 8, Theories and Stages of Personality Development, an infant is a unique being who is born with a certain disposition or temperament determined by his or her physical inheritance. For example, he or she may have a quiet, easygoing disposition, be irritable and difficult to please, or be very alert and inquisitive.

Just as the infant has his or her own unique disposition, so too do the parents. Depending on the fit in disposition between a child and his or her parents, there may be a higher capacity for trust or for anxiety-producing tension or conflict. As an example, consider the experience of a cranky, irritable infant who is born to a frequently anxious mother versus an easygoing, confident mother. The psychological "fit" between a parent and child can be an important factor in the development of a child's self-esteem.

A family is a very complex social structure. Countless factors shape its development and that of each of its members. **Family system** is a term that describes the characteristics of a family. These characteristics include the roles in a family, such as mother, father, oldest child, and so on. Other characteristics include the ways that a family interacts, such as boundaries, open and closed patterns of communication, and so on. These characteristics are described afterward in this chapter.

**Adaptation** is the process of adjusting to one's environment in such a way that the growth and development potential of that individual in his or her life and the general balance in the family are enhanced. **Maladaptation** in the family is often the result of chronic ineffective coping on the part of one or both parents. Maladaptation can result in dysfunctional patterns of responses to stress within one or more family members. A dysfunctional family system is one in which one or more members of the family communicate in a way that diminishes the general emotional health of all members of the family. Children usually acquire these dysfunctional social and communication patterns in their socialization within the family. Maladaptive characteristics in the family system can contribute to the development of mental disorders in one or more family members.

**Socialization** is the shaping of an individual to the communication style, beliefs, and emotional patterns of a social group. The internal and external stresses and forces that affect the child, both parents, and every child in the family shape the growth and development of a child in the family. Most of these family forces, stresses, and dynamics have been examined in order to understand the causes of mental illness.

Personality theorists generally believe that the usual cause of mental illness is the result of two factors: genetic physiologic inheritance and the effect of the family environment on the child during infancy and childhood. In order to understand the importance of the multiple forces and dynamics that occur in families, mental health theorists turned to the scientific field for the terminology to describe family processes. General systems theory has been adopted from the field of biology to explain family processes and their effects on personality development.

## ◆ GENERAL SYSTEMS THEORY

General systems theory is a helpful concept to nurses in the care of clients. Von Bertalanffy developed the original concept of systems theory in the 1920s. In his field, biology, he was constantly impressed by the organization of organisms and the dependence of biological systems on one another. The metabolism and growth of one organism depends on another; for example, photosynthesis by trees requires carbon dioxide given off as a waste product by human metabolism. Conversely, humans use oxygen given off as a waste product by trees in their metabolic process.

As scientists from other fields began to apply von Bertalanffy's general systems concepts to their own disciplines, they began to see that there was, indeed, an interdependence of one system on another. This concept can be applied to the smallest microscopic life form or the solar system and the interactions of the planets.

This idea of interdependence applies very well to the fields of psychiatry and psychology. No human being exists in complete isolation from all others. The infant, for example, depends on others for his or her physical care and nurturing. His or her personality is formed as the result of interactions, primarily with immediate family and later with teachers, peers, and others.

## ◆ SYSTEMS, SUBSYSTEMS, AND SUPERSYSTEMS

What is a system? A **system** is actually a collection of working parts that, when combined, make up a more complex working object or abstract entity. These smaller components are called subsystems. They are essential to the overall functioning of a system. A **subsystem** is a concrete or abstract, essential part of a larger system and relates in specific ways with all parts of the larger entity. Without the subsystem, the system cannot function.

The human psyche is an example of an abstract system. It is made up of three major parts or subsystems: the id, ego, and superego. If one or more of these subsystems is not present, the psyche is unable to function. The cardiovascular system is a concrete example. This system is made up of several working subsystems—the heart, arteries, veins, and so on.

The body itself is a very complex entity made up of a large number of systems. When a number of systems are essential for an entity to function, it is called a supersystem. A **supersystem** is a large complex made up of many systems. A state's department of mental health is also a supersystem; it consists of many hospitals, departments, and groups of workers essential to its functioning.

## THE HUMAN BEING AS A SYSTEM

The human being is a system made up of two main subsystems, the physiologic and psychological. The physiologic subsystem includes many smaller subsystems, such as cardiovascular, neurologic, and musculoskeletal. If one of these subsystems fails, the result is that all the other subsystems will ultimately fail, and death will occur. The human psychological subsystem includes the id, ego, and superego subsystems.

As noted, a human being is part of larger systems that can be called supersystems. A person belongs to several social supersystems. His or her primary social system is the family. It is in the family that he or she acquires basic values, self-image, and the capacity for relating with others throughout his or her lifetime. In addition, a person belongs to social systems through school and work. A person is also a part of the ecologic supersystem; in the environment he or she lives interdependently with other animals, plants, gases, and water.

## SYSTEMS THEORY AND MENTAL ILLNESS

The concept of systems is important for our purposes. It allows us to look for the cause of mental illness somewhere within one of a human's subsystems or supersystems. Identification of the cause, when possible, allows us to plan therapeutic interventions.

## SOCIOCULTURAL ENVIRONMENT

One of the challenges in the delivery of therapeutic nursing care is to find common themes that provide the basis for effective communication. This challenge includes being able to bridge differences in education level, age, social class, and so on. With the increasing diversity of persons from all regions of the world who live in the U.S. society, there is an increasing challenge to deliver culturally competent care. **Cultural competence** is the ability to bring the following components of empathic nursing care into a therapeutic relationship:

Self-awareness

Awareness and acceptance of cultural differences

Understanding of basic differences in personal approaches to health, hygiene, and illness

Basic understanding about a client's culture

Adaptation skills

As an introduction to the types of cultural issues that may create communication barriers between a nurse and client, review the types of questions that appear in Box 9-1.

The development of cultural sensitivity requires three different conditions to be present in the nurse:

- An open-minded attitude about experiencing other world views
- Awareness about one's own biases and attitudes that create barriers to direct interaction with a group
- Willingness to experience culture directly

In order to determine the extent that a client's culture will impact his or her clinical treatment and rehabilitation from a mental disorder, the factors shown in Box 9-2 can be important indicators in delivering culturally competent nursing care.

Negotiating a plan of care and client compliance when there are cultural issues is an important consideration at all times. It is important to know whether you and your client are able to communicate clearly or whether there are language or cultural barriers that prevent or

---

**BOX 9-1. Questions for Eliciting Patients' Explanatory Models of Illness**

What do you call your problem? What name does it have?
What do you think has caused your problem?
Why do you think it started when it did?
What does your sickness do to you? How does it work?
How severe is it?
Will it have a short or long course?
What do you fear most about your sickness?
What are the chief problems your sickness has caused you?
What kind of treatment do you think you should receive?
What are the most important results you hope to receive from the treatment?

Adapted from Kleinman, A., Eisenberg, L., & Good, B. (1978). Culture, illness and care: Clinical lessons from anthropologic and cross-cultural research. *Annals of Internal Medicine, 88*(2), 251–258.

---

### BOX 9-2. Factors Indicating Heritage Consistency

1. Childhood development occurred in the person's country of origin or in an immigrant neighborhood in the United States of like ethnic group.
2. Extended family members encourage participation in traditional religious or cultural activities.
3. Individual engages in frequent visits to country of origin or to the "old neighborhood" in the United States.
4. Family homes are within the ethnic community.
5. Individual participates in ethnic cultural events, such as religious festivals or national holidays, sometimes with singing, dancing, and costumes.
6. Individual was raised in an extended family setting.
7. Individual maintains regular contact with the extended family.
8. Individual's name has not been Americanized.
9. Individual was educated in a parochial (nonpublic) school with a religious or ethnic philosophy similar to the family's background.
10. Individual engages in social activities primarily with others of the same ethnic background.
11. Individual has knowledge of the culture and language of origin.
12. Individual possesses elements of personal pride about his or her heritage.

Reprinted with permission from Spector, R.E. (1991). *Cultural diversity in health and illness*. Norwalk, CT: Appleton and Lange, p. 55.

---

reduce compliance with the nursing care plan. Obtaining assistance to clarify these questions is essential to provide an environment in which the client can begin to recover health. The guidelines in Box 9-3 are important in clarifying the expectations of the translator and communicating clearly the information that is sought from the translator. These guidelines also help to illustrate the unique types of communication issues that occur when there are language barriers in the health care setting.

### ◆ CONCEPTS IN FAMILY SYSTEM FUNCTIONING

#### FAMILY SYSTEM TERMINOLOGY

The immediate family into which a child is born is called the **nuclear family.** It is made up of mother, father, and siblings; it is also known as the **family of origin.** The family members not in the nuclear family—grandparents, aunts, uncles, cousins, and so on—are known as the extended family.

## BOX 9-3. Guidelines for Using a Translator

1. Slow down the communication process.
2. Give one or two sentences at a time to be translated unless the translator has been trained (i.e., U.N. translators) to do simultaneous translation.
3. Orient the patient to the process. Ask him or her to slow down communication. It may be necessary to repeat this request often.
4. Never stand during an interview; situate yourself next to the patient so that you are directly in the line of communication. Communicating with body language and eye contact is also important. This can be controlled by sitting next to the patient. Do not sit with the translator in the middle or the result will be a tennis-match style of communication.
5. Orient the translator about the topics to be covered and why it is important that accuracy be maintained.
6. Allow the translator to let you know when something is difficult to translate so that you can reword it and not be misinterpreted. Sometimes with sensitive topics translators may need coaching to ask the questions, or the translator will have to be changed. For example, a male translating questions about a sexual history may have difficulties with a female patient.
7. Do not have translators ask questions that you would not feel comfortable asking yourself. Also, do not give them the question in an angry or upset manner because they will find it difficult to translate or will want to protect the patient from your anger.
8. To avoid errors, limit the use of medical jargon in your interview. Otherwise you will force more errors as the translator goes from English medical terminology, to English lay language, to the target language. For example, if you use the term renal calculi, the translator has to translate the medical to the lay English, kidney stones; to the Spanish lay, "piedras en los riñones." The more coding and decoding the translator does the greater the chances for error.
9. Give positive praise to the translators and acknowledge their contribution. Review the positive aspects of the translation, and also those that need improvement both from the translator's and the health care provider's perspective.

## DYNAMICS

A **dynamic** is a constantly operating force within a system that results in some type of action or observable result. If, for example, a person was orphaned as a young child or born with a major handicap, it can be said that these factors lying deep within the experience of a person have a constantly operating effect on him or her. Dynamics are usually operating in all of us without our conscious awareness.

There are dynamics that occur within a person's psyche, such as unconscious impulses or drives of the id. In addition, there are social system dynamics that operate in families. These can include defensive avoidance of a family member with an explosive temper or schizophrenia.

## OPEN AND CLOSED FAMILY SYSTEMS

Depending on the openness or closedness of the family, a child's needs are or are not shaped or formed in such a way that is healthy and supports his or her continuing social and psychological development.

An **open family** is one in which the members, especially the parents, have had the opportunity to develop as healthy, active, members of society with positive self-esteem. They not only contribute to the society and their families, but also they are able to recognize their needs and have them met by others when necessary. In other words, they know how to receive or take from others whatever they need to develop as actualized human beings in a socially responsible manner. An open family allows for flexibility in the roles of its members.

A **closed family,** on the other hand, is rigid and allows little change in the roles and patterns in the family. Usually one of the parents (frequently both) has moderate to high levels of psychopathology. The climate in the home does not support the development and ultimate healthy separation of the child from the family when he or she reaches adulthood.

The majority of people we work with in psychiatric settings come from the latter type of family. The dynamics in the closed family frequently contribute to inadequate or pathologic personality development in the developing child. These traits evolve into the adult's personality. Remember that an individual's personality has been shaped over a long period of time. The shaping of a child's personality usually is the result of the family's needs but without their conscious awareness of the profound effects that family communication patterns and dynamics may have on the developing personality of the child.

## ◆ EFFECTS OF MENTAL ILLNESS ON FAMILY DYNAMICS

Accordingly, when this family member becomes mentally ill, it is a worsening of a mental state to which the family has become accustomed. The family's dynamics are changed significantly if the person is treated in a mental health setting and his or her normally dysfunctional pattern is eliminated. A simple example of this is a woman who has a violent temper even when she is only mildly angry. Her family unconsciously knows her boiling point. They relate as a family in a way that will not upset her. Conversely, when the family is upset about something, she expresses the emotion that others feel, and it helps to clear the air.

This is the normal communication style of this particular family. Equilibrium in the family is maintained by the dynamic of the mother's anger. If her boiling point were to change permanently to a better, healthier level, it would dramatically change the way the family members interact. The other family members would unconsciously work to restore communications to their former normal style.

All families, open or closed, relate in a way that maintains their normal communication patterns. When the behavior of one person is changed, it disrupts these patterns and causes increased anxiety in all the other members. Accordingly, if people admitted to a mental health facility are treated with no attention to the family, their chances for long-term recovery are diminished. Family patterns that may have contributed to the development of the client's dysfunctional symptoms must be examined and, if necessary, modified. This requires that the family meet with a family therapist, usually one or more times weekly, during the client's hospitalization. The types of patterns and dynamics that exist in families are described in the following.

## SIBLING POSITION IN FAMILY OF ORIGIN
Studies of all types of families have found that birth order, or **sibling position,** strongly influences the way a person communicates and behaves in a family. In addition, a person carries these interpersonal traits into adulthood, and they become part of the way he or she relates in any social setting. Generally, the oldest child is more responsive to criticism, is more responsible, achieves consistently, and functions behaviorally in a more rigid manner than younger brothers or sisters. These traits result from the parents' tendencies to demand more of oldest children and expect them to assist with the care of younger siblings.

The youngest child frequently is more dependent, less achievement-oriented, and often quite charming. This results from the love and attention received by the youngest child. If his or her needs were easily met, he or she did not learn to tolerate frustration in pursuit of goals.

The middle child, because of his or her position between the oldest and youngest children, frequently is more flexible and independent. He or she also tends to be more easygoing than is the oldest or youngest child. A client's interaction style in the hospital setting, both with caregivers and other clients, frequently reflects his or her sibling position.

## FAMILY RULES
**Family rules** are the unwritten expectations about what types of roles or behavior are acceptable or unacceptable to the family. Remember

that most people behave in ways that ensure approval by those they care about. As we grow older we tend to conform to the expectations of others in order to maintain their love and acceptance. These rules are often based on the value system that each partner brings into a marriage. Remember that we inherit many of our values from our families. Most people tend to marry individuals with similar values or expectations. It is in this way that family patterns, rules, and expectations tend to remain somewhat similar from one generation to the next.

## BOUNDARIES

Boundaries are the rules that keep the role of one family member separate from another within a family system. Staying within one's role in the family is often the key to acceptance in the family. Boundaries develop as the result of family rules. For example, if women in a family have traditionally been passive, a daughter from such a family may be passive as well. She will most likely marry a man who enjoys his role as sole decision maker. This type of family pattern of relationships teaches the children to go to the father automatically when a decision needs to be made. If the mother uncharacteristically makes a major decision, conflict usually results. She has, in effect, overstepped her customary **boundary** and altered her normal role in the family.

When a mentally ill person is successfully treated and reenters the family, the role he or she filled before treatment is changed. Accordingly, his or her normal boundaries of functioning are also different. A family therapy process, in conjunction with inpatient psychiatric hospitalization, is designed to renegotiate and reestablish boundaries and role patterns so that the newly discharged person's different (and healthier) style of functioning will not be reshaped by the family to his or her preadmission family role.

## HOMEOSTASIS

The concept of a system is helpful when we look at homeostasis or equilibrium within a family. It can be helpful to visualize a mobile with a number of objects hanging from it as a symbol of homeostasis. Compare the mobile with a family system. When it is in balance it maintains perfect equilibrium. If one of the objects is tapped, all the other objects are affected and jostled. If one object is removed, there is an even stronger effect; the entire mobile loses its balance.

**Homeostasis** is a dynamic, ever-changing state in which a system constantly works to maintain balance. As one subsystem or person changes, the other members alter their patterns of communication or behavior to maintain the balance of the family. When a person becomes mentally ill, the family struggles to counter the effects of his or her worsening symptoms. If admission to the hospital becomes necessary, it triggers a crisis. The removal of the person from the family can allow the family to work toward equilibrium or homeostasis. Remember, however, that without the return of the ill member to the family, true family homeostasis is disrupted.

The concept of general systems theory applies to all systems. It encourages us to view physically or mentally ill clients holistically. We are aware of the interaction of physical illness on the psyche, and conversely, of the psyche on physical illness. It also allows us to evaluate the interaction of the overall social system and family on the etiology, diagnosis, and treatment of illness.

## K E Y   P O I N T S

■ The family is the first social group that each person experiences. Patterns of behavior in a family that contribute to mental illness are referred to as the family system.

■ A system is a collection of working parts that, when combined, make up a more complex working object or entity.

■ A subsystem is a small but essential part of the system that relates to all parts of the larger system and is an integral part of it.

■ A supersystem is a large complex made up of many systems.

■ Human beings are made of two major interdependent systems, the physiologic and the psychological.

■ Identifying the cause of mental illness within one of the human systems, subsystems, or supersystems helps caregivers plan therapeutic interventions.

■ Major concepts in family systems functioning include:
  —*Family system terminology:* nuclear and extended family and family of origin
  —*Dynamics:* constantly operating forces within a system
  —*Open family system:* family members have flexible roles; helps produce healthy, active people
  —*Closed family system:* family members have rigid roles; does not support healthy development

■ Treatment of a mentally disordered person needs to include attention to family dynamics. When the family is not considered, the client's chances for long-term improvement are diminished.

■ Family dynamics that affect mental health and mental illness are sibling position in family of origin, family rules (expectations about roles and behavior), and boundaries (rules that keep one person separate from another).

■ Homeostasis is a dynamic state in which a system constantly works to maintain balance. Families attempt to maintain homeostasis, or equilibrium, in response to changes in their system or subsystem.

## SELF-AWARENESS ACTIVITY

- What do you think has been the most important contribution of your family to your development?
- Where on the continuum between open and closed family does your original family operate most of the time?
- How do you respond to that style of communication?
- What are the conscious choices you make to contribute to your own homeostasis?

## QUESTIONS

1. Understanding the concepts of systems, subsystems, and supersystems is important in nursing because:
   a. Supersystems can function well, even when some subsystems are dysfunctional.
   b. Understanding the role of human systems in mental illness can help caregivers plan therapeutic interventions.
   c. A closed family system produces adaptive family patterns of communication that can contribute to mental illness.
   d. All of the above.
2. It is important that caregivers assess the family of a person treated in mental health facility because:
   a. It improves the person's long-term chances for recovery.
   b. Family behavior patterns often contribute to the client's dysfunction.
   c. The way that the family interacts with the client may need to be modified.
   d. All of the above.
3. Sibling position in a family
   a. has little or no influence on communication and behavior.
   b. impacts interpersonal traits into adulthood.
   c. has not yet been studied.
   d. controls all communication and behavior.
4. Homeostasis means that
   a. a family system constantly works to maintain balance.
   b. families need just one familiar mode of communication.
   c. each individual is separate, so a change in one family member does not affect another family member.
   d. mentally disordered people should be permanently removed from their families to maintain the family balance.

## BIBLIOGRAPHY

Barry, P.D. (1996). *Psychosocial nursing: Care of physically ill patients and their families* (3rd ed.). Philadelphia: Lippincott-Raven.

Bernal, H. (1996). Delivering culturally competent care. In Barry, P. (Ed.). *Psychosocial nursing: Care of physically ill patients and their families* (3rd ed.). Philadelphia: Lippincott-Raven.

Boyd, M. & Nihart, M. (1998). *Psychiatric nursing: Contemporary practice.* Philadelphia: Lippincott-Raven.

Carpenito, L.J. (2000). *Nursing diagnosis: Application to clinical practice* (8th ed.). Philadelphia: Lippincott Williams & Wilkins.

*Diagnostic and statistical manual of mental disorders* (4th ed.). (1994). Washington, DC: American Psychiatric Press.

Kaplan, H.I., & Sadock, B.J. (1998). *Comprehensive textbook of psychiatry* (6th ed.). Baltimore: Williams & Wilkins.

Lefley, H. (1998). Families, culture, and mental illness: Constructing new realities. *Psychiatry, 61*(4), 335–355.

Madsen, W., & Nichols, M. (Eds.) (1999). *Collaborative therapy with multi-stressed families: From old problems to new futures.* New York: Guilford Press.

McGoldrick, M. (Ed.). (1999). *Genograms: Assessment and intervention.* New York: W. W. Norton.

Nichols, M., & Schwartz, R. (Eds.). (2000). *Family therapy: Concepts and methods.* Boston: Allyn & Bacon.

Sadock, B., & Kaplan, H. (1998). *Synopsis of psychiatry: Behavioral sciences/clinical psychiatry.* Philadelphia: Lippincott-Raven.

Toman, W. (1976). *Family constellation: Its effects on personality and social behavior* (3rd ed.). New York: Springer.

## DEVELOPING CRITICAL THINKING SKILLS THROUGH CLASS DISCUSSION

### UNIT 2 Case Study
## Foundations of the Therapeutic Relationship

Gloria is 28 years old. She and her husband Tom have a 1-month-old infant. Almost as soon as Gloria arrived home from the hospital, she began to have difficulty coping with her baby. She became acutely depressed and suicidal, with frequent waves of anxiety about taking care of the infant. Gloria was referred by her obstetrician to a psychiatrist. She was admitted to an inpatient psychiatric unit for treatment.

### DISCUSSION QUESTIONS

1. According to Maslow's Hierarchy of Human Needs, what would be your nursing priorities when caring for Gloria? What nursing interventions could you employ to ensure that these needs are met?
2. Erikson identified eight stages of personality development. In what stage would Gloria be? What nursing interventions could you employ to facilitate Gloria's development?
3. What are some of the key components of a therapeutic relationship? What could you do to foster a therapeutic relationship?
4. How will you know whether you have developed a therapeutic relationship with Gloria?
5. Gloria may have difficulty discussing her feelings with nursing staff. What techniques could you use to enhance communication? Why would these techniques be helpful?
6. What impact might this diagnosis and hospitalization have on Gloria's family?

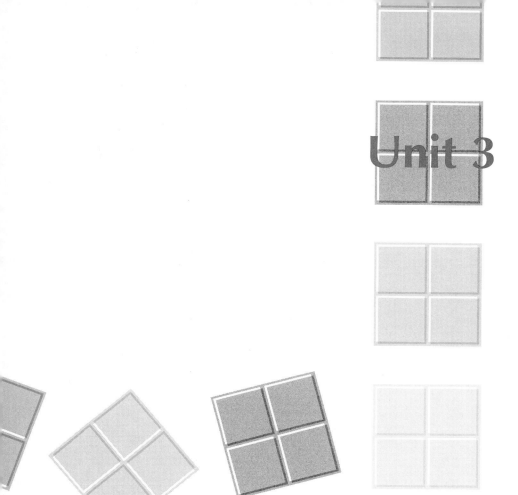

# Unit 3

# FOUNDATIONS OF DECISION MAKING IN THE MENTAL HEALTH SETTING

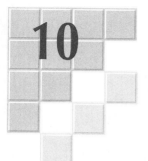

# Nursing Process in the Mental Health Setting

## Behavioral Objectives

*After reading this chapter the student will be able to:*

- Name the five steps of the nursing process.
- Name the number of nursing diagnoses identified by the North American Nursing Diagnosis Association.
- Name three reasons why the use of nursing diagnoses in clinical practice was developed.
- Describe why the use of a formal assessment tool is important in reviewing the range of potential health problems of a newly admitted client.
- Describe five of the patterns of human functioning (response) that are used in assessing and diagnosing clinical problems that nursing is prepared to diagnose and treat.
- Explain why the assessment review of these patterns can assist the nurse in developing a comprehensive care plan.
- Name the three preliminary steps to effective nursing care planning.
- Describe the five elements of a nursing care plan.
- Describe how problem solving is used in the planning phase of the nursing process.
- Explain why contracting with the client is an essential part of the nursing care plan.
- Use systems theory to explain why a nursing care plan is essential to a therapeutic outcome for the client.
- Explain the association between a nursing goal and the interventions designed to address the nursing diagnoses.

## K e y   T e r m s

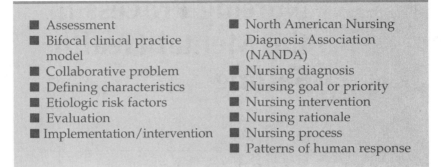

- Assessment
- Bifocal clinical practice model
- Collaborative problem
- Defining characteristics
- Etiologic risk factors
- Evaluation
- Implementation/intervention

- North American Nursing Diagnosis Association (NANDA)
- Nursing diagnosis
- Nursing goal or priority
- Nursing intervention
- Nursing rationale
- Nursing process
- Patterns of human response

Interacting therapeutically with clients demands a capacity for relating well with people. In addition, the nurse must understand nursing theories, physical and psychosocial assessment, and specific nursing tasks. Nurses must also possess the cognitive skills of analyzing, decision making, and evaluating—indeed, a nearly limitless number and range of skills. Caring for clients is a complex process.

It is important to give structure to this process in order to be able to practice nursing skills in an organized manner. The term **nursing process** has been coined as a title for the steps involved in organizing and implementing nursing care of clients. The five steps are as follows:

1. Assessment
2. Nursing diagnosis
3. Planning
4. Implementation/intervention
5. Evaluation

These steps are the same whether the nurse is in the home, community, or hospital setting. Increasingly, mental health care is occurring out of the hospital in the community and at home. These alternative care sites provide positive client outcomes and more cost-effective care. The steps in the nursing process are shown in Figure 10-1. This diagram demonstrates that the different steps of the nursing process are dynamic and interactive with each other. At no time is any one of the steps in the nursing process considered close. Each step is open-ended and open to continuing assessment, intervention, and evaluation criteria.

## ◆ ASSESSMENT

**Assessment** is the first step of the nursing process. Assessment includes gathering all the information needed to diagnose the specific

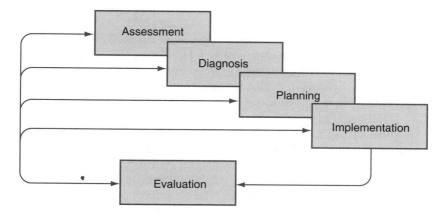

FIGURE 10–1. Relationships between the steps of the nursing process. (Alfaro, R. [1998]. *Applying nursing process: A step-by-step guide* [4th ed.] Philadelphia: Lippincott-Raven.)

problems that require nursing care and to develop a care plan. The care plan is specifically designed to meet the client's unique needs; it results in a therapeutic outcome. This type of information seeking includes an initial interview session with the client in which the information listed in the following should be obtained. Frequently it may take more than one session to complete the collection of data. Depending on the information given in response to questions, additional questions might be useful in order to reach a good comprehension of the client's situation. In addition, while talking, the areas of mental functioning described earlier (see Chapter 14, The Mental Status Exam) can be observed. The evaluation of mental status should be included under this section. The types of questions to be asked are as follows.

1. *Tell me what was going on that caused you to feel this way?* This information helps the nurse to understand the client's perception of his or her problem. A client commonly misinterprets the actual reason for admission and will relate the problem differently.
2. *Was there something specific that caused things to come to a crisis?* Frequently, the client's level of emotional stress has been increasing for a number of days, weeks, or months. There has been an accompanying deterioration in his or her ability to cope with this stress. There is usually a precipitating event

that causes the client to go into crisis (see Chapter 24, Crisis Intervention).

3. *With whom do you live?* This information describes the client's immediate support system or lack of it. He or she could be living with family or friends or may live alone. Watch emotional responses as the question is answered; it can give clues as to the quality of the client's living situation. If a quick answer is given and eye contact is avoided, it could be an indication to explore this subject to obtain more information.

4. *How have things been for you with them?* One of the greatest factors in successful coping is the availability of a support system. Frequently, the members of the client's support system, whether family, friends, or some other type of support person or group, have been under stress or, for some reason, have been unavailable during the critical period before the crisis.

5. *What type of work do you do?* The answer to this question can give many types of information, including his or her capacity for role functioning in a job, psychosocial status, and level of education.

6. *Have you been working up until this admission?* If the answer is no, then determine how recently the client was able to work and what happened to lead him or her to stop working.

7. *Have you and your family (or whomever the client lives with) been under any unusual stress during the past year?* Describe the type of stress being asked about. For example, *Has anyone in the family died? Been very sick? Has there been a divorce in the family?* Review the life-change events in the Holmes and Rahe scale that appears in Chapter 12, Stress: Effective Coping and Adaptation, in order to be aware of the significant events that impose stress on individuals.

8. *When you are under stress, what do you usually do to help yourself?* This indicates the client's level of coping ability, as well as his or her problem-solving capacity and current reality orientation.

The answers to these questions provide an understanding of the issues concerning the client. Other important sources of information during the assessment step are family members, current and former charts, and the reported observations of caregivers from nursing and other disciplines.

## ◆ NURSING DIAGNOSIS

### HISTORY OF DEVELOPMENT
### OF NURSING DIAGNOSES

A **nursing diagnosis** is a statement of a specific type of patient care problem that a nurse is clinically prepared to diagnose and treat. In

1973 a group of nurses met in St. Louis in order to identify the types of health problems that nurses are clinically prepared to diagnose and treat. This group of nurses called their organization the **North American Nursing Diagnosis Association (NANDA)**. Their guiding principles in selecting a list of nursing diagnoses included the following:

1. Identify all clinical problems that nurses identify and diagnose in clients.
2. Develop specific and consistent names for the different problems that nursing care can address.
3. Classify the different diagnoses into groups and subgroups in order to study the relationships between the different diagnoses, as well as the specific patterns that contribute to the clinical problem.
4. Develop a numeric code for the various diagnoses, groups, and subgroups of diagnoses so that the codes can be entered into computer systems.

The original number of nurses that met in 1973 has expanded to include an international group of nurses from clinical, academic, and research settings. They meet every 2 years to review, analyze, and add to the list of nursing diagnoses. The list of approved nursing diagnoses is called Taxonomy I—Revised. Taxonomy is a word that describes the laws and principles covering the classification of items into natural and related groups. The most recent meeting of NANDA was held in 2000. There are 155 approved nursing diagnoses, plus seven new NANDA-approved nursing diagnosis categories approved at the most recent conference. The core list of approved nursing diagnoses is located in Appendix B.

## THE SELECTION OF NURSING DIAGNOSES AS THE FOCUS OF CARE

When an adequate amount of information has been collected, it can be used to formulate nursing diagnoses as the basis for the planning of care. The American Nurses Association Social Policy Statement has defined the use of nursing diagnoses in planning care as an essential part of the practice of nursing. It has also been included in nurse practice acts written into law in many states. One of the implicit expectations of the diagnostic and treatment process is that the goal of the specific interventions designed in the planning stage must be identified so that a basis for evaluating nursing care outcomes is established.

A registered nurse, using the criteria developed by the institution in which he or she works, performs the formal selection of a nursing diagnosis. The information gathered by members of the nursing care team and given to the registered nurse further expands the information known about the client. Effective care planning depends on a reliable database and proper identification of problems appropriate for nursing intervention. These nursing problems are then classified into the nursing diagnoses developed by NANDA.

## PATTERNS OF HUMAN RESPONSE

Whenever nursing assessment occurs and a nursing diagnosis assessment model is used, specific **patterns of human response** (functioning) are evaluated. They include the following:

*Exchanging.* This pattern includes the clinical problems present when normal physical functioning is altered. Many types of physical functions can be altered as a response to different types of mental disorders. For example, the acutely anxious person may have poor nutrition, normal sleep may be disrupted, normal digestion may be disrupted, resulting in diarrhea, and so on.

*Communicating.* This pattern includes the clinical problems present when the capacity for verbal communication is altered. Most of the mental disorders have the potential to contribute to altered communication.

*Relating.* This pattern includes the clinical problems present when normal, effective interpersonal processes are altered. Changes in mental functioning often cause significant alterations in normal interpersonal processes.

*Valuing.* This pattern includes the clinical problems associated with the meaning of significant personal events such as illness and death.

*Choosing.* This pattern includes the clinical problems present when there is ineffective coping, compliance, decision-making, or health-seeking behavior.

*Moving.* This pattern includes the clinical problems present when health status is altered by changes in physical mobility or body coordination.

*Perceiving.* This pattern includes the clinical problems present when perception of the self or the environment is altered because of acute or chronic psychological or physical distress.

*Knowing.* This pattern includes the clinical problems present when cognitive processes are altered because of a psychiatric disorder, organic brain deficit, knowledge deficit in an otherwise well-functioning individual, or knowledge deficit owing to below-normal intellectual functioning.

*Feeling.* This pattern includes the clinical problems present when distressing affect or mood results in ineffective coping.

A questionnaire format that covers a broad range of psychosocial and physical functions can assist in assessing the problems that may be present within these patterns. The Barry Psychosocial Assessment

Interview Schedule in Appendix A demonstrates the types of questions that provide assessment data for use in the mental health setting. The list of nursing diagnoses shown in Appendix B is further classified within each of the Patterns of Human Response shown above. Appendix B also indicates those categories that may be more prevalent in the mental health setting.

## HOW NURSING DIAGNOSES ARE CHOSEN

The nursing diagnosis categories are described in a manual published by NANDA. Information about the categories can also be found in a variety of nursing textbooks. Some of these are listed in the bibliography at the end of the chapter. (See also holistic health care priorities discussed in Chapter 3, Inpatient Hospitalization: The Mental Health Treatment Team and the Therapeutic Milieu.)

Definitions accompany each of the nursing diagnoses. These definitions have been developed and researched in clinical practice by nurses across the United States and Canada. Each nursing diagnosis category contains sections that describe the elements of the nursing problem or diagnosis. These sections are the etiologic risk factors and the diagnosis' defining characteristics.

The **etiologic risk factors** of an actual nursing diagnosis include the contributing factors to a diagnosis, such as Ineffective Individual Coping. These factors may include losing a job, getting a divorce, or moving to a new city. These same risk factors may *potentially* place the person under increased stress and require psychosocial nursing interventions.

The **defining characteristics** of a nursing diagnosis are the signs or symptoms that the person is manifesting or describing related to the nursing problem. There are two categories of criteria that must be met for the diagnostic label to be applied. *Major* signs or symptoms *must* be present in order to use a particular nursing diagnosis. For example, for the nursing diagnosis Impaired Adjustment, at least one major defining characteristic must be present in order for the diagnostic criteria to be met: "verbalization of nonacceptance of health status change or inability to be involved in problem-solving or goal-setting."

*Minor* signs or symptoms *may* be present. Minor defining characteristics in the diagnosis of Impaired Adjustment are "lack of movement toward independence; extended period of shock, disbelief, or anger regarding health status change; lack of future-oriented thinking."

## THE DEVELOPMENT OF A NURSING DIAGNOSIS

Following the assessment step of the nursing process, the registered nurse analyzes the assessment data and one or more nursing diagnosis statements are developed. Each nursing diagnosis statement describes the specific clinical problems that need to be addressed by nursing interventions. A nursing diagnosis statement also includes the cause of the problem. This statement then guides the nursing care plan for all members of the nursing staff on a 24-hour basis.

The following are examples of nursing diagnosis statements that may be seen in the mental health setting. The actual nursing diagnosis category is printed in italics. It is followed by the words "as evidenced by" and "related to." The defining characteristics or symptoms follow the words "as evidenced by" and are shown in bold type. The causative factor or factors follow the words "related to" and is indicated in bold type. Examples of nursing diagnoses that can be seen in the mental health setting are:

> *Social isolation* as evidenced by **expressed feelings of aloneness and lack of meaningful relationships** related to **death of father and beginning college away from home**
>
> *Sensory perceptual alterations* as evidenced by **auditory hallucinations,** related to **psychosis**
>
> *Noncompliance* as evidenced by **not taking psychotropic medication,** related to **lack of insight into mental illness**

The diagnosis states the problem, the defining characteristics or symptoms of the problem, and the primary cause or causes of the problem. Nursing care planning and interventions are developed around the defining characteristics and cause or causes of the problem. It is important that the nursing diagnosis and resulting care plan are in agreement with the client's admitting diagnosis and the therapeutic goals of the multidisciplinary mental health team.

## ◆ COLLABORATIVE PROBLEMS

Nursing diagnoses can be developed within two primary types of clinical problems experienced by mental health clients:

> A type of problem that registered nurses can identify and treat without medical approval
>
> A type of problem that involves collaborative care planning with a physician or other licensed health care provider

A **collaborative problem** is developed in conjunction with a medical diagnosis or diagnosis by a licensed health care provider from another health discipline. There is a related treatment plan developed by the other health care provider. The nursing diagnosis rounds out and completes the care ordered by a physician or other health care provider. Table 10-1 shows examples of nursing diagnoses that are collaborative with other disciplines.

---

**TABLE 10–1. Examples of Nursing Diagnoses Useful for Other Disciplines**

| *Physical Therapy* | *Speech Therapy* |
|---|---|
| Self-Care Deficits | Impaired Communication |
| High Risk for Injury | Impaired Swallowing |
| Impaired Physical Mobility | Altered Thought Processes |
| Noncompliance | |
| Unilateral Neglect | |
| Fatigue | |
| | |
| *Occupational Therapy* | *Nutritional Therapy* |
| Diversional Activity Deficit | Altered Nutrition |
| Fatigue | Impaired Swallowing |
| Impaired Home Maintenance | Feeding Self-Care Deficit |
| Instrumental Self-Care Deficit | |
| | |
| *Social Service* | *Respiratory Therapy* |
| Caregiver Role Strain | High Risk for Aspiration |
| Ineffective Family Coping | High Risk for Altered Respiratory Function |
| Decisional Conflict | Ineffective Airway Clearance |
| Altered Family Process | Dysfunctional Weaning Response |
| Impaired Home Maintenance | |
| Instrumental Self-Care Deficit | |
| Social Isolation | |

Carpenito, L.J. (2000). *Nursing diagnosis: Application to clinical practice* (8th ed.) Philadelphia: Lippincott-Raven.

---

In psychiatric settings, the diagnostic codes developed by the American Psychiatric Association are used to describe the condition for which a client is admitted to the inpatient setting. These are the same codes used in outpatient mental health care. In the mental health setting, all nursing diagnoses should be developed in conjunction with the identified mental disorder admitting diagnosis. The mental disorder diagnostic codes are published in the *Diagnostic and Statistical Manual of Mental Disorders,* fourth edition (DSM-IV). This book can be found in all mental health settings.

The division of nursing care problems into two types—one that the registered nurse can identify and treat independent of other licensed health care providers, and one that requires collaboration and care planning with one or more other licensed health care disciplines-is called a **bifocal clinical practice model.**

The nursing care plan is always developed to address the specific nursing diagnosis, as well as the added nursing interventions that are standard accepted nursing roles in the mental health setting. These include nursing assessment for physical safety, administration of medications, and so on.

The nursing diagnosis statements are presented in the multidisciplinary team meetings attended by all members of the unit clinical staff. By discussing the nursing diagnoses in these meetings, all members of the team are aware of the specific problems, unique for each client on the unit, that the nurse will be addressing. The use of nursing diagnoses assists the nurse in organizing the nursing care plan so that therapeutic and time-effective nursing care is ensured. The nursing diagnosis step of the nursing process is essential to therapeutic nursing care. Properly ′selected nursing diagnoses provide the foundation of stating client problems so that therapeutic clinical outcomes can be achieved.

Whenever possible, the nurse should discuss with the client the selection of a nursing diagnosis and the nursing care planning associated with decreasing or resolving the nursing problem associated with the diagnosis. The agreement of the client with the rationale used in naming the diagnosis and the goals to be used in evaluating the outcome of the nursing intervention is an important step in obtaining patient compliance in resolving the identified health problem. A **contract** is the name of the informal agreement made between nurse and client to achieve wellness or therapeutic clinical outcomes.

## ◆ PLANNING

The planning stage involves a problem-solving process. The steps are as follows:

1. Analyze the data.
2. Identify and rank the significant problems (stated in Nursing Diagnosis terminology).
3. Examine the possible causes of each.
4. Consider the possible interventions for each.
5. Rule out the interventions that are not possible to implement.
6. Consider the possible outcome of each of the possible interventions.
7. Choose one or more interventions for the identified nursing diagnosis. The identified problems and the interventions that will help resolve the client's problem are then discussed with the client. Usually he or she will agree with the plan. The client may also request that the plan be modified. In either case, the nurse and client should agree about the final plan. This is also known as a contract.

These mental states are presented in association with a case description in which the mental state is prominent. The nursing care planning format presented above uses fundamental concepts in presenting the nursing care problems and their associated nursing diagnosis with each of the mental states. The format includes the following components:

Nursing diagnosis—A statement of a nursing problem selected from the list of NANDA—approved nursing diagnoses. The nursing diagnosis also includes a brief statement about the cause of the nursing problem.

Nursing goal or priority—A statement about the expected measurable client behavior that demonstrates that the original clinical problem has been resolved or is decreased so that discharge is possible.

Nursing intervention—A statement about the nursing behavior or action that can alter the client's clinical problem and achieve the nursing goal or priority.

Nursing rationale—A statement developed in conjunction with each nursing intervention that provides the reasoning to support the nursing plan for each diagnosis.

Evaluation—A statement that describes the change in behavior that can be used as a measure of whether the nursing intervention is effective.

A written nursing care plan that is based on nursing diagnosis of client problems is the guide used by all members of the nursing staff so that the client receives consistent care. The use of such a plan ensures that all nursing members of the multidisciplinary team are working toward common goals on a 24-hour basis. The plan can also indicate the direction of the therapeutic plan of nursing to the other clinical team members from psychiatry, social work, psychology, and so on. Examples of nursing care plans that can be seen in mental health settings are included in each of the chapters in Unit 4: Nursing the Client With a Mental Disorder. Box 10-1 shows the different steps in the nursing process as prepared in a formal nursing care plan.

## ◆ IMPLEMENTATION AND INTERVENTION

In this step, the nursing care plan is put into practice. It is the *action* part of the nursing process in which interventions are begun. The goal of the **implementation/intervention** phase of the nursing process is to decrease or eliminate the symptoms of the specific problems that have been identified. A critical aspect of the implementing step is that all members of the nursing care team should use the care plan consistently. If not, the client's progress toward wellness will be undermined by inconsistent care approaches.

*(text continues on page 138)*

## BOX 10-1. Sample Nursing Care Plan

Pedro Perez, a 59-year-old widowed man, has been admitted to the inpatient psychiatric unit with a DSM-IV diagnosis of Major Depressive Disorder (296.23) or Schizoid Personality Disorder (301.20). Refer to the clinical vignette in Chapter 15 for additional information on Pedro's presenting symptoms.

When developing a nursing care plan, the nurse must evaluate the individual client and write the plan according to the client's needs. After a thorough nursing assessment is completed, appropriate nursing diagnoses are identified. The nurse then prioritizes the diagnoses and determines nursing interventions and criteria for evaluation of the interventions. A nursing care plan is best completed in conjunction *with* the client so that both client and nurse work together to meet the client's needs. Throughout Pedro's hospitalization, the nurse and Pedro continuously evaluate the plan of care and revise the expected outcomes or interventions as needed. The following is an example of a nursing care plan that might be implemented by the nurse working with Pedro. It provides basic information that should be considered and included in a nursing care plan, although it is not all-inclusive.

### NANDA DIAGNOSIS
Ineffective Individual Coping (5.1.1.1)

#### Definition
Inability to form a valid appraisal of the stressors, inadequate choices of practiced responses, and/or inability to use available resources.

#### Defining Characteristics

| *Subjective* | *Objective* |
|---|---|
| Change in usual communication patterns | Decreased use of social support |
| Fatigue | Inability to meet role expectations |
| Verbalization of inability to cope or to ask for help | Inadequate problem-solving |
| | Poor concentration |
| | Sleep disturbance |

#### Related Factors
High degree of threat
Inadequate level of perception of control
Inadequate social support created by characteristics of relationships
Situational crisis
Uncertainty

*(continues)*

## BOX 10–1. Sample Nursing Care Plan *(Continued)*

### Expected Outcomes
*Pedro will*
Identify personal strengths that may promote effective coping.
Participate in decision making regarding treatment for diagnosed prostate cancer.
Initiate conversations with staff and clients on the unit.

### Evaluation
1. Pedro identified his "work ethic" and "determination" as personal strengths. Applying these strengths to his inpatient treatment he identified and met his goals.
2. Pedro sought information on treatment options for prostate cancer, met with his family, and decided on a treatment regimen.
3. Pedro was initially reticent when interacting with staff and client on the unit. By discharge he was responsible for orienting new clients to the unit.

### Nursing Interventions with Rationales
Develop a trusting relationship with Pedro. *A trusting relationship encourages a client to be honest and receptive to nursing staff and others.*

Assist Pedro in identifying his personal strengths and abilities. *Knowing one's skills increases self-esteem and encourages the use of those skills.*

Encourage independence in the completion of personal responsibilities. Give positive reinforcement for use of adaptive coping and problem solving skills. *Positive reinforcement and success increases self-esteem and encourages the repetition of similar behaviors.*

Offer to remain with Pedro during initial interactions with others on the unit. *The presence of a trusted person increases one's sense of security when participating in new or difficult tasks.*

### NANDA DIAGNOSIS
Dysfunctional Grieving (9.2.1.1.)

### Definition
Extended, unsuccessful use of intellectual and emotional responses by which individuals, families, [and] communities attempt to work through the process of modifying self-concept based upon the perception of loss.

### Defining Characteristics
| *Subjective* | *Objective* |
|---|---|
| Alteration in libido | Alteration in activity level |
| Denial of loss | Alteration in eating habits |
| Sadness | Alteration in sleep patterns |
| | Difficulty in expressing loss |
| | Interference with life functioning |

*(continues)*

## BOX 10–1. Sample Nursing Care Plan *(Continued)*

### Related Factors
Loss of wife and contact with family
Chronic illness

### Expected Outcomes
*Pedro will*
Verbalize feelings of grief and sadness.
Identify and use social support available to him.
Take in adequate food and fluids to maintain physiological function.

### Evaluation
1. Pedro is able to verbalize feelings of grief, loss, and sadness about the death of his wife. Additionally, he is able to discuss his fears about his diagnosis of prostate cancer.
2. Pedro has improved communication with his children and converses with them regularly. His children have arranged to provide physical and emotional support while Pedro undergoes treatment for prostate cancer.
3. Pedro is eating 90% to 100% of all meals and snacks. He verbalizes understanding of the importance of an adequate intake of food and fluid. He has gained 3 pounds since admission.

### Nursing Interventions with Rationales
Develop a trusting relationship with Pedro. Demonstrate empathy and caring. *Within a trusting relationship the client is more likely to express real emotions.*

    Assist Pedro in problem solving and identification of social support systems. Provide positive feedback for decisions. *Increases self-esteem and self-efficacy and encourages repetition of desired behaviors.*

    Monitor Pedro's food and fluid intake, and weigh regularly. *Provides best information on client's nutritional status and when additional interventions are indicated.*

### NANDA DIAGNOSIS
Decisional Conflict regarding treatment of prostate cancer (5.3.1.1)

### Definition
The state of uncertainty about course of action to be taken when choice among competing actions involves risk, loss, or challenge to personal life values.

### Defining Characteristics
*Subjective*
Verbalized uncertainty about choices
Verbalized feeling of distress while
   attempting a decision

*Objective*
Delayed decision making
Physical signs of distress or
   tension

*(continues)*

## BOX 10–1. Sample Nursing Care Plan *(Continued)*

### Related Factors
Lack of experience or interference with decision making
Lack of support system

### Expected Outcomes
*Pedro will*
Participate in decisions regarding healthcare and treatment of prostate cancer.
Evaluate available choices in relation to personal values.
Use problem-solving skills to achieve desired treatment and outcomes.

### Evaluation
1. Pedro sought information on treatment options for prostate cancer, met with his family, and decided on a treatment regimen.
2. Pedro evaluated treatment options for prostate cancer based on his religious beliefs and personal values. His values and beliefs guided his treatment decisions.
3. Pedro reports that he "feels good" about his treatment decisions and is hopeful that the treatment he selected will result in a desired outcome.

### Nursing Interventions with Rationales
Assess Pedro's understanding of treatment options and provide information regarding treatment options for prostate cancer as indicated. *To assure that the client understands treatment options and potential outcomes. Provides a basis for decision making.*

Facilitate family communication and collaborative decision making. *Enhanced family communication allows the client to process his treatment options within a personal and familial frame of reference. It also increases his social support.*

Provide reinforcement for decisions Pedro makes regarding treatment. *Positive reinforcement encourages the repetition of desired behaviors.*
Support Pedro's informed choices and decisions. Assist him in articulation of his choices to others. *Reinforces the client's ability and right to make personal choices regarding healthcare. Facilitates communication and clarifies decisions.*

The successful implementation of a nursing care plan typically results in the desired outcomes for the client. In this situation, on discharge Pedro would have the confidence and support he needs to make decisions regarding treatment of his prostate cancer. He would also have a better sense of himself and would be more confident in accessing and using social support systems.

Boyd, M.A., & Nichart, M.A. (1998). *Psychiatric nursing: Contemporary practice.* Philadelphia: Lippincott-Raven; Townsend, M.C. (2001). *Nursing diagnoses in psychiatric nursing* (5th ed.). Philadelphia: F.A. Davis Company; Wilkinson, J.M. (2000). *Nursing diagnosis handbook* (7th ed.). Upper Saddle River, New Jersey: Prentice-Hall Health.

Another important aspect of the implementing stage is that ongoing assessment of the client's problem or problems should be part of daily nursing care. In addition, obtaining more detailed information about the client's life, relationships, experiences, and so on can further refine the database. As more specific information about the client's problem is gathered, it may be necessary to alter the plan and at the same time notify other nursing colleagues about the change in approach and the new knowledge leading to the modification in the care plan.

To promote a systems approach, the care plan should be shared with the other members of the nursing staff and, in most instances, with the family. If a family therapist is working with the family, review the plan with him or her in case there are differences in the care approaches of nursing and the family therapist. The family therapist is usually aware of complex family dynamics that may have been detrimental to the hospitalized family member.

When clients and family members receive conflicting messages from two different care disciplines they become confused. Accordingly, they may be noncompliant with the recommendations they receive. Ultimately, the client may lose the social support that could contribute toward more rapid resolution of his or her problems.

When the nursing care plan is shared with the family, they experience a greater sense of security about their family member's prognosis. In addition, it is an opportunity to explain the interventions designed to support their loved one's mental disorder and model a beneficial type of caregiving behavior. Specific interventions for the various psychiatric disorders are described in Unit 5, Intervention and Treatment of Mental Disorders.

## EVALUATION

Evaluation is the final step of the nursing process. The outcome of nursing care usually can be observed during and after the intervention step. Is there a decrease in the symptoms that originally caused the plan to be implemented?

Evaluating involves obtaining verbal or nonverbal feedback from the client about the results of interventions. Verbal feedback is also known as subjective information; the client directly describes how he or she feels. Nonverbal feedback includes those clues the client gives, frequently without conscious awareness. These include facial or body gestures and observable emotional states, such as tenseness, anger, sadness, depression, and so on. This type of information is called objective; in a way, the client is the object being observed.

The nurse's objective observations can, on occasion, differ from the subjective comments the client makes about himself or herself. For example, the client may say that he or she is feeling much better and more cheerful. On several occasions throughout the day, however, the client may be observed sitting alone, silently weeping.

The evaluation stage is actually similar to the original step in the nursing process. The final step of the nursing process involves collecting data that will determine whether the goals of the nursing care plan were achieved. When an evaluation of any type of intervention process occurs, it is important to base the evaluation on criteria or standards that determine whether the goal was reached. This means that the symptoms of the problems originally identified should be decreased or entirely relieved. When the evaluation determines that some or all of the symptoms remain, the nursing process should be reinitiated. A reassessment of the *current* symptoms should occur, and a new or modified care plan should be instituted.

## ◆ THE IMPORTANCE OF DOCUMENTING NURSING ACTIONS IN THE NURSING CARE PLAN AND PATIENT NOTES

It is important to document all nursing actions in the mental health setting. Because of the distressed state of the client, there can be rapid changes in mental status that are important to monitor. The nurse is the individual who spends the most time with clients in the mental health setting. All members of the mental health team scan the nurses' notes to determine what changes have occurred in the client's status. In addition, to the documentation of nursing actions in the patient notes, it is also essential to note all nursing care on the nursing care plan. Other nurses who follow on subsequent shifts seek information about the progression of the nursing care plan. It is suggested that the nurse in the mental health setting follow the institutional guidelines for documenting in the nursing care plan. The general guidelines for nursing documentation are shown in Table 10-2.

## KEY POINTS

- Psychiatric nurses need the following skills and knowledge: interpersonal communication, nursing theory, and the nursing process.
- Nursing process refers to the five steps involved in organizing and implementing client care. The steps are assessment, nursing diagnosis, planning, implementation/intervention, and evaluation.
- Assessment includes gathering all information needed to diagnose a client's specific problems. A nursing diagnosis can be formed when an adequate amount of information has been gathered. This diagnosis serves as the basis for planning the client's care.

## TABLE 10–2. Documentation of Nursing Outcomes

Documentation of the outcomes of nursing interventions provides ongoing information to the treatment team about the effects of nursing interventions.

Symptom relief through the use of medication or therapy

Improved ability to cope with stress

Improved ability to function

Decreased risk of further disability

Physical, mental, emotional, and spiritual well being

Appropriate expression of feelings

Improved interactions and communication with family members, friends, and staff

After documenting nursing interventions, a follow-up note should be written with the following guidelines in mind:

Use objective language.

Document the client's mood, level of anxiety, and thought processes.

Use concrete examples, such as client's statements and action, when appropriate.

Adapted from Eggland, E. (1997). Charting tips: Documenting psychiatric and behavioral outcomes. *Nursing 97, 27,* 25.

■ Nursing care planning is a problem-solving process that includes seven steps:

1. Analyze data.
2. Identify and rank significant problems.
3. Examine possible causes of each problem.
4. Consider possible interventions for each problem.
5. Rule out interventions that cannot be implemented.
6. Consider the outcome of each possible intervention.
7. Choose one or more interventions for the identified diagnosis.

The result of the nursing care planning process is a written care plan that guides all of the nursing care and is compatible with the plan of the unit mental health team.

■ The goal of the implementation or intervention stage is to decrease or eliminate the symptoms of the specific identified problems.

■ Evaluation involves gathering data (subjective and objective feedback) about whether the goals of the plan have been met.

■ Guiding principles for NANDA for selecting and approving nursing diagnoses include:

—Identify all clinical problems that nurses identify and diagnose.

—Develop specific and consistent names for these problems.

—Classify diagnoses to study the patterns that contribute to clinical problems.

—Review research findings related to proposed diagnostic categories.

—Develop a numeric code for the diagnoses, to be used in computer data entry.

■ The approved list of nursing diagnosis categories, issued by NANDA in 2000, contains 155 previously approved diagnoses and seven newly approved additional diagnoses.

■ In nursing assessment, specific patterns of human functioning that are evaluated include exchanging, moving, communicating, perceiving, relating, knowing, valuing, feeling, and choosing.

■ Each nursing diagnosis category contains etiologic contributing risk factors and the defining characteristics of the diagnosis.

■ Etiologic contributing risk factors are those factors that may potentially place the person under increased physical and psychosocial stress and require nursing interventions.

■ Defining characteristics of a nursing diagnosis are the signs or symptoms a person is manifesting or describing related to the nursing problem. These characteristics are categorized as major or minor.

■ A nursing diagnosis statement describes the specific clinical problem to be addressed and the cause of the problem. The statement is used to guide all nursing staff members in client care.

■ The nursing diagnosis is always developed in conjunction with a medical diagnosis and related medical treatment plan.

■ Planning inpatient nursing care in mental health nursing is based on three steps:
—Admission to inpatient setting with DSM-IV diagnosis
—Nursing assessment of all physical and mental patterns
—Development of nursing diagnosis statements

■ The nursing care plan format consists of five parts:

1. *Nursing diagnosis*—statement of nursing problem and its cause
2. *Nursing goal or priority*—expected measurable client behavior showing the original clinical problem has been resolved or decreased enough for the client to be discharged
3. *Nursing intervention*—nursing behavior action that can alter the client's clinical problem and achieve the nursing goal or priority
4. *Nursing rationale*—the reasoning to support the nursing plan for each diagnosis, used in conjunction with each nursing intervention
5. *Evaluation*—a description of the change in behavior that can be used to measure whether the nursing intervention is effective

## SELF-AWARENESS ACTIVITY

This chapter is the "how to organize nursing care" section of the book. It describes the structure or working foundation on which specific information is added in order to create nursing care plans that provide an environment of care and safety to persons with mental disorders.

- How did you feel as you were reading this chapter? Did you begin to get a sense of what the structure of nursing is about?
- Did the information make sense to you?
- Did the steps in the nursing process have a logical flow?
- Were you able to envision yourself in the hospital or in a client's home while using these concepts?
- How realistic did it seem to you to imagine yourself actually working with these steps of the nursing process?

## QUESTIONS

1. The nurse is meeting with a client and asks, "Are you feeling less anxious after taking the Ativan I gave you?" This is an example of what step of the nursing process?
   a. Implementation
   b. Assessment
   c. Planning
   d. Evaluation
2. The nurse identifies a nursing diagnosis of Sleep Pattern Disturbance related to depression. This nursing diagnosis is related to which pattern of human response?
   a. Exchanging
   b. Relating
   c. Perceiving
   d. Feeling
3. The most important reason that nursing care plans should be shared with members of the health care team, clients, and sometimes family is to
   a. protect the nurse from legal liability.
   b. validate the essential role of the nurse.
   c. prove to governmental and accrediting agencies that appropriate care has been planned.
   d. facilitate the provision of consistent, quality care.
4. NANDA nursing diagnosis categories were developed to
   a. identify all clinical problems that nurses identify and diagnose in clients.
   b. provide specific, consistent names for the problems nursing care can address.
   c. classify the diagnoses and study their relationships and patterns.
   d. All of the above.

## BIBLIOGRAPHY

Barry, P.D. (1996). *Psychosocial nursing: Care of physically ill patients and their families* (3rd ed.). Philadelphia: Lippincott-Raven.

Boyd, M., & Nihart, M. (1998). *Psychiatric nursing: Contemporary practice.* Philadelphia: Lippincott-Raven.

Carpenito, L.J. (2000). *Nursing diagnosis: Application to clinical practice* (8th ed.). Philadelphia: Lippincott Williams & Wilkins.

*Diagnostic and statistical manual of mental disorders* (4th ed.). (1994). Washington, D.C.: American Psychiatric Press.

Eggland, E. (1997). Charting tips: Documenting psychiatric and behavioral outcomes. *Nursing 97, 27,* 25.

Gordon, M., Avant, K., Herdman, H., Hoskins, L., Lavin, M., Sparks, S., & Warren, J. (2001). *NANDA nursing diagnoses: Definitions and classification.* Philadelphia: North American Nursing Diagnosis Association.

Latvala, E., Janhonen, S., & Wahlberg, K. (1999). Patient initiatives during the assessment and planning of psychiatric nursing in a hospital environment. *Journal of Advanced Nursing, 29*(1), 64–71.

*Nursing's Social Policy Statement.* (1995). Washington, D.C.: American Nurses Association.

Rosdahl, C. *Textbook of basic nursing* (7th ed.). Philadelphia: Lippincott-Raven.

Sadock, B., & Kaplan, H. (1998). *Synopsis of psychiatry: Behavioral sciences/clinical psychiatry.* Philadelphia: Lippincott-Raven.

Timby, B.K. (2000). *Fundamental skills and concepts in patient care* (7th ed.). Philadelphia: Lippincott Williams & Wilkins.

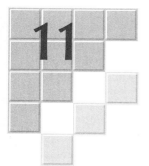

# Human Emotions

## Behavioral Objectives

*After reading*
*this chapter*
*the student*
*will be able to:*

- Describe the physiologic changes caused by emotions such as anger and fear.
- Explain the "fight or flight" syndrome.
- Explain three ways that a child may handle or repress unacceptable feelings.
- Describe anxiety and tell how it is experienced.
- Describe how a small child expresses aggression and learns to control this feeling.
- Identify the different types of anger.
- Describe the differences among the experiences of control, powerlessness, and hopelessness.

## Key Terms

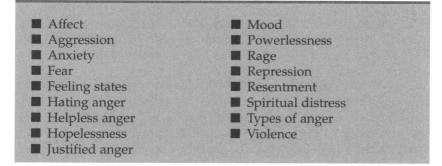

- Affect
- Aggression
- Anxiety
- Fear
- Feeling states
- Hating anger
- Helpless anger
- Hopelessness
- Justified anger
- Mood
- Powerlessness
- Rage
- Repression
- Resentment
- Spiritual distress
- Types of anger
- Violence

Emotions are **feeling states** that involve both physiologic and psychological changes. If a need is satisfied, the resulting emotion tends to be pleasant. For example, when babies are hungry, they make their needs known. When they are fed, they relax in satisfied, contented emotional states; conversely, if a need is blocked or ungratified, the resulting emotions are unpleasant. Thus, if babies are not fed when they make their needs known, they become tense and frustrated, usually showing their frame of mind by loud, angry crying.

### ◆ PHYSIOLOGIC RESPONSES

Emotional stress, whether it is pleasantly or unpleasantly experienced, is often accompanied by physical changes. When a person is angry, heart and pulse rates speed up, the face flushes, breath quickens, and hands tremble. When struck by fear, some of the preceding symptoms may occur, as may blanching or turning pale; in addition, the mouth may become dry, lips may tremble, pupils may dilate, the breath may be held, the digestive tract may slow down (peristalsis may actually reverse itself), and small hairs on the body may stand erect. Even a feeling of delight tends to produce physiologic changes, although they usually are not as intense as those evoked by anger, hatred, fear, or anxiety.

The *fight or flight response* in the body is the result of sympathetic nervous system activation. As may be recalled from anatomy and physiology principles, the major division of the nervous system that controls all body functions is the autonomic nervous system. This system has two major branches, the parasympathetic and sympathetic. The parasympathetic nervous system maintains the normal homeostasis of all organs and body systems. When the individual is threatened or challenged, the sympathetic nervous system overrides the parasympathetic nervous system physiology in order to prepare the body for survival. The concept of "fight or flight" is the normal physiologic shift that gives the body the fullest potential strength to overcome the challenge or threat.

In the "fight or flight" syndrome, the physical reactions that accompany emotions of anger and fear are readying the body for addressing the challenge or threat by creative thinking, active aggression, or escape from what is feared (hence, the name fight or flight syndrome). The adrenal glands pour out adrenaline into the bloodstream. The result is increased mental vigilance and extra physical strength or power available for quick or lifesaving action.

All people feel both pleasant and unpleasant emotions. Humans have needs they want filled; when a need is met they feel good, but when a need is unmet they feel unpleasant emotions. Humans are creatures torn among many conflicting emotions, which run the range between the extremes of love and hate, childlike trust and paranoid suspicion, self-sacrificing bravery and lowly cowardice. Emotions are powerful motivators of behavior. It is important to note that unpleasant emotion is often the underlying cause of positive growth and change; unpleasant emotion usually results in an attempt by the individual to become free of the emotional distress by creating changes in behavioral response or the cognitive interpretation of the cause of the unpleasant emotion. The outcome can be a more adaptive form of coping.

## ◆ CONTROL OF EMOTIONS

One of every person's major struggles is learning to control his or her emotions. Even in early childhood, one learns ways to express emotions or repress them. **Repression** is a defense mechanism created by the unconscious mind in order to minimize the negative effects of emotion on both mental and physical functioning. Repression is an important mechanism in the process of adaptation. Some emotions are acceptable in a social group; others are not. Each culture defines its own standards of behavior, and its citizens must conform to these standards in order to be socially accepted.

Some cultures impose more control over emotions than do others. As an example of this, contrast the lack of emotionalism that is a valued personality characteristic in some ethnic groups with one that embraces a rich range of emotional responses.

A child raised in the former type of culture may be taught to repress expression of emotion, to become stoic. This is not to say that he or she is unemotional. He or she has the same strong urges to express joy, love, hatred, and fear as any other human being, but social acceptance by the immediate and extended family may depend in part on whether expression of emotion is controlled. Family custom may demand a deadpan facial expression even when experiencing intense fear, joy, or pain.

The child raised in an emotionally open culture may grow up in a highly charged atmosphere. He or she is highly verbal and is encouraged to express likes and dislikes freely; laughter and tears may succeed each other quickly. Surging anger often results in aggressive behavior.

All too often, a child learns that the expression of certain emotions is unacceptable. Repression may occur in one way or another because he or she feels these emotions—such as jealousy, hatred, anger, and fear—and punishment may occur for showing them. Repression is a defense mechanism that pushes unpleasant thoughts or feelings into the unconscious (see Chapter 13, Stress: Ineffective Coping and Defense Mechanisms).

Although a child may no longer be consciously aware of these repressed feelings, they can strongly influence his or her conscious choices. These buried feelings may cause a person to experience guilt, depression, hostility, or other unexplainable negative feelings. The child may displace these feelings onto toys, pets, or belongings; for example, he or she may break or destroy his or her possessions or mistreat a pet.

Mature, enlightened parents should encourage their children to feel their emotions fully and verbalize their feelings when it is appropriate. They should help them find ways of expressing their feelings that damage neither society nor the child.

## ◆ COMMONLY EXPERIENCED EMOTIONAL STATES

The following list includes many of the emotional states experienced by human beings. As you are reading the names of each of the states in the following, notice if you experience the feeling associated with it. Where in your body do you experience the feeling? Is it in your mind or in your chest, stomach, or some other part? Feeling or emotion is usually experienced in the body rather than the mind. Feelings are very much intertwined with the body and somatic sensations, rather than in the head, thinking, or cognitive realm. Other names for feelings are **affect** and **mood**. Affect and mood are the internal or subjective feeling states. Affect is also used to describe the feeling state that can be seen by an observer making an objective assessment.

| | |
|---|---|
| Aggression | Hate |
| Anger | Homesickness |
| Anxiety | Hopefulness |
| Bitterness | Hopelessness |
| Boredom | Jealousy |
| Complacency | Joy |
| Curiosity | Love |
| Cynicism | Peace |
| Depression | Powerlessness |
| Despair | Relief |
| Disillusionment | Resignation |
| Elation | Reverence |
| Enthusiasm | Shame |
| Envy | Shyness |
| Fear | Smugness |
| Fury | Spiritual distress |
| Grief | Trust |
| Guilt | Wistfulness |

### ANXIETY

**Anxiety** is a vague and unpleasant feeling that produces many somatic effects or physical sensations in the body: tenseness, tremors, cardiovascular excitation, gastrointestinal tightening, and/or restlessness. It causes feelings of apprehension, helplessness, and general distress. Anxiety differs from the emotion of fear, in which there is a specific, identifiable cause. When a person is anxious, he or she is not able to identify the focus or reason for the emotional distress. Until the cause of anxiety is identified, the feeling will continue as an unspecific and unpleasant physical and mental state.

## FEAR

**Fear** is a feeling of dread associated with a specific cause that is identifiable. The feeling is accompanied by a subjective experience of psychological distress. If the fear is acute, normal problem-solving abilities often are diminished. A person may feel overwhelmed about being able to engage in problem solving to address the cause of the fear and to modify or change the contributing conditions.

The physiologic responses to fear include an increase in heart rate and blood pressure; dilation of pupils; and vasoconstriction of peripheral blood vessels, resulting in whitening or blanching of the skin accompanied by a decrease in skin temperature. With acute fear, the person's neuromuscular responses may be "frozen," disorganized, or uncoordinated. The change in body coordination and organization is matched by a mental state of disorganization.

## AGGRESSION

Just what is aggression? Karl Menninger, in his book *Man Against Himself*, defines **aggression** as an emotion compounded of frustration and hate or rage. It is an emotion deeply rooted in every one of us, a vital part of our emotional being that must be either projected outward on the environment or inward, destructively, on the self.

Menninger likens hate to an ugly, gray stone wall that is softened in time by love. Love is compared to a creeping mantle of green ivy that covers the ugly starkness of the stone, turning it into a thing of beauty. He postulates that hate and frustration appear first in personality growth, followed by the appearance of love as we mature. Hate never completely disappears, however. It shows itself in various aggressive disguises and even, on occasion, in frankness when our controls slip.

Aggression becomes apparent in the infant shortly after birth. In the child's prenatal life all of its needs are met, but with the advent of birth its comfort is violently shattered. It is this birth trauma that supposedly sets the pattern for all subsequent frustration anxieties. As the infant becomes hungry, cold, wet, and uncomfortable, he or she exhibits rage by crying, stiffening, and contracting muscles. The skin flushes a deep red color, and the infant may hold his or her breath.

As the baby grows older, he or she exhibits increasing rage when needs are not met. He or she may have temper tantrums, scream, hold his or her breath, scratch, strike out, throw and smash toys and other articles within reach, bite, pinch, kick, whine, and refuse to comply with instructions or admonitions. Still later, he or she may run away, use angry or abusive language, spit, or soil himself or herself intentionally. The child is self-centered and wants his or her own way. This is common, frequently encountered behavior in the normal small child. It is a display of frank, uninhibited aggression.

The mind begins to defend itself by using defense mechanisms that operate at an unconscious level to control the unpleasant feelings of anxiety and anger. Depending on the developing emotional strength of the child, these mechanisms can either help or hinder further personality development.

Progressively, these manifestations of aggression are met by environmental controls, such as parents, other family members, and caregivers who start curbing temper tantrums and destructive behavior. As early as the first year of life, the infant whose angry behavior is met with harsh responses by caregivers experiences the early effects of shame. The child resents restrictions and demands and his or her hostility builds. This feeling of hostility is accompanied or followed by a deep feeling of guilt. In clarifying the difference between shame and guilt, the feeling of shame is one in which a person feels badly about one's self. With guilt, a person feels badly about something he or she has done.

In addition to guilt feelings, the child fears the loss of love and approval of those who are significant to him or her. Additionally, the child expects to be punished when he or she is disobedient. The small child learns to modify his or her behavior to conform to the demands of family and, later, to conform to the expected norms of society. Slowly he or she learns to build up a set of inner controls, and as self-judgment or conscience develops in the child, he or she learns to differentiate between right and wrong.

## ANGER

**Anger** is an inborn emotional reaction to loss or violation. In its most basic response, it stimulates the individual to retrieve or recover what was lost or obtain what he or she wants to have. This can include the newborn infant who "loses" the nipple while nursing; the 6-month-old infant who drops his or her toy; the 2-year-old child who wants a cookie; the adolescent who is angry about not being trusted to borrow the family car; the family that must go on welfare; or the individual who is forced into early retirement.

The physiologic responses to emotion depend on the type of anger being experienced. There are six predominant patterns of anger:

- Justified anger
- Rage
- Hating anger
- Resentment
- Violence
- Helpless anger

**Justified anger** is a physical and mental state in which the individual feels in control and energized to use the angry feeling to correct the "wrong" or to retrieve what was lost. The person experiences the loss as a challenge that he or she has the power or strength to address. During the state of active or organized anger a person feels in mental control, there is a heightening of skin color, respirations become fuller, and the blood pressure and pulse are decreased.

**Rage** is a state of expressed anger marked by disorganization and loss of control. Rage is most commonly expressed outwardly toward the person or situation that is perceived to have violated the person's well being. It is common for the person to experience shame after the rage is expressed. Shame is an emotion that causes a person to feel badly about oneself. It is often accompanied by a sense of worthlessness.

**Hating anger** is a type of animosity or intense dislike that can operate at two different levels: resentment/hostility or violence. The feeling of hating anger is held within an individual toward another person or situation that is perceived, accurately or inaccurately, to have caused harm or personal injury to the one who feels the hatred. Hating anger that is experienced internally and not actively expressed is called resentment or hostility. When hating anger is expressed externally, it is theorized that it is at the core of violent behavior or violence.

**Resentment** is a feeling of hostility and dislike expressed toward another person as the result of an actual or perceived violation. The hostility is expressed either nonverbally or verbally. Nonverbal cues include the following:

- Avoiding the presence of the person towards whom the resentment is felt
- Averting eyes and avoiding eye contact when in the presence of the person toward whom the resentment is felt
- Increased body tension
- Nonverbal behaviors such as folding of arms over chest, body avoidance, or leaning away from the person towards whom the resentment is felt. There is a "chip on the shoulder" body posture in the presence of the person toward whom the resentment is felt.

Resentment is expressed verbally by curt, abbreviated answers, frequently accompanied by a tense tone of voice.

**Violence** is an unjust or unwarranted exertion of power that is fueled by anger. Violence is expressed by one person toward another person. It can also be expressed by one person toward one or more persons associated with an institution toward which the violent person harbors anger and resentment. Violence results in emotional and physical injury.

**Helpless anger** is a cause of marked personal distress. The individual perceives that he or she is unable to address the cause of his or her anger and feels disempowered. This experience is similar to that of powerlessness described below. In the state of helpless anger, the individual feels emotionally overwhelmed and disorganized. Breathing becomes rapid and shallow; the pupils dilate; systolic and diastolic blood pressure are elevated; the person appears pale because skin temperature is decreased owing to vasoconstriction of the peripheral capillaries. Helpless anger is believed to be at the heart of the victim response.

## HOPELESSNESS

**Hopelessness** is a self-perception in which individuals believe that they have no choices or alternatives in their current life situations. The belief that they are helpless to meet their own needs and change their circumstances continues to support the experience of hopelessness.

One of the adaptive needs of human beings is to feel that they have some measure of control over their own feelings as well as their functioning in the environment in which they live. Hopelessness is a state of perceiving that one has no control. It becomes a very limiting factor in having the energy to change or the belief that change from the current state is possible.

It is normal for all individuals to experience feelings of hopelessness occasionally. Usually, however, the perception motivates the person to view his or her current experience from a different perspective. The ability to change perspective in most cases increases the level of energy to change, as well as the belief that change is possible.

When a feeling of hopelessness persists beyond 2 weeks, depression often results. The symptoms of depression are described in Chapter 15, The Client With a Mood Disorder. Many of the factors described in the experience of hopelessness are also present in the state of powerlessness. Box 11-1 shows the continuum from feeling in control to feeling the loss of control characterized by powerlessness and hopelessness.

## POWERLESSNESS

**Powerlessness** is a self-perception that one's own actions cannot change the outcome of a current negative life situation. Usually a person can recognize that change is needed, but feels incapable of making it happen. The feeling is often accompanied by a physical and mental

---

### BOX 11–1. The Continuum of Control

**PERCEPTIONS OF CONTROL**

**In Control**
The perception that one has choices and is able to create change in his or her psychological state or current life circumstances

**Powerlessness**
The perception that one's actions cannot effect changes in outcome

**Hopelessness**
The perception that one's needs have no potential to be met

experience of lacking the energy or strength to create a different outcome.

The differences between the subjective states of hopelessness and powerlessness, showing the continuum from the experiences of control to powerlessness and hopelessness, are shown in Box 11-1.

## SPIRITUAL DISTRESS

**Spiritual distress** is a fundamental distress within the self that leads one to question the meaning of one's life. As with other forms of emotional distress, this type of deep personal questioning is a normal human response. This type of personal introspection often motivates personal growth and development. When the process consumes a significant amount of one's day and persists for a period beyond a few weeks, it is possible that it can undermine effective coping and lead to prolonged spiritual distress.

When spiritual distress occurs, a person expresses concern about the meaning of one's life, for example, the presence or absence of a belief in God, the meaning of suffering and pain, or the value of living. The normal religious practices that may previously have been valuable and meaningful may now be perceived as meaningless.

Prolonged spiritual distress that does not gradually move to deeper understanding or acceptance can eventually lead to the experience of hopelessness, described earlier. As with hopelessness, if the experience of spiritual distress does not lead to a different level of understanding or insight, depression can occur.

## K E Y   P O I N T S

- Emotions are feeling states that involve both physical and psychological changes. They are powerful motivators of behavior.
- The fight or flight syndrome is a physical response to emotions related to challenge or threat. It prepares the body for aggression (fight) or escape from the perceived danger (flight).
- Learning to control emotions is a major human task.
- Children learn to repress emotions that they learn are unacceptable. Even though the emotion is no longer visible, it can continue to exert an influence on the child's behavior.
- Anxiety is a vague, unpleasant feeling that produces physical sensations such as tension and increased heart rate. An anxious person often cannot identify the reason for the emotional distress.
- Fear is the result of a specific, identifiable cause. The physiologic reactions may be very similar to anxiety.
- Anger is an inborn, instinctive emotional reaction to violation or loss.

■ Aggression is a combination of frustration and hate or rage. Outward manifestations of this emotion in children are usually met by the controls of family; children learn to modify the aggressive behavior.

■ Directing aggression inward is often the result of strong guilt feelings and is theorized to be a possible causative factor in both physical and psychological disorders.

■ Pathologic forms of inwardly directed aggression include antisocial behavior, sexual impotence and frigidity, criminality, and various forms of self-mutilation.

■ Three perceptions people have about control are: in control (one has choices), powerlessness (one's actions cannot effect changes), and hopelessness (one's needs have no potential to be met).

■ All people occasionally have a sense of powerlessness; however, if these feelings persist, they often lead to depression.

### SELF-AWARENESS ACTIVITY

As you were reading this chapter, were you aware of feeling many of the emotions discussed in the text?

• What were some of those feelings?

• Did some of them cause you to feel uncomfortable?

In the field of psychiatry it is common that as one reads about different emotional states or observes them in a clinical setting, unexpected and unpleasant feelings or old memories of distressing events may emerge. If this happens, you are encouraged to talk to your instructor, spiritual advisor, or some other trusted person so that these feelings can be adequately explored.

## Q U E S T I O N S

1. The client expresses that he has no other option but to commit suicide in order to deal with his current life situation. The nurse recognizes this as
   a. hopelessness.
   b. fear.
   c. powerlessness.
   d. anxiety.

2. It is important that the nurse understands that physiologic reactions to emotional stress
   a. are minor and not relevant to nursing care in psychiatric settings.
   b. are a result of parasympathetic nervous system stimulation.

   c. are the result of pleasant or unpleasant emotional experiences.

   d. all of the above.

**3.** The nurse could best explain the primary difference between fear and anxiety to a client as:

   a. relating only to the degree of psychological distress experienced.

   b. fear causing a physiologic response, whereas anxiety does not.

   c. fear resulting from a specific, identifiable cause, whereas anxiety is vague; its cause often cannot be identified.

   d. anxiety is a more serious concern.

**4.** Anger is an inborn emotional reaction to

   a. loss

   b. birth

   c. siblings

   d. shame

## BIBLIOGRAPHY

Barry, P.D. (1991). An investigation of cardiovascular, respiratory, and skin temperature changes during relaxation and anger inductions. *Dissertation Abstracts International, 52-09-B*, 5012.

Barry, P.D. (1996). *Psychosocial nursing: Care of physically ill patients and their families* (3rd ed.). Philadelphia: Lippincott-Raven.

Biringen, Z. (2000). Emotional availability. *American Journal of Orthopsychiatry, 70*(1), 104–114.

Boyd, M., & Nihart, M. (1998). *Psychiatric nursing: Contemporary practice.* Philadelphia: Lippincott Williams & Wilkins.

Carpenito, L.J. (2000). *Nursing diagnosis: Application to clinical practice* (8th ed.). Philadelphia: Lippincott Williams & Wilkins.

Cassem, N., & Bernstein, J. (1997). Depressed patients. In N. Cassem (Ed.). *Massachusetts General Hospital handbook of general hospital psychiatry.* St. Louis: Mosby.

Gerow, J., & Bordens, K. (2000). *Psychology: An introduction.* Carrollton, TX: Alliance Press.

Harris, P. (1999). Individual differences in understanding emotion: The role of attachment status and psychological discourse. *Attachment and Human Development, 1*(3), 307–324.

Kubler-Ross, E. (1981). *Living with death and dying.* New York: Macmillan.

Ogden, J. (2000). *Health psychology: A textbook.* Buckingham, England: Open University Press.

Rathus, S. (2000). *Psychology: The core.* Fort Worth, TX: Harcourt College Publishers.

Rosenbaum, J., Pollack, M., Otto, M., & Bernstein, J. (1997). Anxious patients. In N. Cassem (Ed.). *Massachusetts General Hospital handbook of general hospital psychiatry.* St. Louis: Mosby.

Sadock, B., & Kaplan, H. (1998). *Synopsis of psychiatry: Behavioral sciences/clinical psychiatry.* Philadelphia: Lippincott Williams & Wilkins.

Timby, B.K. (2000). *Fundamental skills and concepts in patient care.* Philadelphia: Lippincott Williams & Wilkins.

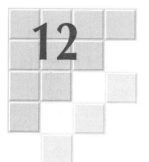

# Stress: Effective Coping and Adaptation

---

## Behavioral Objectives

*After reading this chapter the student will be able to:*

- Define coping and name the three stages of the coping process described by Lazarus.
- List the three ways the mind evaluates events or occurrences in its monitoring process.
- Describe the action of neurotransmitters as they relate to stress.
- Describe the three major realms of psychological functioning that are affected by stress and name five responses under each.
- Explain why an event that causes a change in a person's life causes stress.

---

## Key Terms

- Adaptation
- Coping
- Emotion focused coping
- Maladaptation
- Neurotransmitters
- Problem focused coping
- Primary appraisal
- Psychopathology
- Reappraisal
- Secondary appraisal
- Stress
- Stressor

---

**Stress** is a word in common use today. Many people believe that the world is becoming increasingly stressful. Indeed, it seems that the rapid changes in the world have had a strong impact on social systems and the individuals who compose them. The word stress is used in two ways. The first refers to the subjective feeling of tension experienced in the physiologic, mental, and/or spiritual realms as a response to environmental events that are perceived as threatening. Table 12-1 shows the different types of physical, mental, and spiritual responses that can occur during times of stress. The second use of the word commonly refers to those environmental events that result in internal feelings of stress. Actually, the correct word to use when describing a threatening environmental event is **stressor**.

**Adaptation** is the ability of the human being to perceive reality and respond to it in a way that supports his or her own emotional and physical well being and that of others in the social environment. When some aspect of mental functioning is disordered, it can result in misperceptions of reality and misjudgments that alter effective decision making. Healthy coping processes deteriorate when effective decision making is altered.

**Maladaptation** is the result of ineffective coping. When maladaptation occurs, it is the symptom of disordered perception or cognitive processes. The result of maladaptation is tension and distress in those who share the client's social environment.

---

### TABLE 12–1. General Responses to Stress

*Body Responses*

| | |
|---|---|
| Increased heart rate | Headache |
| Increased blood pressure | Backache |
| Indigestion | Nausea |
| Diarrhea | Constipation |
| Decreased appetite | Increased appetite |
| Tightness in chest | Clenching of jaw, neck, shoulders, and arms |
| Prone to colds, flu | Difficulty breathing |
| Urinary frequency | Sneezing |
| Prone to accidents | Insomnia |

*Mind Responses*

**Cognitive**

| | |
|---|---|
| Forgetfulness | Decreased concentration |
| Math and spelling errors | Blocking |
| Preoccupation | Decreased attention to details |

**Emotional**

| | |
|---|---|
| Anxiety | Being close to tears |
| Depression | Angry outbursts |
| Feelings of worthlessness | Suspiciousness |
| Self-criticism | Jealousy |

*Spiritual Responses*

| | |
|---|---|
| Decreased interest | Loss of sense of inner vitality |
| Decreased hope | Loss of sense of inner calm |
| Decreased connectedness with others | Loss of sense of connectedness to God or higher force |
| Decreased creativity | Loss of enthusiasm or motivation |
| Loss of capacity to feel joy | Withdrawal |
| Isolation | |

Hospital admission occurs when the client or members of his or her social environment determine that the level of distress requires professional intervention that is not available in the home, outpatient, or community mental health care system. It is important to note that the clinical role of nursing, that of assessing the whole-person response to illness, is a unique caregiving perspective. In contrast, other disciplines focus on specific aspects of functioning in their treatment models.

The nurse has the most intimate ongoing contact with the client. Accordingly, he or she can observe the subtle clinical changes that indicate improvement or deterioration in the client's condition. These changes can be the first indicators that the treatment plan is working or needs modification. The role of the nurse is to implement the nursing care plan, and also to be the first observer of clinical changes for the treatment team. Reporting clinical observations can inform the treatment team about the effectiveness of the team assessment and treatment plan. The nursing role is a critical factor in the successful treatment of mental disorders.

## ◆ THE COPING PROCESS

### PSYCHOLOGICAL STRESS
**Coping** refers to the way the mind responds to events that are challenging or threatening. It is important to be aware that an occurrence perceived as threatening by one person may be a challenge to another, and be perceived by a third person as quite normal. For example, an experienced pilot does not usually feel psychological distress when sitting at the controls; an experienced student pilot may feel the challenge of sitting at the controls; and a neophyte student of flying may feel a high level of psychological distress when the time to sit at the controls arrives. It is the difference in these individuals that causes the differences in their responses. In addition to the psychological uniqueness of the meaning of flying a plane to the three pilots, there are differences in their physiologic responses to the event of piloting. These differences create an internal subjective reaction that can never be identical for any two people.

Effective coping is the ability to manage internal or environmental stressors. Adequate physical, psychological, behavioral, or cognitive resources aid effective coping. **Emotion focused coping** and **problem focused coping** are the two most common supports to effective coping. Table 12-2 explains the differences between these two types of coping. Emotion focused coping is a coping style in which a person experiencing stress attempts to relieve it by changing his or her internal reactions to an environmental stressor. Problem focused coping is a coping style in which a person experiencing stress seeks to change the external event that is causing the internal stress reac-

TABLE 12–2. **Differences Between Emotion-Focused and Problem-Focused Coping**

| Emotion-Focused Coping | Problem-Focused Coping |
| --- | --- |
| *Definition* | *Definition* |
| Creating thoughts or actions to relieve situational emotional stress. These thoughts or actions do not change the external event. They change the internal emotional reaction to the event. | Taking action to change the external event that is causing the emotional stress. These thoughts or actions attempt to change the environmental stressor. |
| *Examples* | *Examples* |
| Talking to oneself to reduce worry | Making an appointment with a teacher when a student is having difficulty with a course |
| Having lunch with a friend and talking about the stress | |
| Using food or drink to reduce tension | Sitting down with a family member to attempt to resolve a problem when there is stress occurring within the family |
| | Studying with another student before an exam |

tion. Because of the different subjective experiences of stress, it follows that coping responses are also uniquely different. Coping is the result of the exquisite interplay of perceptions of stressful events, the psychological meaning attributed to them, and the physiologic responses associated with that meaning.

At the same time that the mind is monitoring these external and internal events, it gradually uses a variety of mechanisms to adapt to the stress associated with them. Some of these are unconscious devices, called defense mechanisms; they operate automatically. Defense mechanisms are described in Chapter 13, Stress: Ineffective Coping and Defense Mechanisms. The person also engages in active, conscious problem solving about the distress. These solutions, usually ones that have worked in the past, are called coping devices.

As a person adapts to his or her internal feelings of stress, the mind modifies its awareness of both internal and external steps that make up the coping process. The mind constantly monitors the environment in order to provide safety. Another word for monitoring is appraising.

Richard Lazarus has described the steps involved in the appraisal process. The three possible outcomes of **primary appraisal** are as follows:

1. The event is unimportant and can be ignored.
2. The event is good and contains no threat.

3. The event is potentially or already threatening owing to one or more causes:
   a. It is harming the psyche or has resulted in a significant change in self-esteem, relationships, role, or physical health.
   b. It contains a threat that one of the events described in the preceding could occur.
   c. It may be a challenging rather than a threatening event if mastery results in a positive outcome.

The next step in this process is called **secondary appraisal.** During this stage, the mind decides whether it is all right or in trouble. If the mind experiences anxiety about the situation, then it automatically uses defense mechanisms to regulate the unpleasant emotion associated with the awareness. In addition, during this state the individual can ask, "What can I do to help myself?" This is the time when the person uses conscious coping strategies. For example, a college freshman feeling overwhelmed by all the new experiences may decide on any one of several options to reduce stress—to begin jogging, drop one difficult course, talk it out with his or her parents over the telephone, or any number of other stress-relieving activities.

The mind is continuously evaluating the outcome of its coping efforts and is ready to develop new strategies if those currently in use are not working. This is called **reappraisal.**

## PHYSIOLOGIC STRESS

Adaptation involves both a psychological and physiologic state of well being. With increased research on the effects of neurotransmitters on the body, scientists are rapidly learning that it is impossible to separate the mind and body in assessing a person's health status. The most commonly known neurotransmitter is adrenaline. Think for a moment about what effects adrenaline causes in the body during an extremely angry moment or a close call while driving. Awareness of the danger of a near-accident is experienced through the perceptual sphere of our psychological system. Anger is experienced through the emotional sphere of our psychological system. Both experiences, however, have strong physiologic effects. They include elevations in pulse and respirations, slowing of digestion, and so on.

**Neurotransmitters** are the chemical bridges between the mind and body. They are biochemical substances released in the central nervous system that send messages through both branches of the autonomic nervous system: the parasympathetic nervous system and sympathetic nervous system. These two branches of the autonomic nervous system send messages to all body organs and muscles. Researchers in the field of neurochemistry have currently identified more than 100 such substances, all having different effects within the body. In addition to the interactive effects of neurotransmitters on the stress response, there are neuroendocrine substances produced by the adrenal glands, such as adrenaline, that play powerful roles in the stress response.

The thought processes involved in coping activate the neurotransmitters and neuroendocrine substances. Scientists expect that new types of neurotransmitters and neuroendocrine hormones and new mechanisms of these currently known substances will increasingly be recognized as significant players in the mediation of stress and the development and course of many, if not most, types of illness, both physical and mental.

## ◆ THE EFFECTS OF COPING ON MENTAL AND PHYSICAL HEALTH

As nursing examines the effects of stress on physical and mental disease processes, coping has been identified as a critical factor that influences the potential for wellness or disease. Coping is the response to a demand or threat.

In 1980, the American Nurses Association described nursing as "the diagnosis and treatment of human responses to actual or potential health problems." Since 1980, nursing philosophy and practice have been influenced by a greater elaboration of the science of caring and its integration with the traditional knowledge base for diagnosis and treatment of human responses to health and illness. The word *response* is a term that encompasses the concept of coping. Ideally, when a person is challenged or threatened by environmental stressors, he or she has a variety of resources present that support healthy, effective coping. The resources that assist in an effective coping response include the following:

- Good problem-solving ability
- Prior experience with the stressor
- Adequate knowledge about the cause of the stressor
- Available support systems, such as family, friends, and so on
- Adequate sleep, nutrition, and physical hygiene to support normal mental and physical functioning

If an individual is challenged or threatened by a stressful event and is unable to cope effectively, he or she experiences psychological stress. If the stressful feeling is severe, it is possible that a mental disorder can occur. The primary cause of many types of mental disorders is ineffective coping.

When mental or physical disease is present, the demands on an individual are greater. Effective coping becomes yet another demand on a person who is already weakened by his or her mental or physical condition. The role of a mental health nurse is to provide support that assists with effective immediate and long-term coping.

## ADAPTATION

**Adaptation** is the process of coping effectively with one's social environment so that growth and development proceed in a way that supports healthy social relationships, good self-esteem, and ongoing positive challenge. Psychosocial adaptation, as described in Chapter 7, Communicating in the Therapeutic Relationship, is the ability of an individual to perceive reality and respond to it in a way that supports his or her own emotional and physical well being and that of others in the environment. All of these characteristics of adaptation are built on the foundation of effective coping.

When ineffective coping occurs, it is the foundation of maladaptation. **Maladaptation** is caused by ineffective coping with a significant stressor or set of stressors that results in internal feelings and external behaviors that reduce the quality of life for an individual. Maladaptation usually affects the quality of interpersonal relationships as well. Concepts relating to ineffective coping are addressed in Chapter 13, Stress: Ineffective Coping and Defense Mechanisms. The relationship among stress, coping, and adaptation can be seen in Figure 12-1.

## ◆ LIFE EVENTS THAT CONTRIBUTE TO THE STRESS RESPONSE

An important factor in the level of stress a person feels is the number of events in his or her life that are causing change. A person whose life is more or less routine—whose personal life and working life are stable and without change or conflict—undergoes relatively low levels of stress. In the current world of frequent change in the structure of family and workplace, very few people find this to be so. In fact, it is not uncommon to find that one life change often precipitates other life changes.

With the knowledge that stress is experienced in direct relationship to the number of life changes one is undergoing, it is possible to understand that an accumulating series of changes can intensify until one more new change becomes "the straw that breaks the camel's back." For example, if a woman is promoted to a new position in another city, she usually encounters the following changes:

- Leaving a workplace where she is secure and has many acquaintances
- Moving to a new workplace where she must take on new responsibilities, usually before she is fully oriented and before she knows her new supervisors, peers, or subordinates

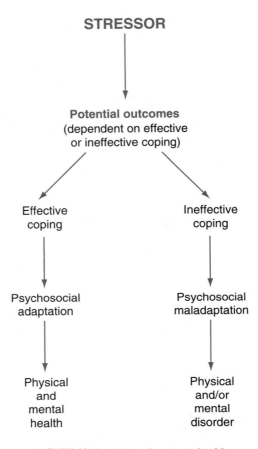

FIGURE 12–1. Effects of stress on health.

- Leaving a home that she may need to sell or breaking a lease
- Hunting for a new home, which is usually more costly
- Moving her possessions
- Leaving her friends and moving to a new area with no immediate family or other sources of support
- Arranging for new telephone installation, changes of addresses to all friends, creditors, magazines, and so on

Can you see that what initially sounds like a positive event can actually cause an individual to experience increasing levels of stress? Robert Rahe, a researcher in the field of stress, developed an assessment scale in which point values were established for the specific events the study participants reported as most stressful. The events and the points assigned to each appear in Table 12-3. The researchers found that when the study participants' stress points totaled more than 250, they frequently encountered minor life crises. You may be interested in reviewing the life events in this questionnaire to determine your own current life stress score.

## TABLE 12–3. **Life-Changing Event Questionnaire**

| Social Area | Life Event and Life Change Unit (LCU) Value* |
|---|---|
| Family | Death of spouse (105) |
| | Marital separation (65) |
| | Death of close family member (65) |
| | Divorce (62) |
| | Pregnancy (60) |
| | Change in health of a family member (52) |
| | Marriage (50) |
| | Gain of a new family member (50) |
| | Marital reconciliation (42) |
| | Spouse begins or stops work (37) |
| | Son or daughter leaving home (29) |
| | Trouble with in-laws (29) |
| | Change in number of family gatherings (26) |
| Personal | Jail term (56) |
| | Sex difficulties (49) |
| | Death of a close friend (46) |
| | Personal injury or illness (42) |
| | Change in living conditions (39) |
| | Outstanding personal achievement (33) |
| | Change in residence (33) |
| | Minor violations of the law (32) |
| | Begin or end school (32) |
| | Change in sleeping habits (31) |
| | Revision of personal habits (31) |
| | Change in eating habits (29) |
| | Change in church activities (29) |
| | Vacation (28) |
| | Change in schools (28) |
| | Change in recreation (28) |
| | Christmas (26) |

*(continues)*

---

TABLE 12–3. **Life-Changing Event Questionnaire**

| Social Area | Life Event and Life Change Unit (LCU) Value* |
|---|---|
| Work | Fired at work (64) |
| | Retirement from work (49) |
| | Trouble with boss (39) |
| | Business readjustment (38) |
| | Change to different line of work (38) |
| | Change in work responsibilities (33) |
| | Change in work hours or conditions (30) |
| Financial | Foreclosure of mortgage or loan (57) |
| | Change in financial state (43) |
| | Mortgage (home, car, etc.) (39) |
| | Mortgage less than $10,000 (26) |
| Directions: | Sum the Life Change Units (LCUs) for life changes during the past 12 months. |
| | Totals between 250 and 400 LCUs: Increased possibility of minor life crisis. |
| | Total over 400 LCUs: Increased possibility of major life crisis. |

Although unvalidated, the author's finding in using this scale in stress workshops is that many people today experience stress at the 400-point level without developing crisis or serious physical or mental illness. This may be the result of general adaptation to the increasing levels of stressors in our society since Rahe's original studies. A word of caution, however. Individuals who are experiencing stress at 400 or higher levels should become familiar with events listed on this questionnaire. They would be wise to review future decisions carefully in order to reduce or delay current or anticipated changes that could introduce further stress and potentially compromise coping abilities.

*Signifies the numerical point value assigned to each stressor.

Adapted from Rahe, R. (1990). Psychosocial stressors and adjustment disorder: Van Gogh's life chart illustrates stress and disease. *Journal of Clinical Psychiatry, 51*(11), 15.

## ◆ EFFECTIVE COPING FACTORS

Researchers who study coping have identified a number of effective coping factors, which are described elsewhere in this chapter. The use of nursing skills that draw on these factors can be helpful to clients with mental disorders.

*The Value of Worry.* The experience of worrying about an upcoming threatening event can often be a trigger to effective coping. The important factor is how much the person is worrying. A moderate level of worry is usually adaptive. For example, a person who is not worried about an upcoming serious event, such as coronary bypass surgery, may not be adequately prepared psychologically and may be overwhelmed just prior to surgery or during the immediate postoperative period because he or she has not had the benefit of the anticipatory worrying that motivates problem-solving and other important aids to effective coping.

The moderately worried person, on the other hand, engages in a variety of adaptive activities to decrease his or her mental distress. These activities include asking questions of the physician, talking with others who have had the surgery, problem solving about how to cope, and expressing concern about the surgery to family members and friends. Accordingly, this person receives extra social support. The highly worried person is usually overwhelmed with anxiety to the point that he or she does few or none of the steps described. Excessive worry frequently contributes to ineffective coping and ultimately to maladaptation.

*Focusing on the Objective, Concrete Aspects of a Current or Anticipated Threatening Event.* Usually, when a person is undergoing a difficult time, it is helpful for him or her to gather as much information as possible about what to expect. The information includes specific elements, for example, answers to specific questions such as: How long will this last? What will be going on around me? What will I see, hear, taste, smell, and so on? What is causing this to happen? What do other people do to cope with this situation?

Generally, it can be helpful for the person to obtain objective, concrete, realistic answers to these questions. Long, involved answers are not necessary. Complicated answers sometimes can generate more anxiety. Brief answers that provide specific elements of information can regulate emotional responses or stimulate problem solving.

The nurse can provide information so that an individual can judge how well he or she can perform or respond to specific types of events. When individuals have information about how to take care of themselves, they usually feel more able to cope with new types of situations. Realistically, in new situations most people do not know what they do not know! Accordingly, an empathic caregiver may be able to anticipate the specific aspects of the new situation that are likely to be anxiety provoking and share that information.

Effective coping is essential to good health, both physically and mentally. The next chapter provides information about what happens when normal coping efforts are not successful.

## KEY POINTS

- Stress refers to the subjective feeling of tension in response to environmental events that are perceived as threatening. These events are called stressors.

■ Coping refers to how the mind responds to awareness of potential threats.

■ An event perceived as threatening by one person may not be threatening to another person. Likewise, coping mechanisms vary from person to person.

■ Defense mechanisms are unconscious and operate automatically. Coping devices are conscious and are usually based on successful previous experience.

■ Neurotransmitters are chemicals released in the body that trigger the changes in physical responses that are the foundation of different emotions.

■ Coping has been identified as a critical factor that influences the potential for wellness or disease. Ineffective coping mechanisms are the primary cause of mental disorders.

■ Resources that assist an effective coping response include the following:
—Good problem-solving ability
—Prior experience with the stressor
—Adequate knowledge of the stressor's cause
—Availability of a support system
—Adequate sleep, nutrition, and physical hygiene

■ Adaptation refers to coping effectively with one's environment, resulting in growth and development that support healthy social relationships and good self-esteem.

■ Stress is experienced in direct relationship to the number of life changes a person is currently undergoing and the availability of personal resources.

■ Effective coping mechanisms include a slight to moderate level of *worrying* and *focusing* on the objective or concrete aspects of a threatening event.

## SELF-AWARENESS ACTIVITY

Have you been aware when your mind is helping you to cope effectively with a difficult event? For example, when you have a challenging exam and you spot a difficult question, do you notice a rise in anxiety—followed by some internal messages to yourself—and then a feeling of internal calm?

- Can you think of three recent times when you have been aware of your own effective coping?

- During these three experiences with effective coping can you identify if they were instances of emotion focused coping or problem focused coping?

## QUESTIONS

1. The client tells the nurse that she has decided to cut back her work hours from 40 to 32 per week to reduce her life stressors. The nurse recognizes that the client *probably*
   a. is in denial about the amount of stress in her life.
   b. has determined an appropriate course of action to reduce her stress.
   c. has not yet completed a primary appraisal of her situation.
   d. does not recognize the source of stress in her life.

2. The nurse is assisting the client to develop effective coping skills. One way the nurse could this would be to
   a. encourage the client to be totally self-reliant.
   b. encourage the client to sleep 5 to 6 hours a night to allow more time during the day.
   c. encourage the client to discuss how he or she has dealt with similar stressors in the past.
   d. encourage the client to discuss only the current stressors.

3. To help the client feel less stress when he or she is hospitalized, the nurse should
   a. not allow the client to be alone at any time.
   b. provide technical and detailed information on every aspect of the hospitalization.
   c. provide objective, concrete, and realistic answers to questions.
   d. discourage any visitors from staying with the client more than 5 to 10 minutes.

4. The nurse is aware that worry is
   a. a way of rehearsing a reaction to an upcoming stressful event.
   b. seldom a trigger for effective coping.
   c. most useful if it is constant.
   d. usually a sign of serious neurosis.

## BIBLIOGRAPHY

American Nurses Association. (1991). *Standards of clinical nursing practice.* (1991). Kansas City, MO: American Nurses Association.

American Nurses Association. (1995). *Nursing social policy statement.* Kansas City, MO: American Nurses Association.

Barry, P.D. (1996). *Psychosocial nursing: Care of physically ill patients and their families* (3rd ed.). Philadelphia: Lippincott-Raven.

Boyd, M., & Nihart, M. (1998). *Psychiatric nursing: Contemporary practice.* Philadelphia: Lippincott Williams & Wilkins.

Carpenito, L. (2000). *Nursing diagnosis: Application to clinical practice* (8th ed.). Philadelphia: Lippincott Williams Wilkins.

Carpenito, L. (1999). *Handbook of nursing diagnosis.* Philadelphia: Lippincott Williams & Wilkins.

Gendolla, G. (2000). On the impact of mood on behavior: An integrative theory and a review. *Review of General Psychology, 4*(4), 378–408.

McDonald, S., & Ahern, K. (1999). Whistle-blowing: Effective and ineffective coping responses. *Nursing Forum, 34*(4), 5–13.

Rahe, R. (1990). Psychosocial stressors and adjustment disorder: Van Gogh's life chart illustrates stress and disease. *Journal of Clinical Psychiatry, 51*(11), 15.

Sadock, B., & Kaplan, H. (1998). *Synopsis of psychiatry: Behavioral sciences/clinical psychiatry.* Philadelphia: Lippincott Williams & Wilkins.

Shaw, C. (1999). A framework for the study of coping, illness behaviors and outcomes. *Journal of Advanced Nursing, 29*(5), 1246–1255.

Wrosch, C., Heckhausen, J., & Lachman, M. (2000). Primary and secondary control strategies for managing health and financial stress across adulthood. *Psychology and Aging, 15*(3), 387–399.

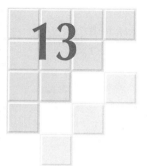

13

# Stress: Ineffective Coping and Defense Mechanisms

---

## Behavioral Objectives

*After reading this chapter the student will be able to:*

- Contrast the differences between effective and ineffective coping.
- Describe the role of ineffective coping in the conditions included in the nursing diagnosis categories.
- Name the primary feeling that triggers the use of defense mechanisms.
- List the four levels of defense mechanisms and the two defense mechanisms within each category.
- Explain the use of denial and give an example of ineffective denial.
- Describe the differences and similarities between repression and suppression.
- Define general adaptation syndrome and name its three progressive stages.

---

## Key Terms

- Conversion
- Coping, effective
- Coping, ineffective
- Defense mechanisms (listed by level)
  Narcissistic defense mechanisms
  —Denial

  —Distortion
  —Delusional projection
  Immature defense mechanisms
  —Acting out
  —Avoidance
  —Projection
  —Regression

Neurotic defense
mechanisms
—Displacement
—Identification
—Isolation
—Rationalization
—Reaction formation
—Repression
Mature defense
mechanisms

—Altruism
—Anticipation
—Humor
—Sublimation
—Suppression
■ General adaptation
syndrome
■ Paranoia
■ Psychosis
■ Psychotic behavior

The American Nurses Association has described nursing practice as the diagnosis and treatment of the human response to illness. The term *response* can be described as a reaction to a stimulus. It also can be generalized to include the concept of coping as a response to a stimulus or event. Effective coping has been identified as a factor that is essential to mental and physical health.

The North American Nursing Diagnosis Association (NANDA), described in Chapter 10, Nursing Process in the Mental Health Setting, meets every 2 years to update the full list of health care problems that nurses address in their nursing care. Currently the list includes nine patterns of human functioning that contribute to overall wellness. Within these nine patterns are a total of 155 categories of conditions that nurses can address.

Of that number, more than half of these conditions are psychosocial in nature. Most of the psychosocial category titles are very specific. They include such names as Social Isolation, Altered Parenting, Self-Esteem Disturbance, and so on. Additional categories include psychosocial factors in the cause or etiology of the condition, for example, Sleep Pattern Disturbance, Altered Health Maintenance, and Altered Sexuality Patterns.

In all of the NANDA categories that involve a problem with psychosocial adaptation, ineffective coping is occurring. Indeed, ineffective coping is an umbrella term or comprehensive concept that is a fundamental factor in all mental disorders and psychosocial-related nursing diagnoses. Box 13-1 includes the NANDA definitions relating to **ineffective coping**.

**Effective coping** is the combination of conscious problem-solving strategies and unconscious defense mechanisms that result in the cognitive and behavioral responses to challenging or threatening events. The factors that compose effective coping were described in the previous chapter. The differences between effective and ineffective coping,

> BOX 13–1. **North American Nursing Diagnosis Association (NANDA) Definitions of Ineffective Coping**
>
> **INEFFECTIVE INDIVIDUAL COPING**
> A state in which the individual experiences, or is at risk to experience, an inability to manage internal or environmental stressors adequately because of inadequate resources (physical, psychological, behavioral, and/or cognitive).
>
> **DEFINING CHARACTERISTICS**
> Verbalization of inability to cope or ask for help
> *Or*
> Inappropriate use of defense mechanisms
> *Or*
> Inability to meet role expectations

as well as the differences in approach between emotion-focused and problem-focused coping, are shown in Table 13-1.

## HOW DEFENSE MECHANISMS FORM A RESPONSE TO INEFFECTIVE COPING

### THE USE AND PURPOSE OF DEFENSE MECHANISMS

**Defense mechanisms** are protective processes automatically developed by the unconscious mind when the conscious coping techniques are unable to manage the anxiety or uncertainty of a threatening event and there is a risk of ineffective coping. Because adaptation is a fundamental requirement of coping with life's demands, it is natural that humans have developed unconscious defense mechanisms that increase their sense of security, protect their self-esteem, and assist in solving their emotional dilemmas. The self-conscious personality, with its intense need for security and self-esteem, evokes protective mental defenses as instinctively as self-preservation prompts protection against physical harm. Anxiety is part of life from the cradle to the grave. Everyone, to a greater or lesser degree, employs defense mechanisms to ensure comfort and defend against anxiety. A study of these mechanisms is essential to understanding human behavior and should lead to a clearer recognition of the forces operating in the psyche.

Some defense mechanisms, if employed within certain adaptive limits, may help to promote a sound or generally "healthy" personality. If used excessively, however, defense mechanisms may lead to a personality distortion. The maladaptive use of defense mechanisms can progressively disorganize the personality.

## TABLE 13–1. Problem-Focused and Emotion-Focused Behaviors

| Behavior | Problem or Emotion Focused | Definition | Effective | Ineffective |
|---|---|---|---|---|
| Goal setting | Problem focused | The conscious process of setting time limitations on behavior | When goals are attainable and manageable, ie, making an appointment with boss to discuss pay raise | When the appraisal of the situation is missed or inaccurately evaluated |
| Information-seeking | Problem focused | Process of learning about all aspects of a problem that provides perspective and reinforces self-control | When situations are complex and additional information is needed, ie, attending a parent effectiveness class because of being unsure about discipline techniques | When the needed information is already obtained and the activity delays action |
| Mastery | Problem focused | Learning of new procedures or skills that facilitate self-esteem, reinforce self-control | When there are new procedures to learn, ie, self-care activities, insulin injection, catheter care | When the situation does not require learning new procedures or they have nothing to do with the stressful situation |
| Help-seeking | Problem focused | Reaching out to others for support; sharing feelings provides an emotional release, reassurance, and comfort | When similar problems are shared by others, ie, in Alcoholics Anonymous, weight loss programs, psychosocial programs | When using help-seeking to avoid action in the current situation |
| Minimization | Emotion focused | The seriousness of the problem is minimized | Useful way of providing needed time for appraisal; ie, a person is told that her child is in an automobile accident and forces herself to think the accident is minor until additional information is received | When the appraisal of the situation is missed or inaccurately evaluated |
| Projection, displacement, and suppression of anger | Emotion focused | When anger is attributed to or expressed toward a less threatening person or thing | When threat is reduced, the individual can deal with the situation; ie, the boss reprimands a worker for submitting a report late—the worker in turn hits his fist on the copying machine as he walks by | When reality is distorted and relationships disturbed, which further compounds the problem; suppression of anger may result in stress-related physical symptoms |
| Anticipatory preparation | Emotion focused | Mental rehearsal of possible consequences of behavior or outcomes of stressful situations | Provides the opportunity to develop perspective as well as to prepare for the worst; ie, when waiting for exam results, the patient develops a plan of action if the results are negative | Anticipation creates unmanageable stress as in anticipatory mourning |
| Attribution | Emotion focused | Finding personal meaning in the problem situation, which may be through religious faith or individual belief | May offer consolation, ie, fate, the will of the divine, luck | When all sense of self-responsibility is lost |

Adapted from Carpenito, L. (1997). *Nursing diagnosis: Application to clinical practice* (7th ed.) Philadelphia: Lippincott.

Defense mechanisms are unconscious and automatic mental maneuvers that decrease the unpleasant feeling of anxiety. These mechanisms begin operating in early childhood. Different types of these adaptive defense mechanisms appear as the child matures.

Depending on the level of stress a person is experiencing, the mind shuts out all or part of a painful awareness. Generally speaking, adults use the defense mechanisms that develop early in life only when severe stress occurs or when a person has a low tolerance for stress. The higher-level, more mature mechanisms develop as the personality matures. They are used when the level of stress being experienced is low to moderate.

## ◆ TYPES OF DEFENSE MECHANISMS

Defense mechanisms are classified by the age at which they appear in the child, the amount of reality they block, and the level of pathology they can cause if used excessively. In this section the defenses seen most commonly in the mental health care setting are discussed. In addition, examples of maladaptive use of these defenses are given to illustrate their effect on personality and potential to cause mental disorder.

### NARCISSISTIC DEFENSE MECHANISMS
### (BIRTH TO 3 YEARS)

The term *narcissistic* is used to refer to a person who is self-centered in an exceedingly immature way. The word is derived from the Greek myth about Narcissus, a very handsome young man who fell in love with the reflection of his face in a pond. It is normal for toddlers and young children to be self-centered, but as the child develops, he or she should gradually develop the capacity to be aware of others as well as self. **Narcissistic defense mechanisms** develop as the earliest defense mechanisms. These defenses are denial, distortion, and delusional projection. They are employed by the healthy adult mind only during periods of extreme stress. When used routinely in the older adolescent or adult, they contribute to the development of severe forms of mental disorders, such as schizophrenia.

**Denial** is the first defense used in infancy. It remains available as the strongest defense for shutting out painful awareness in the environment. The person sees, hears, or perceives an event but the mind refuses to recognize it consciously. Denial and the other two defenses in this category are used when the mind senses a severe threat.

Tom is a married, 53-year-old man with a high-level position in a large organization. The company president told him that his job would be ending in 2 months. He refused to discuss the matter further. Four weeks later he still refused to discuss his termination with his boss. He became increasingly withdrawn. He did not disclose his situation to his wife and family. His superiors at work became increasingly concerned for his well being as he continued to shut out the reality of his employment.

**Distortion** is an automatic unconscious defense mechanism used to reshape external reality to reduce anxiety and restore a feeling of emotional comfort. When present in a mental disorder, it is the basis for hallucinations and nonparanoid types of delusions.

To continue with the story of Tom: He does not have a regular savings program and has limited monetary savings. During his career he continuously told himself that he could never lose his job and would receive a plentiful monetary settlement when he retired. In essence, he deluded himself with a belief that was untrue.

**Delusional projection** is a mechanism by which the mind forms conclusions and beliefs that are not based on reality. These beliefs, when firmly rooted, form the basis of paranoid delusions, in which a person believes that someone is out to get him or her.

After several weeks of using denial and distortion to quiet his unconscious psychological terror about his circumstances, the mental pressure is causing yet another serious defense mechanism to occur. While at work, Tom increasingly believes that his superiors are plotting against him—that they plan to injure and eventually kill him to get rid of him. Beliefs—with no basis in reality—that someone is going to purposely injure another are called **paranoia**.

The effect of chronic use of narcissistic defense mechanisms to shut out reality is often a serious mental disorder. This disorder may require hospitalization when outpatient mental health intervention either does not occur or is not successful.

## MATURE DEFENSE MECHANISMS (AGES 2 TO 4 YEARS)

The immature defenses develop during the toddler stage and are used by healthy adults under moderate to severe stress and people with all types of personality disorders. **Acting out** is the behavioral outcome of conflict between an unconscious need to express anger and a conscious need to deny it.

Ann is a 19-year-old college student who is living away from home for the first time. She has a high level of unconscious anger about emotional abuse she experienced from her mother. She is aggressive and unreasonable in relationships with women authority figures at her school, such as her freshman advisor, one of her instructors, and the dormitory monitor. She is acting out or expressing the anger she feels toward her mother but does not consciously acknowledge.

**Avoidance** causes an individual unconsciously to stay away from any person, situation, or place that might cause unwanted sexual or aggressive feelings to occur.

Because of Ann's unresolved conflict with her mother, she unconsciously avoids close relationships with all women. As a result Ann is increasingly isolated in her new college environment.

**Projection** is a less pathologic form of delusional projection, described in the preceding. It occurs when a person is unable to acknowledge his or her own thoughts or feelings and attributes them to others.

When Ann's freshman advisor asks to meet with her, Ann is quiet and sullen. When her advisor asks what is wrong, Ann looks at her and angrily says, "I know you don't like me."

**Regression** occurs when the mind is unable to tolerate severe intrapsychic or environmental stress. As a way of reducing anxiety, a person's psychosocial functioning returns to an earlier developmental stage.

In her family Ann was very dependent on her father and frequently acted childlike when she was with him. Now that she is away at college, she has begun to visit a senior male student from her hometown. He is becoming irritated with her frequent unexpected visits and her requests for assistance and counsel.

The chronic use of immature defense mechanisms, although not as seriously maladaptive as narcissistic defenses, indicates major developmental and adaptation problems. Without modification of the defenses that Ann is using, she is at risk for depression, anxiety disorder, or other types of mental disorders related to her inability to cope adaptively with her new living conditions.

## NEUROTIC DEFENSE MECHANISMS (AGES 4 AND OLDER)

Neurotic defenses can cause a significant level of psychological distress, but usually do not result in the need for psychiatric hospitalization. If neurotic defenses cause some form of ineffective coping with a significant life event, it is possible that major forms of depression or anxiety may result. Descriptions of neurotic defenses appear in the following.

**Displacement** occurs when feelings about a person or thing are shifted to another, safer object. Although the feelings are shifted, their original cause remains the same. For example, when a person is angry with the boss he or she may go home and become angry with a family member or play an extra hard game of tennis. **Identification** is a defense mechanism that results in a person taking on the thoughts, feelings, or particular circumstances of another person as if they were his or her own. For example, an expectant father may develop symptoms of morning sickness similar to those of his pregnant wife.

**Isolation** is a defense mechanism that separates the emotion associated with a thought; the emotion is repressed, however. For example, a nurse may be working closely with a dying client and be able to acknowledge that the person's symptoms indicate he or she is near death. Although very attached to the client, the nurse may not experience the grief associated with this awareness until a later time. Other names for isolation are *intellectualization* and *rationalization*.

**Reaction formation** is a defense mechanism that is also known as *compensation*. It is used when a thought, feeling, or impulse is unacceptable to the conscious mind. As a result, the defense causes the person to behave in the exact opposite manner. A person who has had an amputation, for example, may feel deep rage toward the surgeon, but when the doctor enters the room, the client is very cordial. **Repression** is sometimes considered to be one of the most important defense mechanisms. It causes the anxiety associated with any distressing internal awareness to be stored away in the unconscious. Without the capacity to repress painful thoughts, feelings, and memories, humans could be overwhelmed by them.

## MATURE DEFENSE MECHANISMS (AGES 6 AND OLDER)

These defense mechanisms are used by the healthy, mature mind when it is under minimal stress. These defenses have a larger conscious component than the defense mechanisms described in the preceding. Because of their conscious component, mature individuals often use them as conscious coping devices when they recognize they are experiencing stress. These mechanisms develop during the middle and later years of childhood. They include **altruism,** which is a defense that channels the desire to satisfy one's own needs into the wish to meet the needs of others. **Anticipation** is a defense by which a person intellectually and emotionally acknowledges an upcoming situation that is expected to provoke anxiety. By acknowledging it and working through some of the anxiety in advance, the event will be less stressful when it occurs.

**Humor** is a defense used when a person cannot fully tolerate a difficult situation. It is used without expense to the self or another person. Humor differs from **wit,** in which the actual anxiety-provoking subject is avoided. **Sublimation** operates in association with the defense of repression. In sublimation, a repressed urge or desire is expressed in a socially acceptable or useful way. **Suppression** is a defense that is similar to repression; it stores thoughts or memories in the subconscious mind where they are easily retrievable. Repression stores thoughts or memories in the unconscious where they usually remain buried and are not retrievable.

## CONVERSION: AN UNCLASSIFIED DEFENSE MECHANISM

Be aware of another defense mechanism that is actually a combination of elements of other defense mechanisms. **Conversion** is a mechanism by which emotional conflicts are channeled into physical symptoms or physical illness. An example is when an individual develops chronic diarrhea or constipation as the result of emotional conflict. The symptoms are real in conversion. Doctors are baffled, however, to explain the cause. When a physiologic basis cannot be found despite a good diagnostic workup, it is important to assess the psychological stress the client has been and is currently experiencing. The interaction between mind and body is increasingly being recognized as an important etiology in the development of physical illness. The field of *liaison psychiatry* addresses the emotional outcomes of physical illness.

## ◆ GENERAL ADAPTATION SYNDROME

When coping efforts are not successful and defense mechanisms are not able to reduce the effects of stress, the result is a subjective feeling of anxiety and concurrent physiologic symptoms created by the stressor. These physical symptoms occur as the result of neurotransmitter stimulation. Hans Selye, known as the "father of stress research," described the physiologic responses to stress in a concept called the **general adaptation syndrome** (GAS). The GAS includes the following three stages:

1. The alarm reaction: The body responds to a stressor with a strong defensive response stimulated by hormones from the adrenal cortex. This decreases to a steady and consistent physiologic stress response. If the stressor is not withdrawn, the body moves to the next stage.
2. The stage of resistance: The body maintains resistance to the stressor until it disappears. If the stressor does not disappear, the body moves to the next stage.
3. The stage of exhaustion: The effects of the continuing stressor cause the body's resistance ability to fail. Ultimately, without medical intervention, death will occur.

The human psyche and body are well designed to endure the effects of stress. Realistically, however, they are limited in their ability to tolerate severe, unremitting stress. Eventually a point arrives at which either the mind or the body is unable to continue providing resistance to either environmental or intrapsychic stress. When this happens, the person can become physically or mentally ill. Table 13-2 shows the different factors that contribute to either effective or ineffective coping.

## ◆ TYPES OF BEHAVIOR

### MALADAPTIVE BEHAVIOR
Maladaptive behavior is the result of ineffective coping and psychosocial maladaptation. When ineffective coping is caused by chronic use of

### TABLE 13–2. **Patient and Family Members' Responses to the Stress of Illness**

Stress

↓

Regression

Possible Outcomes

| **Effective Coping:** Adaptation (factors in outcome) | **Ineffective Coping:** Maladaptation (factors in outcome) |
|---|---|
| **Normal Mental Status** | **Abnormal Mental Status** |
| *Effective Thought Process* | *Ineffective Thought Process Owing to:* |
| Adequate memory | Organic mental disorder |
| Adequate problem-solving ability | Low intelligence level |
| Good judgment | Excessive anxiety or depression |
| | Functional psychiatric disorder |
| | Poor memory |
| | Poor problem-solving ability |
| | Poor judgment |
| *Normal Coping Style* | *Abnormal Coping Style* |
| Patient's intrapsychic defenses are adaptive | Ego unconsciously underuses or overuses certain predictable defense mechanisms |
| Patient is able to use normal stress management to cope adequately with stress | Patient loses ability to use conscious stress management mechanisms |
| Illness is not life threatening | Illness is life threatening or is *perceived* as life threatening |
| Illness is not highly threatening to patient's self-esteem and body image | Illness is threatening to self-esteem or body image |
| Illness is not threatening to normal role functioning | Illness is threatening to normal role functioning |
| *Personality Style* | *Personality Style* |
| Illness does not cause a major change in the way the patient normally interacts with others and environment: personality is strong enough to cope with stress | Depending on the type of illness and its particular threat to the patient, any personality style can be at risk because of the stress of major illness |
| *Family Coping Style* | *Family Coping Style* |
| Family is normally able to adapt to stress | Family's normal response to stress may be chronically inadequate, or the family may be overwhelmed by the catastrophic illness or death of one of its members |
| Illness is not perceived as life threatening or causing major shifts in role of family member | Illness may cause major shift in role functioning within family |
| One or more family members are emotionally detached enough to allow the patient to voice concerns about self | Patient has no family to support him or her |

*continued*

| TABLE 13–2. **Patient and Family Members' Responses to the Stress of Illness** *(Continued)* | |
|---|---|
| *Other Social Relationships in Environment* | *Other Social Relationships in Environment* |
| Caregivers appropriately assess and therapeutically intervene with maladapting patient | Caregivers are unable to assess and intervene with maladapting patient |
| Patient's level of stress is responsive to caregivers' interventions | Patient's level of stress is not responsive to caregivers' interventions |
| Patient's work role is not permanently threatened | Patient's work role is threatened |
| Patient's relationships outside of the family are not permanently threatened | Patient's role in functioning in social and work relationships is chronically or permanently threatened |
| Patient has friends with whom to explore concerns about illness and receive support (close friends are sometimes able to be more objective than family members) | Patient has inadequate or no social relationships for support |
| Physical environment supports homeostasis | Physical environment threatens homeostasis |

From Barry, P. (1996). *Psychosocial nursing: Care of physically ill. Patients and their families* (3rd ed.). Philadelphia: Lippincott-Raven.

narcissistic or immature defenses, there can be serious behavioral problems. Maladaptive behavior usually causes severe strain in family and social relationships. Consider, for example, the behavior of Ann, discussed previously in the chapter.

### PSYCHOTIC BEHAVIOR

**Psychotic behavior** is the most severe manifestation of ineffective coping. It is caused by psychosis. **Psychosis** is the mental state caused by a loss of contact with reality. Usually psychosis occurs when the actual external reality is too threatening or anxiety provoking to be acknowledged. The mind unconsciously uses every defense possible to deny, distort, and avoid reality when it does not have the strength to cope consciously and problem solve about the actual problem or sets of problems that are occurring. The story of Tom illustrates the potential for psychotic behavior because of his need to shut out totally the reality about his job loss. His behavior moves into the psychotic range when he begins to fear that his coworkers are plotting against him.

The cause of mental disorder usually is related to ineffective coping. The reason why individuals with mental disorders are admitted to the hospital is to provide an environment that supports effective coping. The primary purpose of nursing care is to provide an environment where individuals can be restored to their prior effective coping level, receive medications that support coping, or learn new coping methods. The next unit describes how the nursing process in mental health care can assist clients in returning to states of mental health.

K E Y   P O I N T S

---

■ Ineffective coping is a fundamental factor in all mental disorders and psychosocial-related nursing diagnoses.

■ Excessive use of defense mechanisms can lead to personality distortion.

■ Defense mechanisms are classified by the age at which they appear, the amount of reality they block, and the level of pathology they can cause. The major groups of defense mechanisms include narcissistic, immature, neurotic, and mature.

■ Narcissistic defense mechanisms include denial, distortion, and delusional projection.

■ When used routinely, narcissistic defense mechanisms can cause severe forms of mental disorders such as schizophrenia.

■ Immature defense mechanisms include acting out, avoidance, projection, and regression.

■ Neurotic defense mechanisms include displacement, identification, rationalization, reaction formation, and repression.

■ Mature defense mechanisms, used by the healthy, mature person when experiencing minimal stress, include altruism, anticipation, humor, sublimation, and suppression.

■ Conversion is a mechanism in which the mind channels emotional conflict into physical symptoms.

■ The general adaptation syndrome (GAS) developed by Hans Selye includes three progressive stages: alarm, resistance, and exhaustion.

### SELF-AWARENESS ACTIVITY

As you were reading about the different defense mechanisms, were you able to recall times when one or more of these mechanisms was used? Remember that all people experience all or most of these mechanisms at different times in their lives.

- Which mechanisms do you most commonly use?
- Is it possible to know what feeling or feelings these defense mechanisms prevent you from experiencing?
- Are you able to recognize how these defense mechanisms assist you in coping effectively in your everyday life?
- Is there one or more of these defenses that you believe may contribute to ineffective coping?

## Q U E S T I O N S

1. The client says to the nurse "You are incompetent. You are always late" after a disturbing telephone call. The nurse recognizes this as
   a. projection.
   b. reaction formation.
   c. displacement.
   d. distortion.
2. The nurse identifies that she employs some defense mechanisms in her personal life. The nurse should understand that
   a. she must consciously control her use of all defense mechanisms.
   b. any use of defense mechanisms leads to maladaptive behavior.
   c. the use of some defense mechanisms is normal and generally "healthy."
   d. she did not develop healthy coping skills as a child.
3. The nurse may facilitate the development of mature defense mechanisms in a client by
   a. making fun of the client to encourage the use of humor.
   b. discussing upcoming situations with the client to work through some anxiety in advance.
   c. teaching the client how to avoid anxiety-provoking situations.
   d. all of the above.
4. The most severe manifestation of ineffective coping mechanisms is
   a. altruism.
   b. conversion.
   c. psychotic behavior.
   d. repression.

## BIBLIOGRAPHY

American Nurses Association. (1995). *Nursing social policy statement*. Kansas City, MO: American Nurses Association.

Barry, P.D. (1996). *Psychosocial nursing: Care of physically ill patients and their families* (3rd ed.). Philadelphia: Lippincott-Raven.

Boyd, M., & Nihart, M. (1998). *Psychiatric nursing: Contemporary practice*. Philadelphia: Lippincott Williams & Wilkins.

Brooke Army Medical Center. (1973). *Interpersonal skills* (videocassette). Fort Sam Houston, TX: Academy of Health Sciences.

Carpenito, L. (1999). *Handbook of nursing diagnosis* (8th ed.). Philadelphia: Lippincott Williams & Wilkins.

Carpenito, L. (2000). *Nursing diagnosis: Application to clinical practice* (8th ed.). Philadelphia: Lippincott Williams & Wilkins.

Collins, M., Mowbry, C., & Bybee, D. (1999). Measuring coping strategies in an educational intervention for individuals with psychiatric disabilities. *Health and Social Work,* 24(4), 270–290.

Folkman, S., & Moskowitz, J. (2000). Stress, positive emotion, and coping. *Current Directions in Psychological Science,* 9(4), 115–118.

Heim, C., Ehlert, U., & Hellhammer, D. (2000). The potential role of hypocortisolism in the pathophysiology of stress-related bodily disorders. *Psychoendocrinology,* 25(1), 1–35.

Lazarus, R.S. (1992). Coping with the stress of illness. *WHO Regional Publication, European Series,* 44, 11–31.

Sadock, B., & Kaplan, H. (1998). *Synopsis of psychiatry: Behavioral sciences/clinical psychiatry.* Philadelphia: Lippincott Williams & Wilkins.

Weisman, A. (1997). Coping with illness. In N.H. Cassem (Ed.). *Massachusetts General Hospital handbook of general hospital psychiatry* (4th ed.). St. Louis: Mosby–Year Book.

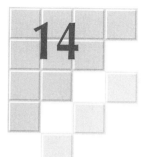

# The Mental Status Exam

## Behavioral Objectives

*After reading this chapter the student will be able to:*

- List the categories of mental status functioning.
- Name the three spheres of orientation.
- Describe three types of facial expressions, posture, and dress.
- Name four categories of affect and give an example of one emotion in each category.
- Describe the differences between thinking, feeling, and perception.
- Describe the differences between thought content and thought process.
- Name and define five types of thought disorders.
- Name and define two types of perception disorders.

## Key Terms

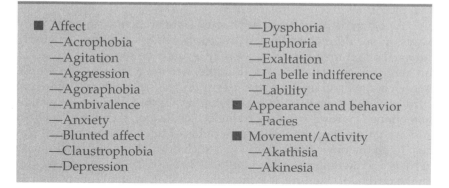

- Affect
  - —Acrophobia
  - —Agitation
  - —Aggression
  - —Agoraphobia
  - —Ambivalence
  - —Anxiety
  - —Blunted affect
  - —Claustrophobia
  - —Depression
  - —Dysphoria
  - —Euphoria
  - —Exaltation
  - —La belle indifference
  - —Lability
- Appearance and behavior
  - —Facies
- Movement/Activity
  - —Akathisia
  - —Akinesia

—Apraxia
—Dyskinesia
—Parkinsonian movement
■ Judgment
■ Memory disorder
—Amnesia
—Confabulation
■ Orientation/Level of
awareness
—Orientation to time,
person, place
—Continuum from
comatose to hypervigilant
■ Perception
—Depersonalization
—Derealization
—Hallucination
—Auditory hallucination
—Hypnagogic
hallucination

—Tactile hallucination
—Visual hallucination
—Illusion
■ Thought content and
process (thinking)
—Blocking
—Circumstantiality
—Déjà vu
—Delusion
—Delusion of grandeur
—Delusion of persecution
(paranoia)
—Delusion of reference
—Flight of ideas
—Loose association
—Neologism
—Obsession of thought
—Preoccupation of thought
—Perseveration
—Phobia
—Tangentiality

To work with clients who are mentally ill, it is important to understand the various ways in which the psyche can dysfunction and to be able to identify the specific symptoms that the client is displaying. First, the symptoms of mental dysfunction must be recognized; only then is it possible to determine the category of mental disorders the client is displaying. The treatment plan of individuals with mental disorders is based on interventions designed to reduce or eliminate the specific symptoms described in this chapter.

A person displays his or her mental state or mental status in many ways. In our normal dealings with people, when we notice something unusual about their behavior, we may actually be seeing symptoms of an abnormal mental state. For example, when we see a person whose speech is slow and unclear, whose eyes do not focus, whose clothes are dirty and disheveled, and whose thoughts are confused, we know that something is wrong. If a person smells like alcohol, then we may begin to form an opinion about the cause of his or her abnormal mental status. If, on the other hand, there is no such odor, then we can eliminate it from a wide range of other possible causes of the person's behavior. In the psychiatric setting, it is important to view mental functioning as comprising many different categories of behavior. **Behavior** is the observable or objective sign of mental functioning.

The categories of mental status functioning are listed below:

Level of awareness and orientation
Appearance and behavior
Speech and communication
Mood or affect
Thinking
Perception
Memory
Judgment

## ◆ LEVEL OF AWARENESS AND ORIENTATION

**Level of awareness** describes the client's wakefulness or consciousness. The levels of awareness range on a continuum from unconsciousness/coma——➤drowsiness/somnolence——➤normal alertness——➤ hyperalertness——➤suspiciousness——➤mania.

**Orientation** is closely related to level of awareness. Depending on a client's level of awareness, he or she may be more or less oriented. Orientation is the person's ability to identify *who* he or she is, *where* he or she is, and the date and approximate time. These three categories of orientation are known as "orientation to time, person, and place" and are often abbreviated to "oriented × 3" to describe the person who is oriented.

Orientation is a major criterion in determining a person's mental status. However, a client, particularly an elderly client, can be cognitively impaired even though he or she is oriented. Orientation by itself does not provide a complete picture of mental status.

## ◆ APPEARANCE AND BEHAVIOR

This category includes observable characteristics of a person, which also can be termed objective data. These include facies or facial expression, posture, dress, physical characteristics, motor activity, and reaction to caregiver.

**Facies** or facial expression includes the following types of characteristics. Pay close attention to whether or not the facies matches the emotions and content expressed by the client during his or her interactions with others. The most common types of facial expressions are as follows:

Animated
Fixed and immobile (also called masked)

Sad or depressed

Angry

Pale or reddened, and so on (coloration of face)

**Gestures** are the subtle physical cues that can indicate what a person is feeling. These can include a flick of a finger or hand that can indicate annoyance, anger, discouragement, and so on; a shrug of the shoulders; a firm shake of the head; and other signs that signify meaning to the observer.

**Posture** is the way a person holds his or her body, and it often indicates how he or she is feeling. Some posture characteristics include the following:

Relaxed

Tense

Erect

Slouching, leaning away from the caregiver

Sitting, lying, and so on

**Dress** refers to the way a person clothes and cares for himself or herself. The way the person dresses usually reflects the appropriateness of his or her social judgment. Some dress characteristics include the following:

Neat

Careless

Eccentric

Foul-smelling, soiled, and so on

**Physical characteristics,** especially the unusual appearance of any part of the body, should be described. For example, the person may have had his or her foot amputated and may have long, unkempt hair and a beard.

**Motor activity,** the way a person moves his or her body, is another important indication of mental status. The various types of movement include the following:

Agitation, restlessness, and so on

Tremors

Motor retardation (slow movement)

Apraxia, or inability to carry out purposeful movement to achieve a goal

Abnormal movement

**Akathisia:** extreme restlessness

**Akinesia:** complete or partial loss of muscle movement

**Dyskinesia:** excessive movement of mouth, protruding tongue, facial grimacing (a common side effect of the major tranquilizers)

**Parkinsonian movement:** fine tremor accompanied by muscular rigidity

**Reaction to caregiver:** the way that a client relates with or responds to a caregiver; can include:
Friendly
Hostile
Suspicious

## ◆ SPEECH AND COMMUNICATION

In this category we are evaluating *how* the client is communicating, rather than *what* he or she is telling us. What the client is telling us is actually a reflection of his or her thinking process, which is described below. The ways in which a person's speech should be evaluated are as follows:

Rate: usually consistent with overall psychomotor status
Volume: quietness or loudness
Modulation and flow: lively or dispirited
Production: ability to produce words

Also included in this section are nonverbal forms of communication. These include facial expression, gesture, and posture, described in the previous section. It is a matter of choice whether they are described under communication or behavior.

## ◆ MOOD OR AFFECT

**Affect** refers to a person's display of emotion or feelings he or she is experiencing. **Mood** is the subjective way a client explains his or her feelings. Actually, the two words can be used interchangeably to describe the feelings associated with thoughts about situations. The following list with accompanying descriptions includes only those emotional states that are considered beyond the normal range.

Inappropriate affects
Unexpected responses to a given situation
Discussion content that does not fit with accompanying emotions
Pleasurable affects
**Euphoria:** excessive and inappropriate feeling of well being
**Exaltation:** intense elation accompanied by feelings of grandeur
Unpleasurable affects **(dysphoria)**
**Depression:** hopeless feeling of sadness; grief or mourning; prolonged and excessive sadness associated with a loss
**Anxiety:** feeling of apprehension that is caused by conflicts that the client is unable to identify
**Fear:** excessive fright of consciously recognized danger
**Agitation:** anxiety associated with severe motor restlessness

**Ambivalence:** alternating and opposite feelings occurring in the same person about the same object

**Aggression:** rage, anger, or hostility that is excessive or seems unrelated to a person's current situation

Mood swings (also called **lability**): alternating periods of elation and depression or anxiety in the same person within a limited time period

Lack of affect

**Blunted or flat affect:** normal range of emotions is missing; commonly seen in people with depression, some forms of schizophrenia, and some types of organic brain syndrome; can be seen in people whose personalities are tightly controlled, where it is termed **constricted** to describe both feeling and the whole personality

**La belle indifference:** of French derivation, meaning "the beautiful lack of concern" and used to describe lack of worry in a difficult situation that ordinarily warrants it

## ◆ THINKING

A person's thinking ability is the way he or she functions intellectually. It is his or her process or way of thinking; his or her analysis of the world; his or her way of connecting or associating thoughts; and his or her overall organization of thoughts. Some of the major disorders in thinking are outlined in the following.

I. Disturbance in thought process (how a person thinks)
   A. **Loose associations:** poorly connected or poorly organized thoughts
      1. **Circumstantiality:** frequent digressions on the way to eventual conclusion
      2. **Tangentiality:** frequent digression until initial reason for beginning a discussion is forgotten
   B. **Flight of ideas:** rapid speaking with quick changes from one thought to another connected thought; frequently seen in manic clients
   C. **Perseveration:** repetition of the same word in reply to different questions
   D. **Blocking:** cessation of thought production for no apparent reason
II. Disturbance in thought content (what a client is thinking)
   A. **Delusion:** inaccurate belief that cannot be corrected by reasoning
      1. **Delusion of grandeur:** exaggerated belief about own abilities or importance

    2. **Delusion of reference:** client's false belief that he or she is the center of others' attention and discussion

    3. **Delusion of persecution:** client's false belief that others are seeking to hurt or in some other way damage him or her either physically or by insinuation

  B.  **Preoccupation of thought:** connecting all occurrences and experiences to a central thought, usually one with strong emotional overtones

  C.  **Obsessive thought:** unwelcome idea, emotion, or urge that repeatedly enters the consciousness

  D.  **Phobia:** strong fear of a particular situation

    1. **Claustrophobia:** fear of being in an enclosed place

    2. **Agoraphobia:** fear of being in an open place, such as outdoors or on a highway

    3. **Acrophobia:** fear of high places

  E.  Other disturbances of thought, or memory impairment—any type of change in ability to recall thoughts from the unconscious into consciousness in an accurate manner

    1. **Amnesia:** complete or partial inability to recall past experiences

    2. **Confabulation:** filling in gaps in memory with statements that are untrue

    3. **Déjà vu:** feeling of having experienced a new situation on a previous occasion (Note: This can normally occur in all individuals when they are fatigued or stressed.)

## ◆ PERCEPTION

**Perception** is the way that a person experiences his or her environment and how he or she perceives his or her frame of reference within that environment. It is equivalent to the person's sense of reality. Perception derives from the senses of vision, hearing, touch, smell, and taste. The information perceived through the senses is monitored by the mind and its defenses. Mental dysfunction can result in distortion of reality that can range from mild to severe.

A hallucination can be the result of serious mental dysfunction. **Hallucinations** are false sensory perceptions that do not exist in reality. The most common types of hallucinations are as follows:

  **Visual hallucination:** seeing object(s) not present in reality

  **Auditory hallucination:** hearing sounds not present in reality

  **Hypnagogic hallucination:** sensing any type of false sensory perception during the twilight period between being awake and falling asleep

Another type of sensory dysfunction, called an **illusion,** is a misinterpretation or distortion (by the ego) of an actual stimulus. Two other terms relating to perception of self or the environment are used to describe mental status dysfunctioning:

**Depersonalization:** feeling detached from one's surroundings

**Derealization:** ranging from a mild sense of unreality to a frank loss of reality about one's environment

## ◆ MEMORY

**Memory** is the mind's ability to recall earlier events. The two types of memory are recent, for events that happened during the previous few days, and remote, for events that occurred from the first recollections of childhood through adolescence, adulthood, and up until the current week.

Memory loss is one of the most important signs of cognitive disorders. The two types of cognitive disorders are delirium and dementia. Memory loss occurs in both delirium, which is an acute brain disorder that is usually reversible, and dementia, a chronic usually irreversible brain disease (see Chapter 21, The Client With a Personality Disorder).

## ◆ JUDGMENT

**Judgment** is the final outcome of the processes described above. It is a person's ability to form conclusions and behave in a socially appropriate manner. If the psyche is functioning properly in the thinking and feeling spheres and a person has good awareness of his or her surroundings, then he or she will form valid conclusions about appropriate conduct.

## ◆ MENTAL STATUS EXAM IN OUTPATIENT CARE

An increasing number of clients are treated as outpatients and monitored by home health or community-based nurses. This means the nurses must make critical assessments of the client's mental status, without the supervision or consulting resources available in a hospital setting. In the case of an elderly client, the nurse may also need to consider the mental status of the client's caregiver (often an elderly spouse) and his or her ability to accurately report on the client's status or be responsible for medications and other care. In addition, the time the nurse spends with clients is brief, which may make assessing mental status more challenging.

A key component of the mental status exam is the nurse's subjective assessment of the mental status categories noted above. These subjective assessments should be backed up by careful observation and charting of specific behaviors. In addition, the nurse should listen carefully to and document the changes reported by the primary caregiver, and try to verify those behaviors as part of the mental status exam. (The mental status exam also can be given to members of the caregiver group.) Finally, all medications, past and present, need to be carefully charted, because medications or interactions between medications can significantly affect mental status.

## KEY POINTS

- Behavior is the observable sign of mental functioning. Nurses can observe a client's behavior to assess his or her mental status.
- Level of awareness refers to the client's wakefulness or consciousness. Orientation is closely related to level of awareness and is measured by clients' ability to identify who they are, where they are, and the date and approximate time (person, place, and time).
- Appearance and behavior that can be observed include facial expression, gestures, posture, dress, physical characteristics, motor activity, and response to caregiver.
- Evaluating speech and communication means noting how the client is communicating. This includes rate of speech, its volume, whether it is lively or dispirited, and the client's ability to produce words.
- Nurses can observe clients' affect, or display of emotions or feelings. Generally, the nurse is looking for affect that is outside the range of normal emotion, such as lack of or inappropriate affect; euphoria; depression, anxiety, fear, aggression; or la belle indifference.
- The client's thinking process reveals how the client is functioning intellectually. A nurse can observe disorders in thought process (loose associations, flight of ideas, and blocking) and disorders in thought content (delusions, obsessive thoughts, and phobias).
- Perception, how clients experience their environment, derives from the five senses. A false sensory perception, or a perception of something that does not exist in reality, is called a hallucination.
- Memory is the mind's ability to recall earlier events. Recent memory is for events that happened in the past few days. Remote memory is for events that occurred from childhood up until the current week.
- A common feature of two major cognitive disorders, dementia and delirium, is loss of memory.
- Judgment is the person's ability to form conclusions and behave in a socially appropriate manner. It is the result of level of awareness, affect, thinking, perception, and memory.

## SELF-AWARENESS ACTIVITY

The mental status exam is a carefully observed assessment of how one's mind is operating at any given moment. In reviewing the different categories, once again, it is quite natural to examine one's own mental functioning and to wonder how and why we feel and behave the way we do. Sometimes we also look at the behavior of those around us—family, friends, and social acquaintances—and seek to change their behavior. Here are some points to consider:

- We can change our own behavior. We have choice and control over our own behavior.
- Changing the behavior of others is a complex process. It can occur only with their choice and participation.
- Unconscious mental processes and defense mechanisms powerfully drive both our own behavior and the behavior of others.
- Are there thoughts, feelings, or behaviors that you experience and wish that you did not? Is it possible that there are unconscious mechanisms that contribute to these experiences?
- When there appear to be unconscious mechanisms that contribute to distressing thoughts, feelings, or behaviors, counseling can be a valuable investment in order to relieve the emotional patterns that may contribute to them.

# QUESTIONS

1. To best assess a client's orientation, the nurse should say to the client:
   a. "Do you know where you are?'
   b. "Can you tell me where you are?"
   c. "Tell me where you are."
   d. "How are you feeling today?"
2. Which of the following statements is *not* true?
   a. A client's gestures can indicate what he or she is feeling.
   b. A nurse can observe whether facial expression matches emotions expressed.
   c. Clients seldom relate with or respond to caregivers.
   d. Facial expression, gestures, and posture are nonverbal ways of communicating.
3. The client says to the nurse "I used to live in Denver. John Denver died in a plane crash. The stock market crashed in the 1930s. I turned 30 two years ago." The nurse recognizes this as

a. circumstantiality.
b. delusions of grandeur.
c. flight of ideas.
d. confabulation.
4. The client is experiencing a disturbance in perception. The nurse expects to observe
   a. loose associations and perseveration.
   b. delusions and obsessive thoughts.
   c. déjà vu and amnesia
   d. depersonalization and illusions.

## BIBLIOGRAPHY

Barry, P.D. (1996). *Psychosocial nursing: Care of physically ill patients and their families* (3rd ed.). Philadelphia: Lippincott-Raven.

Boyd, M., & Nihart, M. (1998). *Psychiatric nursing: Contemporary practice.* Philadelphia: Lippincott Williams & Wilkins.

Carpenito, L.J. (2000). *Nursing diagnosis: Application to clinical practice* (8th ed.). Philadelphia: Lippincott Williams & Wilkins.

Dubin, S. (1998). Hospital extra: The mini mental state exam. *American Journal of Nursing, 98*(11), 16d.

Gerow, J., & Bordens, K. (2000). *Psychology: An introduction.* Carrollton, TX: Alliance Press.

Mezey, M., Mitty, E., & Ramsey, G. (1997). Assessment of decision-making capacity: Nursing's role. *Journal of Gerontological Nursing, 23*(3), 28–35.

Ogden, J. (2000). *Health psychology: A textbook.* Buckingham, England: Open University Press.

Rathus, S. (2000). *Psychology: The core.* Fort Worth, TX: Harcourt College Publishers.

Sadock, B., & Kaplan, H. (1998). *Synopsis of psychiatry: Behavioral sciences/clinical psychiatry.* Philadelphia: Lippincott Williams & Wilkins.

Timby, B.K. (2000). *Fundamental skills and concepts in patient care* (7th ed.). Philadelphia: Lippincott Williams & Wilkins.

# DEVELOPING CRITICAL THINKING SKILLS THROUGH CLASS DISCUSSION

UNIT 3 Case Study
## Foundations of Decision Making in the Mental Health Setting

John is a 48-year-old engineer whose job in the aerospace industry has been eliminated. He does not believe that he can locate
another job in his geographic area. He also believes that his boss
"had it in for him" and that is why his position was eliminated.
He is married and has two children ages 19 and 17. His family is
accustomed to a comfortable middle-class lifestyle. His wife does
not work outside the home and does not cope well with stress.
His 19-year-old son is a sophomore in college and lives at home.
His 17-year-old daughter has already submitted college applications to five private universities in other states. John is angry and
bitter.

## DISCUSSION QUESTIONS

1. What would you assess if John were referred to a mental
   health clinic? How would you assess him?
2. What symptoms of ineffective coping patterns might you
   expect John to manifest? What defense mechanisms might he
   employ?
3. Identify potential nursing diagnoses for each of the patterns of
   human response, according to NANDA.
4. What types of activities would you encourage John to engage
   in to support effective coping?
5. After implementation of effective coping strategies, how
   would you evaluate John's progress?
6. How should John's family be included in this process?

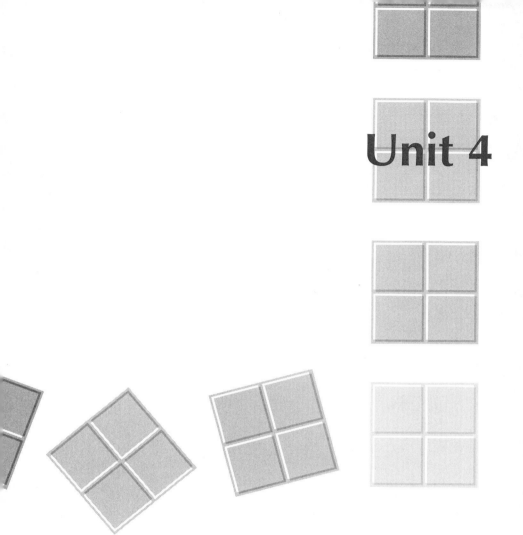

# Unit 4

# NURSING THE CLIENT WITH A MENTAL DISORDER

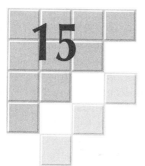

# The Client With a Mood Disorder

---

**B e h a v i o r a l   O b j e c t i v e s**

---

*After reading this chapter the student will be able to:*

- List the major symptoms of the client with a major depressive episode and the client with a manic episode.
- Tell the difference between the symptoms of a person with a bipolar disorder and a person with a cyclothymic disorder.
- Name the medication most commonly prescribed for people with a bipolar disorder.
- Explain the importance of accurately documenting a client's mental and physical status.

---

**K e y   T e r m s**

---

- Bipolar disorder
- Bipolar disorder—Type I
- Bipolar disorder—Type II
- Catatonic symptoms
- Cyclothymic disorder
- Dysthymic disorder
- Grandiosity
- Hypersomnia
- Hypomanic episode
- Libido
- Major depressive disorder
- Major depressive episode
- Mania
- Manic episode
- Melancholic symptoms
- Mood disorder
- Mood episode
- Neurovegetative signs of depression
- Postpartum onset
- Psychomotor agitation or retardation

The affective mental disorders include those mental conditions that cause a change in a person's mood (also known as affect) or emotional state for a prolonged period of time. The changed emotional state may be depression, elation, or a combination occurring in alternate cycles. It is estimated that depressive disorders occur in 10% to 25% of women over their life span. The incidence of depression in men over their life cycle is estimated at from 5% to 12%.

The cause of depression is generally the result of a life event that results in emotional changes and a sense of helplessness about being unable to change the circumstances of one's life or one's feelings about those circumstances. It is recognized that the underlying cause of depression and bipolar disorder is related to changes in neurotransmitter levels. The specific cause of the changes in neurotransmitter levels has not yet been identified.

These conditions are not caused by another physical or mental disorder. It is important to note that a variety of physical illnesses or disorders and side effects of medication can result in depressive symptoms. Such physiologically induced conditions are not included in this category; rather, they are classified under the cognitive disorders category (see Chapter 17, The Client with Delirium, Dementia, Alzheimer's, and Other Cognitive Disorders). It is recommended to the student that psychiatric terms included in this chapter that are not defined can be found in Chapter 14, The Mental Status Exam, or in the Glossary at the back of the book.

The major categories of disorder under this classification of mood disorders are mood episodes, depressive disorders, and bipolar disorders. They include the following major categories:

1. Mood episodes
   a. Major depressive episode
   b. Manic episode
   c. Other
2. Depressive disorders
   a. Major depressive episode
   b. Dysthymic disorder
3. Bipolar disorders
   a. Bipolar I and II disorder
   b. Cyclothymic disorder

## ◆ MOOD EPISODES

**Mood episodes** are periods of alteration in an individual's normal range of emotions for a period of time that is less than those in the mood disorders. The symptoms may be those of depression or mania, similar in fact to the mood disorders. It is the period of time that these symptoms are present that distinguishes mood episodes from mood disorders.

**Mania** is a distinct period of abnormally and persistently elevated mood, characterized by extreme excitement, restlessness, talkativeness, inflated self-esteem, and decreased sleep. The American Psychiatric Association has developed the following criteria for major depressive and manic episodes.

## MAJOR DEPRESSIVE EPISODE

A **major depressive episode** is a period of altered emotional state in which five (or more) of the following symptoms have been present during the same 2-week period and represent a change from previous functioning; at least one of the symptoms is either depressed mood or loss of interest or pleasure.

1. Depressed mood most of the day, nearly every day, as indicated by either subjective report or observation made by others
2. Markedly diminished interest or pleasure in all, or almost all, activities most of the day, nearly every day
3. Significant weight loss when not dieting, or weight gain
4. Insomnia or **hypersomnia** (excessive sleep) nearly every day
5. Psychomotor agitation or retardation nearly every day
6. Fatigue or loss of energy nearly every day
7. Feelings of worthlessness or excessive or inappropriate guilt nearly every day
8. Diminished ability to think or concentrate, or indecisiveness, nearly every day
9. Recurrent thoughts of death, recurrent suicidal ideation without a specific plan, or a suicide attempt or a specific plan for committing suicide

The classic signs of depression that often indicate the need for antidepressant medication are called neurovegetative signs or symptoms. They are included in the previous list of symptoms. The **neurovegetative signs of depression** are specific changes in physical functions, the basis of which are neurotransmitter alterations driven by the depression. It is important to remember that all mental disorders are biologic in nature.

The neurovegetative signs address appetite, sleep, and normal energy level. The level of activity in one's normal daily activities is addressed in the symptoms **psychomotor agitation or retardation.** These psychomotor symptoms describe one's rate of activity—either agitated/speeded up, or retarded/slowed. Normal energy level is also known as **libido.** Libido also includes one's interest in sex. When a person is depressed, the normal sexual drive is usually decreased in conjunction with the decreased libido. The neurovegetative signs include the following:

- Significant weight loss when not dieting, or weight gain
- Insomnia or hypersomnia nearly every day
- Psychomotor agitation or retardation nearly every day
- Fatigue or loss of energy nearly every day

## MANIC EPISODE

A **manic episode** is characterized by a distinct period of abnormally and persistently elevated, expansive, or irritable mood, lasting at least 1 week (or any duration if hospitalization is necessary). During the period of mood disturbance, three (or more) of the following symptoms have persisted and been present to a significant degree:

1. Inflated self-esteem or **grandiosity** (an exaggerated sense of one's importance and power)
2. Decreased need for sleep
3. More talkative than usual or pressure to keep talking
4. Flight of ideas or subjective experience that thoughts are racing
5. Distractibility
6. Increase in goal-directed behavior and psychomotor agitation
7. Excessive involvement in pleasurable activities that have a high potential for painful consequences*

At the beginning of a manic episode, the client's physical appearance becomes increasingly disheveled as he or she speeds up physically, intellectually, and emotionally. The client becomes increasingly restless and aggressive. Underlying urges and impulses seem to take over, and the person's normal judgment appears to lose control. The client's thoughts speed up so that he or she becomes easily distractible. This gives rise to flight of ideas, as the client's mind darts from subject to subject, and accelerated speech flits from one idea to another.

The client's mood becomes euphoric, then shifts into exaltation, and finally, at the peak of the half-cycle, into frenzy. The client in this state sleeps and eats very little, losing weight rapidly. He or she frequently smashes or breaks things unintentionally. When restrained from doing something he or she wants to do, extreme anger outbursts may occur.

## OTHER MOOD EPISODES

Other categories of mood episodes include mixed episode and hypomanic episode. In the mixed episode, criteria are met for both a manic and a major depressive episode. The **hypomanic episode** is a distinct period of elevated mood that is clearly different from a person's usual nondepressed mood, but the behavior and mental state do not classify as a manic episode.

*From *Desk reference to the diagnostic criteria from DSM-IV*. (1994). Washington, D.C.: American Psychiatric Association, pp. 161–164.

Hypomanic clients are usually happy-go-lucky, friendly, bossy, and highly verbal. They have delusions of grandeur and feel possessed of great charm, power, abilities, and wealth. If a manic person is with a group of people, he or she actually has a stimulating effect on the group by causing them to interact better. However, manic persons also tend to offend others, because their language and actions are often coarse, lewd, and suggestive. Moral values again settle into place, and behavior becomes more acceptable with the gradual subsiding of hyperactivity.

## ◆ DEPRESSIVE DISORDERS

### MAJOR DEPRESSIVE DISORDER

**Major depressive disorder** includes the presence of a major depressive episode (symptoms outlined above) without exhibition of a manic episode. A major depressive disorder may be a single or recurrent episode. It can also be further specified according to other features displayed, such as with catatonic or melancholic symptoms or with postpartum onset. **Catatonic symptoms** are those in which a person appears to be in a stupor and may be mute. These symptoms are an extreme form of psychomotor retardation. **Melancholic symptoms** are those in which there is strong evidence of sadness, crying, and despondence. In general, one of the significant differences between extreme sadness and depression is that depressed persons usually do not cry. They often explain that their feelings are "beyond crying." **Postpartum onset** implies that the symptoms of depression develop after childbirth.

For a client experiencing a major depressive episode, speech becomes slow, halting, and anxious as harsh judgment and an increased need for control take over, and the client becomes increasingly self-accusative. In a typical depressive episode, the client paces slowly, later sits on a chair, rocking back and forth and moaning dejectedly, and finally takes to the bed or the floor, where he or she slowly and restlessly moves in a small, circumscribed area. The client is very dejected, has a fixation about his or her worthlessness, the magnitude of his or her sins, and the need for punishment. The client directs all aggression inward and eventually takes the blame for all the difficulties in the world. His or her misery is very great. Just before or immediately after reaching the bottom of this cycle, the client may attempt suicide. Chapter 19, The Client Who Is Contemplating Suicide, addresses the clinical issues of suicide risk assessment and intervention.

### DYSTHYMIC DISORDER

**Dysthymic disorder** is marked by depressed mood for most of the day, more days than not, and has existed for at least 2 years for adults and

1 year for children and adolescents. The symptoms are not as severe, however, as those of a major depressive episode. Two or more of the following symptoms of depression are present: poor appetite or overeating, low energy level or fatigue, insomnia or excessive sleeping, low self-esteem, poor concentration or difficulty making decisions, and feelings of hopelessness.

## ◆ BIPOLAR DISORDER

**Bipolar disorder** is a condition in which a person demonstrates strong, exaggerated, and cyclic mood swings. All normal people are subject to a moderate degree of mood swing. Another term used for mood swings is lability. The form of mood swings found in this type of mental illness is very exaggerated and lasts for weeks or months at a time. There is a slow but steady increase in mood elevation and hyperactivity up to a climax of frenzy, then a slow decrease in activity down to normal behavior again. Then, as a rule, the client starts into the opposite cycle of decreased activity, also called hypoactivity, accompanied by depression, only to swing slowly through this cycle and back to balance once more. Figure 15-1 shows the cycles and the terminology used to describe them.

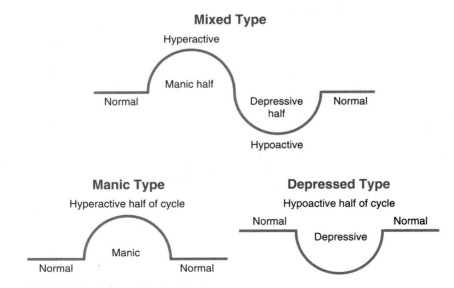

FIGURE 15–1. Cycles of bipolar disorder.

These episodes tend to recur several times within the client's lifetime. It is not unusual for a client to experience only one-half of the cycle, that is, only the hyperactive (manic) phase of behavior or recurrent episodes of hypoactive (depressive) behavior. Whether the client shows the entire cycle or only half of it, he or she will, even without treatment, return to normal and may be normal for several months or years, then repeat the cycle (or half-cycle) again. Modern pharmaceutical therapy helps speed up the rate of recovery greatly. Currently, bipolar disorders are categorized according to whether the predominant characteristic is the presence of manic behavior, which constitutes **Bipolar Disorder—Type I**, or depressive behavior, which is the basis of **Bipolar Disorder—Type II.**

### BIPOLAR I AND II DISORDERS

Bipolar I disorder is characterized by the presence of manic episodes, although a client with this type of disorder can experience a depressed episode. Categories of bipolar I disorder are the single manic episode, most recent episode hypomanic, most recent episode manic, most recent episode mixed, most recent episode depressed, and most recent episode unspecified. Bipolar II disorder is characterized by recurrent major depressive episodes with hypomanic (but not manic or mixed) episodes.

## ◆ CYCLOTHYMIC DISORDER

A person with **cyclothymic disorder** tends to swing between moods of exhilaration and depression, but not to pathologic extremes. However, he or she may develop manic-depressive psychosis in stressful life situations or, in some cases, for no apparent reason. (Changes in brain chemistry have been postulated.) Two subforms are often seen, in which the person shows one of the moods much more than the other. The client who shows exhilaration much of the time is classified as a hypomanic person. Typically, hypomanic clients are outgoing, cheerful, and thoroughly enjoy life; they are vivacious, buoyant, confident, aggressive, and optimistic. Many would make excellent salespeople because they are gregarious, with a high energy level and few inhibitions. Sometimes, however, they are too easily swayed by new impressions. A few of this type are blustering, argumentative, and hypercritical. They all seem to have ready excuses for their failures and can usually talk themselves out of their difficulties. When these people become psychotic, they tend to become manic.

A client who shows a depressed pattern is classified as a melancholic person. This is the cyclothymic personality at the opposite pole from the hypomanic. The melancholic client tends to be easily depressed, although he or she is often kindly, quiet, sympathetic, and even-tempered. He or she is seldom eccentric. In moody periods, the melancholic client is a lonely person, solemn, submissive, gloomy, and self-deprecating. He or she often has feelings of inadequacy and hopelessness, becomes discouraged easily, suffers in silence, and weeps readily, although not in the presence of others. The melancholic client tends to be overly meticulous, conscientious, and preoccupied with work. He or she is fearful of disapproval and feels responsibility keenly. Indecisiveness and caution indicate feelings of insecurity. Under stress, the melancholic client tends to develop a psychotic depression of the manic-depressive type.

## ◆ NURSING CARE OF CLIENTS WITH MOOD DISORDERS

### BIPOLAR DISORDER, MANIC EPISODE
**Nursing Diagnoses**
The nursing diagnoses that are most frequently identified in the care of a client with a manic episode are listed in Box 15-1.

The client with bipolar disorder may be seen in the hospital during either an acute manic or depressive episode. During the manic phase of the illness, the client openly and sometimes aggressively tests

---

**BOX 15–1. Nursing Diagnoses Used in the Care of a Client with Manic Episode Mood Disorder or Manic Phase of a Bipolar Disorder**

- Risk for Violence, self-directed or directed at others, related to poor impulse control or cognitive and perceptual changes
- Altered Nutrition: Less Than Body Requirements related to increased metabolic rate, distractibility, and poor attention span
- Sleep Pattern Disturbance related to hyperactivity and perceived lack of need for sleep
- Altered Social Interaction related to impulsive behavior, distractibility, impaired judgment, cognitive or perceptual changes, and paranoid ideation
- Self-Esteem Disturbance related to delusions and grandiosity
- Sensory–Perceptual Alterations related to decreased ability to concentrate, racing thoughts, distractibility, flight of ideas, hallucinations, delusions, sleep deprivation, or anxiety
- Powerlessness related to feelings of hopelessness and perceived lack of control over life situations and illness
- Altered Family Processes related to role changes, economic crisis, or lack of knowledge about the client's illness

the limits imposed by the therapeutic milieu and specific caregivers. The client's critical tendencies and fault finding challenge the vulnerable aspects and self-esteem of others. Although many of the mental status changes of the manic client may be similar to those of clients with schizophrenia, the personality traits of each have different qualities. The manic client is generally more engaging and warm than the schizophrenic client, who is detached and emotionally cold. Ideally, a primary nursing approach should be implemented.

Major areas of assessment and intervention include attention to the client's hyperactive state and monitoring of the effectiveness and side effects of medications. Additional nursing interventions should be based on the client's mental status and physical and nutritional needs as noted in the list of nursing diagnoses. The energy level of the manic client is almost limitless. The strain on his or her physical well being is severe if not appropriately managed. The major tranquilizers frequently are used to decrease hyperactive status and reduce the delusions, hallucinations, and disorientation that accompany the peak of manic excitement.

In addition to the major tranquilizers, lithium carbonate therapy is used to reduce the cyclic effects of the disorder. It is very effective in the treatment of bipolar disorder. This drug is described in more detail in Chapter 28, Psychopharmacology and Electroconvulsive Treatment of Mental Disorders.

The monitoring of serum lithium levels and titration of dosage, based on mental status and physical symptoms, is of particular importance to the client's treatment. Lithium promotes a therapeutic response in 6 to 10 days. Accurate and descriptive charting of the client's mental and physical signs is important in arranging the dose of lithium at an optimum therapeutic level. Although the medication gradually decreases the frantic activity level of the client, other nursing measures can assist in maintaining his or her well being.

When it is perceived as reasonable by the client, limit setting increases his or her sense of control and trust in the caregiving system. The specific approach to limit setting should be documented in the nursing care plan so that all caregivers will be consistent and effective. Communication with other members of the care team about nursing interventions can assist in the overall therapeutic effectiveness of the nursing and general treatment plan of the mental health team. The client needs frequent showers because hyperactivity increases perspiration. He or she is motivated to eat if foods are provided that can be eaten while standing or moving. Ideally, the environment should not further stimulate the client's level of excitement. Keep noise and light levels low. Provide opportunities for physical activity so the client has an outlet and purpose for his or her hyperactivity.

## MAJOR DEPRESSIVE DISORDER OR BIPOLAR DISORDER, DEPRESSED EPISODE

### Nursing Diagnoses

The nursing diagnoses that are most frequently identified in the care of a client with a major depressive disorder or a client in the depressed phase of bipolar disorder are listed in Box 15-2.

The depressed client feels hopeless and helpless. He or she is vulnerable and suffers from feelings of worthlessness and futility. The depressed client lacks the mental or physical energy to restore himself or herself or to feel hope for the future. The depressed client depends on the nurse for a number of necessities because of these factors. It is important to prioritize these needs in the assessment and intervention process. The first priority when prioritizing needs in all clinical environments is to safeguard the client's life.

When talking with a client admitted for acute depression or who appears acutely depressed, it is important to assess the degree of hopelessness he or she is feeling and be aware of the risk of suicide. Chapter 19, The Client Who Is Contemplating Suicide, provides the assessment and intervention criteria for this type of psychiatric emergency.

A person who is acutely depressed usually demonstrates slowed thought processes, speech, movement, and so on. He or she may not be

---

BOX 15–2. **Nursing Diagnoses Used in the Care of a Client with Major Depressive Disorder or the Depressed Phase of Bipolar Disorder**

- Ineffective Individual Coping related to depression in response to identifiable stressors
- Risk for Self-Directed Violence related to suicidal ideation
- Hopelessness related to perception of lack of choices
- Risk for spiritual distress related to a disturbance in the value system that provides strength, hope, and meaning to life
- Self-concept disturbance related to low self-esteem caused by depression
- Decisional Conflict related to an inability to concentrate and a need for perfection
- Diversional Activity Deficit related to inability to be gratified because of overwhelming depressive feelings
- Sleep Pattern Disturbance related to neurovegetative effects of depression
- Nutrition, altered: *Note:* Alteration can be either More Than Body Requirements or Less Than Body Requirements, depending on whether the person's response to depression is agitated (speeded up) or retarded (slowed down).

able to engage in conversation. Therapeutic intervention may simply involve sitting quietly with the client. Such a presence can be very supportive.

When the client is able to resume communication, his or her statements can be the guide about his or her most important concerns. The therapeutic response for the nurse is to ask questions based on the client's previous statements and continue to ask questions until the issue has been identified and clarified. The next step in communication about an important issue is to assist the client to problem solve about possible options. Such a response allows the client's most urgent concerns to be discussed. The nurse should avoid making reassuring comments that may seem superficial and cause the client to discontinue the discussion and experience more of a sense of isolation (see Boxes 15-3 and 15-4).

## ACCURATE DOCUMENTATION OF MENTAL STATUS

Another aspect of nursing care of the client with a mood disorder is to accurately document his or her mental and physical states. If the client is experiencing a crisis episode, frequent documentation of mental status and physical states is important in order for caregivers to determine the next treatment options. Another clinical area where documentation is important is that of medications. Medications used for depression and bipolar disorders may sometimes take 2 to 3 weeks to elicit a ther-

---

### BOX 15–3. **Clinical Vignette**

Pedro Perez is a 59-year-old widowed man. His wife, Marie, died 2 years ago from breast cancer. He has recently been diagnosed with prostate cancer. Pedro has two children who live 300 and 1,000 miles away. Before the death of their mother they were in communication with their mother and father every week. Since their mother died they have not been in frequent communication with their father. Pedro has no other relatives who live near him. He has been employed as a foreman at a large vegetable-producing farm. He has always been a shy person and has not actively socialized with people from work. His wife Marie was the social coordinator of the family. Since her death he has become more socially isolated.

Pedro's doctors have presented him with his treatment options. He had not called his children to tell them of his diagnosis or to enlist their assistance with considering his treatment options. He has not told his supervisor about his condition. In the past week he has called in sick at work every day. Pedro has been sleeping most of the day. He has lost his appetite and has lost 8 pounds.

Imagine that you are Pedro's neighbor. You've noticed that his truck hasn't moved all week and you haven't seen Pedro. What would you think is going on? What would you do?

---

**BOX 15–4. Nursing Diagnoses Associated With Clinical Vignette**

Note that the clinical vignette in each chapter is accompanied by three nursing diagnoses related to the specific information in the clinical vignette

**COPING: INEFFECTIVE INDIVIDUAL**
**Definition:** A state in which an individual experiences, or is at risk to experience, an inability to manage internal or environmental stressors adequately because of inadequate resources (physical, psychological, behavioral, and/or cognitive).
**Related Nursing Diagnosis:** Ineffective Individual Coping as evidenced by social isolation and withdrawal from family and lack of attendance at work related to death of wife and recent prostate cancer diagnosis.

**GRIEVING DYSFUNCTIONAL**
**Definition:** The state in which an individual or group experiences prolonged unresolved grief and engages in detrimental activities.
**Related Nursing Diagnosis:** Dysfunctional Grieving as evidenced by lack of social contact with children related to death of wife.

**COMPROMISED FAMILY COPING**
**Definition:** That state in which a usually supportive primary person (family member or close friend) is providing insufficient, ineffective, or compromised support, comfort, assistance, or encouragement that may be needed by the client to manage or master adaptive tasks related to his or her health challenge.
**Related Nursing Diagnosis:** Compromised family coping as evidenced by change in children's frequency of communication with father related to death of mother.

---

apeutic response. These medications have sedative and hypnotic effects or may contribute to increased anxiety, impact sleep, or result in a wide variety of physiologic side effects. Accurately charting the client's changes in mental and physical status at frequent intervals helps the clinician overseeing medications to determine when a therapeutic level of medication is reached or the medication regimen needs to be reevaluated (see Boxes 15-5 and 15-6).

## KEY CONCEPTS

---

■ Mood disorders are mental conditions that cause a change in a person's affect or mood for a prolonged period of time. The changed state may be depression, elation, or a cyclical combination of the two.

---

**₀BOX 15–5. Family Teaching When A Client Has a Mood Disorder**

When a family member has a mood disorder, the following recommendations can provide support for the client and give the family more confidence in knowing how to support their family member. Family members should be encouraged to call the client's mental health caregiver whenever the client appears to be at risk for harm.

The client with a mood disorder experiences depressed feelings and usually feels helpless and, sometimes hopeless about being able to return to mental health. The family responses that are therapeutic to this client include:

- Avoid telling client to "buck up" or "get a grip" or other unrealistic expectations
- Provide supportive environment for nonjudgmental discussion about issues of concern to client
- Ask client what he or she believes would be helpful to do about the issues of concern
- Support and assist with processing decisions when client is indecisive
- Encourage client to plan with family around his or her needs and expectations during recovery
- Support client in seeing mental health care provider and attending groups
- Be familiar with family assessment of suicidal risk in Chapter 19, The Client Who Is Contemplating Suicide
- Maintain respectful approach in order to support self-esteem
- Review medication compliance

When the client has a bipolar disorder and is demonstrating manic symptoms, family support can include:

- Support the use of medications when the client's euphoria results in noncompliance
- Provide foods that are easily available and able to be eaten when the client is in motion
- Overview judgment, or lack thereof, that may put the individual at risk
- Quietly offer recommendations for structure when manic pace creates disorganization
- Review medication compliance

---

- A person with bipolar disorder demonstrates strong, exaggerated mood swings.
- Characteristics of a manic episode include grandiosity, decreased need for sleep, racing thoughts, psychomotor agitation, and excessive involvement in activities with negative consequences.
- Characteristics of a major depressive episode include markedly diminished pleasure in daily activities, significant weight loss or gain, sleep disturbances, fatigue or energy loss, feelings of worth-

BOX 15–6. **Web Resources**

*http://www.depression.com*
A commercial site that offers information about various affective disorders in a straightforward format.

*http://www.psyweb.com*
User-friendly resource giving general information on psychiatric disorders, drugs, testing, treatment, and physiology of the brain. Based on DSM-IV criteria.

*http://www.mentalhelp.net*
Provides information about common psychiatric disorders and treatments, as well as professional resources. Offers links to support groups and other online resources.

*http://www.nami.org*
Sponsored by the National Alliance for the Mentally Ill, a nonprofit organization. Provides education and information on mental illness and treatment, as well as resources and advocacy support for the client or significant others.

lessness, diminished ability to concentrate, and recurrent thoughts of death.

■ Clients with cyclothymic disorder exhibit mood swings without the pathologic extremes of bipolar disorder.

■ Major areas of nursing assessment and intervention for manic clients include attention to the client's hyperactive state, monitoring of medication and serum lithium levels, and limit setting to increase the client's sense of control and trust.

■ Major areas of nursing assessment and intervention for depressed clients include assessment for suicide risk and accurate documentation of mental status. Actively suicidal clients should be monitored at all times.

■ Lithium carbonate is the medication most frequently used to reduce the cyclic effects of bipolar disorder.

## SELF-AWARENESS ACTIVITY

It is normal for all persons to experience times of discouragement when unexpected disappointments occur, a relationship ends, or some other unexpected event occurs.

- If it is all right for you to do so, can you reflect on the most difficult event you have experienced in your life?
- As you recall the event, are you able to recall the feelings of helplessness that you experienced?
- Can you remember the different internal strengths or external supports, such as family members, friends, clergy, or professional persons who were available? Do you recall what the most helpful words or actions were for you during that time?
- If you were to experience a similar event, have you learned new options based on prior experience? What are some of the steps you would take to provide support for yourself during this difficult time?

## QUESTIONS

1. When working with a client with neurovegetative symptoms of depression, the nurse would give which symptom the highest priority?
   a. Significant weight loss
   b. Lack of energy
   c. Psychomotor retardation
   d. Decreased libido
2. The major difference between bipolar disorder and cyclothymic disorder is:
   a. The disorders occur at different times of the year.
   b. People with cyclothymic disorders must be hospitalized.
   c. People with bipolar disorder function better from day to day.
   d. Cyclothymic disorder exhibits less extreme mood swings.
3. When working with a client in a manic state, the nurse would most likely include which of the following in a nursing care plan?
   a. Encourage the client to write in a journal to increase personal awareness.
   b. Provide the client with portable snacks to maintain nutrition.
   c. Give the client a room close to the nursing station where the client will feel involved.
   d. Allow the client to lead large group activities to enhance self-esteem.
4. The nurse recognizes that people with depression may feel hopeless and powerless. The most appropriate nursing intervention in this situation is to provide
   a. the client with significant time alone.
   b. the client with as much control as possible.
   c. a milieu where the client has to make no decisions.
   d. a milieu that is bright and cheery.

## BIBLIOGRAPHY

Barlow, D., & Campbell, L. (2000). Mixed anxiety-depression and its implications for models of mood and anxiety disorders. *Comprehensive Psychiatry, 41*(2 Suppl 1), 55–60.

Boyd, M., & Nihart, M. (1998). *Psychiatric nursing: Contemporary practice.* Philadelphia: Lippincott-Raven.

Carpenito, L.J. (2000). *Nursing diagnosis: Application to clinical practice* (8th ed.). Philadelphia: Lippincott Williams & Wilkins.

Cassem, N., & Bernstein, J. (1997). Depressed patients. In Cassem, N. (Ed.). *Massachusetts General Hospital handbook of general hospital psychiatry.* St. Louis: Mosby.

*Desk reference to the diagnostic criteria from DSM-IV.* (1994). Washington, D.C.: American Psychiatric Association.

*Diagnostic and statistical manual of mental disorders* (4th ed.). (1994). Washington, D.C.: American Psychiatric Press.

Frank, E., & Thase, M. (1999). Natural history and preventative treatment of recurrent mood disorders. *Annual Review of Medicine, 50,* 453–468.

Krupnick, S., & Wade, A. (1999). *Psychiatric care planning.* Springhouse, PA: Springhouse Corporation.

Minarik, P. (1996). Psychosocial intervention with ineffective coping responses to physical illness: Depression related. In Barry, P. *Psychosocial nursing: Care of physically ill patients and their families* (3rd ed.). Philadelphia: Lippincott-Raven.

Sadock, B., & Kaplan, H. (1998). *Synopsis of psychiatry: Behavioral sciences/clinical psychiatry.* Philadelphia: Lippincott-Raven. *From *Desk reference to the diagnostic criteria from DSM-IV.* (1994). Washington, D.C.: American Psychiatric Association, pp. 161–164.

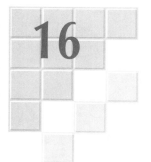

# 16

# The Client With an Anxiety Disorder

*After reading
this chapter
the student
will be able to:*

- Describe the different types of symptoms that occur in anxiety and fear.
- List several possible causes of anxiety.
- Name five subjective and five objective signs of anxiety.
- List the four levels of anxiety described by Peplau and describe the mental state accompanying each.
- Name three categories of anxiety disorders and describe one condition in each category.
- Name three categories of somatoform disorders and describe the psychological process occurring in each.

# K e y   T e r m s

- "Acting out" behavior
- Acute stress disorder
- Agoraphobia without history of panic disorder
- Anxiety
- Body dysmorphic disorder
- Comorbid
- Conversion disorder
- Depersonalization
- Derealization
- Dissociative amnesia
- Dissociative symptoms
- Dysphoria
- Fear
- Generalized anxiety disorder
- Hypochondriasis
- Immobilization
- Medication efficacy
- Objective criteria
- Obsessive–compulsive disorder

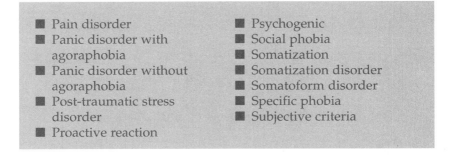

- Pain disorder
- Panic disorder with agoraphobia
- Panic disorder without agoraphobia
- Post-traumatic stress disorder
- Proactive reaction
- Psychogenic
- Social phobia
- Somatization
- Somatization disorder
- Somatoform disorder
- Specific phobia
- Subjective criteria

One of the most common dysphoric emotions known to mankind is anxiety. **Dysphoria,** or dysphoric feeling, is an unpleasant emotion that causes psychological distress or conflict. The North American Nursing Diagnosis Association (NANDA) described **anxiety** as "a state in which the individual or group experiences feelings of uneasiness (apprehension) and activation of the autonomic nervous system in response to a vague, nonspecific threat" (Carpenito, 2000, p. 121). As described in Chapter 11, Human Emotions, anxiety is different from fear.

**Fear** is an uneasy feeling owing to a *known* cause. The basic cause of anxiety is an unconscious conflict between the mind and environment or within the mind itself. Conflicts within the mind are related to tension or disagreement between two or more of the dimensions of the mind. The mind dimensions include judgment, inborn impulses and drives, and ego—the internal monitor of all consciousness and the home of conscious and unconscious defenses. For example, one of the inborn drives may cause a person to feel sexually attracted to another. The judgment dimension may judge the desire to be immoral. If the desire continues and the ego is unable to mediate the conflict, then the result may be anxiety.

The following are some specific causes of anxiety that also have been described in the NANDA nursing diagnosis category of Anxiety: unconscious conflict about essential values or goals of life; threat to self-concept; threat of death; threat to or change in health status; threat to or change in role functioning; threat to or change in environment; threat to or change in interaction patterns; situational/maturational crises; interpersonal transmission/contagion; and unmet needs.

Hildegard Peplau, a psychiatric nurse theorist, proposed four different levels of anxiety, ranging from mild to panic. These levels of anxiety are shown in Box 16-1.

Peplau believed that an individual has the intellectual capacity to learn from anxiety and adapt his or her behavior accordingly. For people in the mild-to-moderate range, Peplau believed that if individuals

> ### BOX 16–1. Levels of Anxiety Proposed by Peplau
>
> #### MILD
> Person is hyperalert and is sharply aware of the environment. His or her perceptual abilities of vision, hearing, and smell are increased.
>
> #### MODERATE
> Person's perceptual abilities are decreased. The person can maintain his or her concentration on one activity, however (selective inattention).
>
> #### SEVERE
> Person's perceptual abilities are markedly diminished. His or her attention span is scattered.
>
> #### PANIC
> Person is either paralyzed or severely agitated. He or she is filled with terror. The object of anxiety is overwhelming in its intensity.

have well-developed coping abilities, they are able to observe the situation causing the anxiety, describe and analyze it, formulate meanings and relations, discuss it with another person to obtain feedback and validation, and benefit from the experience by adapting.

A person with severe anxiety (panic level) is unable to apply the intellectual skills described above. Instead, he or she seeks immediate relief in the easiest way possible to reduce anxiety. This initially easy escape from anxiety may not prove adaptive in the more distant future, however.

The behavior exhibited by a person in flight from anxiety usually falls into one of four categories:

- **"Acting out" behavior** is behavior in which a person projects anger and blame onto others.
- **Somatization** is the defense mechanism of converting mental awareness of stress into actual, physical symptoms or illness.
- **Immobilization** is a reactive state of paralysis in response to crisis or a significant threatening event. Depression or withdrawal can be outcomes of immobilization.
- **Proactive reaction** in which the energy generated by anxiety is used to seek other growth-producing solutions.

Peplau believed that anxiety is a normal part of the human condition. It is the necessary impetus to change and develop better coping skills. Her recommendations for nursing care of the client with anxiety appear later in this chapter.

The North American Nursing Diagnosis Association described the characteristics of anxiety using two types of criteria: subjective, which include symptoms described by the client, and objective, which list the symptoms that can be observed by the nurse. They appear in Table 16-1.

**Subjective criteria** are those characteristics or symptoms that the client describes. Subjective criteria are different from objective criteria. **Objective criteria** are those characteristics or symptoms that are assessed by a nurse or caregiver that may or may not be apparent to the client.

## ◆ ANXIETY DISORDERS

Many categories of anxiety disorder were formerly called neuroses or neurotic disorders. The term neurosis was discontinued in 1987 and replaced with the new category of anxiety disorder. Box 16-2 outlines family teaching when a client has an anxiety disorder. The subcategories of anxiety disorder are as follows:

---

**TABLE 16-1. Subjective and Objective Symptoms Experienced by the Client with Anxiety**

| Subjective Symptoms | Objective Symptoms |
|---|---|
| 1. Increased tension | 1. Sympathetic stimulation cardiovascular excitation, superficial vasoconstriction, pupil dilatation |
| 2. Apprehension | 2. Restlessness |
| 3. Painful and persistent increased helplessness | 3. Insomnia |
| 4. Uncertainty | 4. Glancing about |
| 5. Fearful | 5. Poor eye contact |
| 6. Scared | 6. Trembling hand tremors |
| 7. Regretful | 7. Extraneous movement (foot shuffling, hand/arm movements) |
| 8. Overexcited | 8. Facial tension |
| 9. Rattled | 9. Voice quivering |
| 10. Distressed | 10. Focus on "self" |
| 11. Jittery | 11. Increased wariness |
| 12. Feelings of inadequacy | 12. Increased perspiration |
| 13. Shakiness | |
| 14. Fear of unspecific consequences | |
| 15. Expressed concerns re: change in life events | |

Adapted from Carpenito, L. (2000). *Nursing diagnosis: Application to clinical practice* (8th ed.). Philadelphia: Lippincott Williams & Wilkins.

> **◦BOX 16–2. FAMILY TEACHING WHEN A CLIENT HAS AN ANXIETY DISORDER**
>
> When a family member has an anxiety disorder, the following recommendations can provide support for the client and give the family more confidence in knowing how to support their family member. Family members should be encouraged to call the client's mental health caregiver whenever the client appears to be at risk for harm.
>
> The individual with an anxiety or panic disorder is experiencing rapid shifts in mood that can feel as though they are "going crazy." This is a disorder that can be frightening for the individual and his or her family. The family responses that are therapeutic to this client include:
>
> - Encourage client to plan with family around his or her needs and expectations during recovery
> - Support client in seeing mental health care provider and attending groups
> - Ask the nursing staff to teach the family the anxiety-reducing techniques that have been taught to the client during hospitalization
> - Enlist client's ability to identify the feared object or situation
> - Support the client's use of relaxation and thought-stopping techniques
> - Encourage client to say what he or she is feeling, wants, or needs
> - Assist the client to develop short-term achievable goals
> - Review of medication compliance

1. Panic disorder
   a. With agoraphobia
   b. Without agoraphobia
2. Agoraphobia without history of panic disorder
3. Social phobia
4. Specific phobia
5. Obsessive–compulsive disorder
6. Post-traumatic stress disorder
7. Generalized anxiety disorder
8. Anxiety disorder not otherwise specified

## PANIC DISORDER

Panic disorders are conditions that affect two to three times as many women as men. The lifetime incidence of panic disorders is estimated to be between 2% and 5% of the general population. The continuum in levels of development from anxiety to panic are shown in Table 16-2.

A **panic disorder** is a condition in which the person experiences intense fear or discomfort in which four (or more) of the following symptoms develop abruptly and reach a peak within 10 minutes:

## TABLE 16-2. Degrees of Anxiety

| Degree of Anxiety | Effects on Perceptual Field and on Ability to Focus Attention | Observable Behavior |
|---|---|---|
| Mild | Perceptual field widens slightly. Able to observe more than before and to see relations (make connection among data). | Aware, alerted, sees, hears, and grasps more than before. Usually able to recognize and name anxiety easily. |
| Moderate | Perceptual field narrows slightly. Selective inattention: does not notice what goes on peripheral to the immediate focus but can do so if attention is directed there by another observer. | Sees, hears, and grasps less than previously. Can attend to more if directed to do so. Able to sustain attention on a particular focus; selectively inattentive to contents outside the focal area. Usually able to state "I am anxious now." |
| Severe | Perceptual field is greatly reduced. Tendency toward dissociation: to not notice what is going on outside the current reduced focus of attention; largely unable to do so when another observer suggests it. | Sees, hears, and grasps far less than previously. Attention is focused on a small area of a given event. Inferences drawn may be distorted due to inadequacy of observed data. May be unaware of and unable to name anxiety. Relief behaviors generally used. |
| Panic (terror, horror, dread, uncanniness, awe) | Perceptual field is reduced to a detail, which is usually "blown up," ie, elaborated by distortion (exaggeration), or the focus is on scattered details; the speed of the scattering tends to increase. Massive dissociation especially of contents of self-system. Felt as enormous threat to survival. | Says, "I'm in a million pieces," "I'm gone," "What is happening to me?" Perplexity, self-absorption. Feelings of unreality. Flights of ideas, or confusion. Fear. Repeats a detail. Many relief behaviors used automatically (without thought). The enormous energy produced by panic must be used and may be mobilized as rage. May pace, run, or fight violently. With dissociation of contents of self-system, there may be very rapid reorganization of the self usually going along pathologic lines, eg, a "psychotic break" is usually preceded by panic. |

From Peplau, H. (1989). Theoretical constructs: Anxiety, self, and hallucinations. In A. O'Toole & S. Welt (Eds.). *Interpersonal theory in nursing practice. Selected works of Hildegard E. Peplau.* New York: Springer.

Palpitations, pounding heart, or accelerated heart rate
Sweating
Trembling or shaking
Sensations of shortness of breath or smothering
Feeling of choking
Chest pain or discomfort
Nausea or abdominal distress
Feeling dizzy, unsteady, lightheaded, or faint
**Derealization** (feelings of unreality) or **depersonalization** (being
    detached from oneself)
Fear of losing control or going crazy
Fear of dying
Paresthesias (numbness or tingling sensations)
Chills or hot flushes

According to the *Diagnostic and Statistical Manual of Mental Disorders*, 4th edition (DSM-IV), there are two subtypes: panic disorder with agoraphobia and panic disorder without agoraphobia. **Panic disorder with agoraphobia** describes a person who is fearful of being in open areas or public places or of being alone where escape is difficult or help is unavailable. He or she avoids the feared locations. **Panic disorder without agoraphobia** is a condition that meets the criteria for panic disorder, but the afflicted person does not experience agoraphobia. **Agoraphobia without history of panic disorder** is another category. An individual with this form of panic disorder experiences agoraphobic symptoms but has no history of panic symptoms. Table 16-3 shows the common physical, cognitive, and emotional symptoms of panic disorders.

### Nursing Care of Clients With Panic Disorders
It is rare for clients with anxiety disorders to be admitted to the hospital or inpatient setting. Because of the rapid action of antianxiety medications, most individuals with one or another type of panic disorder are treated in the outpatient setting with ongoing assessment of the efficacy of the medication in managing the mental status symptoms of the panic disorder. **Medication efficacy** is the ability of a medication to work effectively with the unique biochemistry of the effects of the panic disorder and reduce the client's unique emotional symptoms.

The treatment for each type of panic disorder is individual psychotherapy in which the therapist and client gradually explore developmental experiences that may have contributed to the disorder. Frequently, these experiences have been repressed for many years. As the traumatizing events are uncovered, the symptoms gradually disappear. Special phobia clinics, operating in a number of large cities, report limited success treating the problem using behavior-modification techniques.

## TABLE 16-3. Key Diagnostic Characteristics for Panic Disorder With or Without Agoraphobia

| Diagnostic Criteria | Target Symptoms |
|---|---|
| *Panic Disorder Without Agoraphobia* | *Panic Attacks* |
| Recurrent unexpected panic attacks and 1 month or more (after an attack) of one of the following: | Discrete period of intense fear or discomfort with four (or more) of the following symptoms that develop abruptly and reach a peak within 10 minutes: |
| • Persistent concern about additional attacks<br>• Worry about the implications of the attack or its consequences<br>• Significant change in behavior related to the attacks | • Palpitations, pounding heart, or accelerated heart rate<br>• Sweating<br>• Trembling or shaking |
| Absence of agoraphobia | • Sensations of shortness of breath or smothering |
| Not a direct physiologic effect of a substance or medical condition | • Feelings of choking<br>• Chest pain or discomfort |
| *Panic Disorder With Agoraphobia* | • Nausea or vomiting |
| Meets criteria for panic disorder, including panic attacks | • Feeling dizzy, unsteady, lightheaded, or faint |
| Experiences agoraphobia | • Derealization (feeling or unreality) or depersonalization (being detached from oneself) |
| Not better accounted for by another mental disorder, such as a specific phobia or social phobia (eg, avoidance limited to social situations because of fear of embarrassment) | • Fear of losing control or going crazy<br>• Fear of dying<br>• Paresthesias (numbness or tingling sensations) |
| *Agoraphobia:* | • Chills or hot flushes |
| Anxiety about being in places or situations from which escape might be difficult (or embarrassing) or in which help may not be available in the event of having an unexpected or situationally predisposed panic attack or panic-like symptoms | Great apprehension about the outcome of routine activities and experiences<br><br>Loss of disruption of important interpersonal relationships<br><br>Demoralization<br><br>Possible major depressive episode |
| Fears typically involve characteristic clusters of situations that include being outside the home alone; being in a crowd or standing in a line; being on a bridge; and traveling in a bus, train, or automobile | *Associated Physical Examination Findings*<br>• Transient tachycardia<br>• Moderate elevation of systolic blood pressure |
| Situations are avoided (eg, travel is restricted) or endured, with marked distress or anxiety about having a panic attack or panic-like symptoms; or the presence of a companion is required | *Associated Laboratory Findings*<br>• Compensated respiratory alkalosis (decreased carbon dioxide and decreased bicarbonate levels with almost normal pH) |
| | *Other Targets for Treatment*<br>• Loss or disruption of important interpersonal or occupational activities<br>• Demoralization<br>• Possible major depressive episode |

From Boyd, M., & Nihart, M. (1998). *Psychiatric nursing: Contemporary practice.* Philadelphia: Lippincott Williams & Wilkins.

Frequently, well-intentioned medical physicians give minor tran-quilizers to people with anxiety. Unless there is a specific, identifiable cause of anxiety related to a major loss, such as threat of death or loss of job or some other stressful event, such medication only prolongs the client's difficulty. When chronic, persistent anxiety is undermining a person's ability to fulfill normal role functions, he or she should seek psychiatric or counseling assistance. These people, despite the dis-abling nature of their conditions, are rarely treated in the inpatient set-ting; however, nursing care of those who are hospitalized is covered in the section, Nursing Care of Clients With Anxiety Disorders.

## SOCIAL PHOBIA AND SPECIFIC PHOBIA

**Social phobia** is a condition in which a person experiences excessive anxiety when exposed to the scrutiny of others—in a classroom, while speaking publicly, or in a social setting. **Specific phobia** is a condition in which a specific object (eg, snakes or spiders) or a situation (eg, flying, receiving an injection, or seeing blood) stimulates overwhelming anxiety.

## OBSESSIVE–COMPULSIVE DISORDER

The word *obsessive* refers to a person's repetitive thoughts. For exam-ple, a woman may have the intrusive and recurring thought that she wants to injure her mother. The word *compulsive* refers to the repetitive, stereotyped act that the person finds himself or herself unable to resist performing. In this example, the woman may need to wash her hands every time she thinks about hurting her mother in order to neutralize the obsession. A person with **obsessive–compulsive disorder** experi-ences thoughts and actions that are repugnant, but his or her attempts to stop the pattern result in extreme anxiety. With this disorder, the obsessions or compulsions are time consuming and may take an hour or more each day. These repetitive actions significantly interfere with normal routine or occupational and social functioning.

Some clients experience relief from this condition by taking anti-depressant medication. Psychotherapy may help when started early in the disorder process. Treatment of fully developed obsessive–compul-sive disorder is quite difficult. An alternative treatment, behavior ther-apy, is described in Chapter 26, Milieu Therapy and Behavior Modifi-cation. Behavior modification therapy aims to stop the obsessive thoughts, urges, or actions of the client.

## POST-TRAUMATIC STRESS DISORDER

**Post-traumatic stress disorder (PTSD)** is a condition in which a person has experienced a catastrophic event—childhood abuse, a plane crash, hurricane, or war—that anyone would perceive as very stressful. A person who develops this disorder is unable to work through and release dysphoric feelings and unpleasant thoughts that follow the trauma, and instead suppresses them in his or her unconscious.

The person with this disorder continues to experience unpleasant feelings and fears about the catastrophe that do not follow the usual course of diminishing with the passing of time. He or she experiences decreased interest in relationships and external events; lack of control over distressing memories or dreams of the event; sudden sensations of the event beginning again; survival guilt; sleep disorder; or difficulties with memory or concentration. Some Vietnam veterans experience this disorder, as do victims of childhood incest and abuse.

When symptoms persist for 3 months or longer, the disorder is considered to be chronic. When symptoms do not occur until 6 months after the event, it is a delayed-onset PTSD. The person with PTSD may discuss some aspect of the traumatic history during home care for another condition. It is rare for a person to be admitted to the hospital because of the emotional effects of a traumatic event. Post-traumatic stress disorder is a common comorbid condition with other mental disorders, such as depressive and anxiety disorders. A **comorbid** condition is a mental condition that exists in the presence of and may contribute to another mental disorder.

## ACUTE STRESS DISORDER

Acute stress disorder is a condition that can be precipitated by the same types of catastrophic stressors as PTSD. The differences between this disorder and PTSD are the following:

1. Acute stress disorder is accompanied by dissociative symptoms. Dissociative symptoms are the result of a protective defense mechanism that dissociates or separates the memory of the catastrophic event from one's conscious mind. In PTSD the individual has distressing memories of the event. In acute stress disorder, the cognitive and emotional memory is separated from one's conscious awareness by the process of dissociation. There are several types of dissociation associated with acute stress disorder. The different types of dissociative symptoms are:

   Numbing, detachment, or absence of emotional responsiveness to the event

   A reduction in awareness of his or her surroundings, as though "in a daze"

   Derealization or a sense of unreality about what has happened or is currently happening

   Depersonalization or a sense of not feeling personally present in the situation, as though one is watching oneself and not feeling the emotions of the experience

   **Dissociative amnesia** or the inability to recall an important aspect of the trauma

**2.** The disturbance lasts for a minimum of 2 days or a maximum of 4 weeks.

### Nursing Care of Clients with Post-traumatic Stress Disorder or Acute Stress Disorder

Nursing intervention includes providing social support interventions such as group and individual counseling. Actively listening to clients' recollections and encouraging them to identify aspects or details of the traumatic event that are troubling is important. By talking about the traumatic event, clients begin to gain some control over their reactions to the troubling memories.

The nurse should avoid judgmental statements that tell clients how or what to think, feel, or do. Instead, the nurse's role is to help clients sort out the traumatic events as well as to assist them with strategies for managing anxiety and feelings of anger that may be associated with the trauma.

### GENERALIZED ANXIETY AND OTHER ANXIETY DISORDERS

A **generalized anxiety disorder** is a condition in which a person experiences excessive and unrealistic worry and anxiety about two or more life circumstances for at least 6 months or longer. During the 6-month period, the individual experiences more days with unrealistic worry than days without the worry and finds it difficult to control the worry. At least three of the following six symptoms are present when the person is anxious:

1. Restlessness or feeling keyed up or on edge
2. Being easily fatigued
3. Difficulty concentrating or mind going blank
4. Irritability
5. Muscle tension
6. Sleep disturbance (difficulty falling asleep or staying asleep, or restless, unsatisfying sleep)

The category termed anxiety disorder not otherwise specified includes anxiety or phobic avoidance symptoms that do not fit the criteria of the anxiety disorders described above.

## ◆ NURSING CARE OF CLIENTS WITH ANXIETY DISORDERS

### ISSUES IN NURSING ASSESSMENT AND INTERVENTION

When a person is hospitalized for anxiety, he or she initially is relieved to be in a safe environment. Because these clients do not customarily require hospitalization, their admission is an indication of how acutely they are terrorized by feeling out of control.

The person who has a mild-to-moderate level of anxiety continues to retain intellectual ability. During the counseling process, this client can use intellectual skills to define the problem, analyze it, and begin the problem-solving process. The role of the nurse is to listen actively and ask perceptive questions that help the client analyze and solve his or her problem. Solutions should not be recommended because such recommendations ultimately take control away from the client and promote his or her dependence on the caregiver. The goal of nursing care and hospitalization is to encourage autonomy and independence.

The nursing care of these clients should follow the treatment plan of the multidisciplinary care team. Hildegard Peplau proposed that people experiencing excessive anxiety or panic lack the capacity to decrease the anxiety when it is occurring because their ability to cope has been diminished as a reaction to the anxiety and the inability to control it. She recommended incorporating into the nursing care plan a process that teaches these coping skills.

The client whose anxiety is at the severe-to-panic level initially requires anxiety relief. A counseling approach that encourages intellectual reasoning may cause further anxiety. Instead the client can be encouraged to describe the "here and now" of what is happening. The client may be so emotionally scattered that it is difficult to make simple decisions. Simple directions can be given in a calm, reassuring manner. The nurse does not touch the client or give advice or encouragement about the future. Nursing assessment of the client's fluctuating anxiety state should be documented with specific times so that appropriate medication management is ensured.

Antianxiety medication is an important aspect of caring for people with high levels of anxiety. The minor tranquilizers listed in Chapter 28, Psychopharmacology and Electroconvulsive Treatment of Mental Disorders, are the drugs of choice when there are no symptoms of psychosis accompanying the anxiety. The major tranquilizers are used only when psychotic thinking is present. In both instances, the dosage of these drugs should be gradually decreased and discontinued as soon as the person's anxiety becomes tolerable. Both classes of drugs can cause drug dependence.

## ◆ SOMATOFORM DISORDERS

**Somatoform disorders** are mental conditions that cause physiologic symptoms. They occur through an unconscious mental process. Somatoform disorders are included in this chapter because this type of disorder may manifest as different types of physical reactions to anxiety that is repressed or held in the body at the unconscious level. Often, the etiology of somatoform disorders is related to stress responses that are mediated within the physical state of the body, rather than through symptoms of stress and anxiety. The conditions in this category are as follows:

Body dysmorphic disorder
Conversion disorder
Hypochondriasis
Somatization disorder
Pain disorder
Undifferentiated somatoform disorder
Somatoform disorder not otherwise specified

## BODY DYSMORPHIC DISORDER

**Body dysmorphic disorder** is a condition in which a normal-appearing person is preoccupied with an imagined physical defect. It can also occur in an individual who grossly exaggerates a slight physical defect. This disorder is not as severe as a delusional disorder, somatic type, which is described in Chapter 18, Schizophrenia and Other Psychotic Disorders.

## CONVERSION DISORDER

**Conversion disorders** frequently mimic neurologic disorders. The most common symptoms are paralysis of one or more body parts, anesthesia (loss of feeling) or paresthesia (abnormal sensations, such as tingling, numbness, or heightened sensation), blindness, and so on. Frequently, the body part affected is related to an inner psychological conflict the client is experiencing. For example, a couple may have serious marital discord. The husband can possibly be denying his awareness of the difficulties, but may be experiencing deep hatred at an unconscious level and want to kill his wife. He could experience a paralysis of his right arm, without any idea of its cause. Medical physicians usually see these people initially; a very thorough diagnostic process should rule out any physical etiology before a psychogenic cause is suspected.

A person with a severe conversion disorder develops a rigid denial defense, having been denying inner conflict most of his or her life. Such a client requires special care when he or she is hospitalized. Attempts to crack through the denial will result in higher levels of denial and increased anxiety. Consult with the clinician in charge of directing the client's care to learn the exact approach he or she is using and to obtain specific recommendations about nursing interventions so that your efforts are not countertherapeutic.

You will observe increased anxiety as the client's level of denial gradually diminishes. When this occurs, follow the recommendations for nursing care of anxious clients described earlier in this chapter.

## HYPOCHONDRIASIS

People with **hypochondriasis** magnify mild, vague physical symptoms into more severe symptoms of potentially serious illnesses. The person is preoccupied with thoughts about his or her imagined disease over a period of 6 months or more. The client remains preoccupied with his or her fears even though physical examination finds no evidence of physical pathology.

## SOMATIZATION DISORDER

**Somatization disorder** is a condition that usually strikes a person before the age of 30. The person has a history of vague symptoms related to a specific body system. These occur as chronic illnesses that cause him or her to see a variety of physicians. Often the client is hospitalized for diagnostic workup and may also have a pattern of multiple surgeries. The most common symptom complexes are related to gastrointestinal, sexual/reproductive, and neurologic body systems. The client may also have vague, unexplained pain in these organs or in the head, chest, or back. Sexual dysfunction also may be present. Depression and anxiety frequently accompany these symptoms. No physical cause can be found for these conditions.

## PAIN DISORDER

**Pain disorder** is a condition in which a client is consistently preoccupied with pain for a period of over 6 months. Thorough physical examination reveals no physiologic basis for the pain or finds that although there is some pathology, the pain is beyond what should normally be expected.

## SOMATOFORM DISORDERS NOT
## OTHERWISE SPECIFIED

Conditions in this category fit the general criteria of somatoform disorders, but lack the distinct symptom presentation of the other disorders in this category. Symptoms are of less than 6 months' duration.

## ◆ NURSING CARE OF CLIENTS WITH SOMATOFORM DISORDERS

People with these disorders are rarely seen in inpatient psychiatric settings. Instead, they are much more commonly admitted to medical units where their persistent physical symptoms and lack of physical findings frustrate the medical and nursing staffs. These clients are usually unaware of the emotional basis of their disorders and strongly resist understanding the psychological basis for their difficulties. When presented with the suggestion that there may be a psychogenic cause, they frequently become angry and change physicians, only to begin their search for care anew. A **psychogenic** cause is one that results in a physical disorder whose etiology is related to painful or conflicting emotions that are held at the unconscious level (Boxes 16-3 and 16-4).

---

### BOX 16–3. Clinical Vignette

Martha Janney is a 31-year-old single woman. Martha lives alone in Sioux Falls, South Dakota, and is estranged from her family who lives in St. Paul, Minnesota. She is a 7th grade teacher. She was originally attracted to South Dakota several years earlier because the city of Sioux Falls was offering special financial incentives to teachers who were recent college graduates and seeking careers in teaching. Despite living in the area for over 8 years, Martha has not involved herself in community or church-related activities. Other teachers were initially friendly to her and invited Martha to their homes and family activities. Because she did not appear to be interested in friendships with her fellow teachers, they eventually ceased inviting her to join them in social activities.

During the past 2 months Martha's father, who was emotionally and physically abusive to her in childhood, died with little warning as the result of a heart attack. Martha's family attempted to invite her to the funeral and to re-establish relations with her. She refused to attend the funeral. In addition to the loss of her father and her resistance to resuming a relationship with her family, Martha has been under administrative review at school because of an increasing tendency to lose her temper in the classroom. For the past month Martha has been having difficulty sleeping and has been drinking several cups of caffeinated coffee a day to remain alert in the classroom.

Two days ago while driving to work Martha began to experience her heart beat pounding rapidly in her chest. She felt dizzy and light-headed. She was highly anxious and her thoughts alternated between the overwhelming thought "I could be dying" and the thought, "I must be going crazy." She couldn't figure out what was happening.

Do you have an idea of what is happening to Martha?

What recommendations would you make to Martha?

---

### BOX 16–4. Nursing Diagnoses Associated With Clinical Vignette

Note that the use of nursing diagnostic statements must be verified by discussion with the client about those factors that may be contributing to emotional distress. Accordingly, these diagnostic statements are based on defining characteristics and related factors that will need to be reviewed and verified by the client. Notice how the nursing diagnosis statements below and their defining characteristics and related factors appear to be strongly related to one another.

*(continues)*

> **BOX 16–4. Nursing Diagnoses Associated With Clinical Vignette** *(Continued)*
>
> **ANXIETY**
> **Definition:** A state in which the individual experiences feelings of uneasiness (apprehension) and activation of the autonomic nervous system in response to a vague nonspecific threat.
> Related nursing diagnosis: Anxiety related to recent death of father and possible activation of unresolved childhood abuse as evidenced by dizziness, apprehension, and hyperattentiveness
>
> **POST-TRAUMA RESPONSE**
> **Definition:** A state in which the individual experiences a sustained painful response to one or more overwhelming traumatic events that have not been assimilated.
> Related nursing diagnosis: Post-Trauma Response related to emotional and physical abuse in childhood as evidenced by social withdrawal from family and work colleagues
>
> **SELF-CONCEPT DISTURBANCE**
> **Definition:** The state in which the individual experiences or is at risk of experiencing a negative state of change about the way she feels, thinks, or views herself. It may include a change in body image, self-ideal, self-esteem, role performance, or personal identity.
> Related nursing diagnosis: Self-concept disturbance related to increased self-defensiveness as evidenced by anger outbursts.
>
> From *Desk reference to the diagnostic criteria from DSM-IV.* (1994). Washington, D.C.: American Psychiatric Association, pp. 199–200, 213.

## KEY CONCEPTS

- Dysphoria is an unpleasant emotion that causes psychological distress or conflict.
- Anxiety is a vague, uneasy feeling whose source is either unspecific or unknown to the individual. Its basic cause is an unconscious conflict between the psyche and environment or within the psyche itself.
- Fear is an uneasy feeling owing to a known cause.
- The four patterns of behavior a person exhibits while trying to flee from anxiety are acting out, somatization, depression or withdrawal, and using energy generated by anxiety to seek other solutions.
- Panic disorder is a category of anxiety disorder in which the person experiences intense fear or discomfort followed by symptoms such

as shaking, faintness, shortness of breath, accelerated heart rate, and sweating.

■ A person with social phobia exhibits excessive anxiety when exposed to scrutiny by others, such as during public speaking, in a classroom, or in a social setting.

■ With specific phobia, a particular object, such as a snake or spider, stimulates overwhelming anxiety.

■ A person with obsessive–compulsive disorder experiences intrusive, recurring thoughts combined with repetitive, stereotyped action, such as hand washing. Attempts to stop the pattern of thought or action result in extreme anxiety.

■ Post-traumatic stress disorder results from experiencing a catastrophic event, then being unable to work through the dysphoric feelings or thoughts and suppressing them into the unconscious. Symptoms include decreased interest in relationships, flashbacks, survival guilt, sleep disorders, and difficulty concentrating.

■ Mental disorders in which one or more aspects of physical functioning are misperceived or distorted include somatoform disorders, body dysmorphic disorder, conversion disorders, hypochondriasis, pain disorder, and somatization disorder.

## SELF-AWARENESS ACTIVITY

While reading about different types of mental disorders it is very natural to think to oneself, "I've had those feelings. I wonder if I might have an anxiety disorder or be depressed." Every medical and nursing student has these types of questions, and it is important to be aware that it is very natural. It actually becomes a part of self-awareness to compare oneself with the symptoms of different types of conditions. You may wonder, "When is it not natural?" Here are some thoughts for your consideration.

- You may find that you do indeed have symptoms of anxiety, depression, or some other type of mental distress. If you do, it is wise to talk with one of your nursing instructors, a trusted clergy person, your personal physician, or someone else who has knowledge of mental health options who can assist you in determining your different choices. There are always choices. One of the important aspects of talking with someone about your concerns is that when going through a difficult time, the depression or anxiety can sometimes block us from being able to recognize the range of available options.

- Avoid "diagnosing" people in your social circle with one or another of the conditions you are reading about. If you have genuine concerns about the emotional stability of someone you know, you can consider approaching him or her and using a gentle approach. Usually, asking questions about the possibility that there may be some type of mental problem works much better than backing the person into a corner and announcing, "You have a problem and you have to do thus and so." The only time that such an authoritative approach should be considered is if the person's life is at risk. Instead, this type of approach may be more effective, "Mom, you've seemed quieter than usual for the past few months. You've also told me that you're not sleeping well and that you've lost weight. Have you wondered if you might be depressed?" This type of approach provides an opening for the person to acknowledge how she is feeling. She is more likely to develop insight about the possibility of depression when she can talk about it and reason out how she is feeling and what her options are.

- Be gentle with yourself regarding your own feelings and thought processes. Most people are very harsh in their self-judgments.

## QUESTIONS

1. When working with a client with post-traumatic stress disorder, the nurse should
   a. encourage the client not to discuss the trauma.
   b. encourage the client "to forget the past" and move on.
   c. provide the client with nonthreatening opportunities to discuss the trauma.
   d. provide a milieu where the client does not need to make any decisions.
2. A client tells the nurse that he or she cannot stop thinking about locking his or her door. The nurse recognizes that this is an example of
   a. hypochondriasis.
   b. compulsion.
   c. obsession.
   d. agoraphobia.
3. The most appropriate nursing intervention for a client experiencing a panic attack is
   a. having the client stay alone in a quiet room.
   b. encouraging the client to go outside and walk.
   c. telling the client to call a close friend.
   d. staying with the client until he or she feels calmer.

**4.** Before being diagnosed with a conversion disorder, the nurse expects that
   a. a thorough medical examination will occur.
   b. the client was abused as a child.
   c. a physician will prescribe an antianxiety medication.
   d. the client will complain of flashbacks.

---

### BOX 16–5. Web Resources

*http://www.mentalhelp.net*
Provides information about common psychiatric disorders and treatments, as well as professional resources. Offers links to support groups and other online resources.

*http://www.nimh.nih.gov/anxiety/anxiety/index.htm*
Sponsored by the National Institutes of Health. Provides general information, publications, and links to other government agencies and programs.

*http://www.nami.org*
Sponsored by the National Alliance for the Mentally Ill, a nonprofit organization. Provides education and information on mental illness and treatment, as well as resources and advocacy support for the client or significant others.

*http://www.psyweb.com*
User-friendly resource giving general information on psychiatric disorders, drugs, testing, treatment, and physiology of the brain. Based on DSM-IV criteria.

---

## BIBLIOGRAPHY

American Nurses Association. (1995). *Nursing social policy statement.* Kansas City, MO: American Nurses Association.

Barry, P.D. (1996). *Psychosocial nursing: Care of physically ill patients and their families* (3rd ed.). Philadelphia: Lippincott-Raven.

Boyd, M., & Nihart, M. (1998). *Psychiatric nursing: Contemporary practice.* Philadelphia: Lippincott Williams & Wilkins.

Carpenito, L. (1999). *Handbook of nursing diagnosis* (8th ed.). Philadelphia: Lippincott Williams & Wilkins.

Carpenito, L. (2000). *Nursing diagnosis: Application to clinical practice* (8th ed.). Philadelphia: Lippincott Williams & Wilkins.

*Diagnostic and statistical manual of mental disorders* (4th ed.). (1994). Washington, D.C.: American Psychiatric Press.

Krupnick, S., & Wade, A. (1999). *Psychiatric care planning.* Springhouse, PA: Springhouse Corporation.

Mendlowicz, M., & Stein, M. (2000). Quality of life of individuals with anxiety disorders. *American Journal of Psychiatry, 157*(5), 669–682.

Minarik, P. (1996). Psychosocial intervention with ineffective coping responses to physical illness: Anxiety-related. In P.D. Barry (Ed.). *Psychosocial nursing: Care of physically ill patients and their families* (3rd ed.). Philadelphia: Lippincott-Raven.

Moreno, F., & Delgado, P. (2000). Living with anxiety disorders: As good as it gets...? *Bulletin of Menninger Clinic, 64*(3), A4–21.

Ninan, P. (1999). The functional anatomy, neurochemistry, and pharmacology of anxiety. *Journal of Clinical Psychiatry, 60*(22), 12–17.

Peplau, H. (1983). *Living and learning* (Lecture). Hartford, CT: Institute of Living, October 28.

Sadock, B., & Kaplan, H. (1998). *Synopsis of psychiatry: Behavioral sciences/clinical psychiatry.* Philadelphia: Lippincott Williams & Wilkins.

Whitley, G.G. (1994). Expert validation and differentiation of the nursing diagnoses anxiety and fear. *Nursing Diagnosis, 5*(4), 143–150.

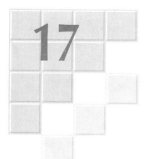

# 17

# The Client With Delirium, Dementia, Alzheimer's, and Other Cognitive Disorders

---

**B e h a v i o r a l   O b j e c t i v e s**

*After reading*
*this chapter*
*the student*
*will be able to:*

- List the causes of cognitive disorders and describe one condition under each category.
- Describe the nursing care of clients with delirium.
- Describe the nursing care of clients with dementia.
- Identify the basic causes that underlie cognitive disorders.
- Explain the difference between acute organic psychoses and chronic organic psychoses.
- Identify the most common degenerative condition that results in significant dementia.

---

**K e y   T e r m s**

- Abrupt or gradual withdrawal
- Alcohol intoxication
- Amnestic disorder
- Aphasia
- Cerebral arteriosclerosis
- Cannabis intoxication
- Cannabis withdrawal
- Cerebrovascular accident
- Cocaine intoxication
- Coma
- Concussion
- Cretinism

- Delirium
- Dementia
- Dementia of the Alzheimer's type
- Diabetes mellitus
- Electrolyte imbalance
- Exophthalmic goiter (Graves' disease)
- Huntington's chorea
- Inhalant intoxication
- MEND A MIND
- Myxedema
- Opioid intoxication

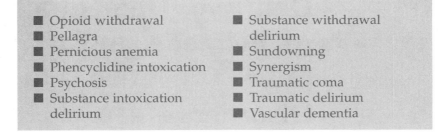

■ Opioid withdrawal
■ Pellagra
■ Pernicious anemia
■ Phencyclidine intoxication
■ Psychosis
■ Substance intoxication
   delirium

■ Substance withdrawal
   delirium
■ Sundowning
■ Synergism
■ Traumatic coma
■ Traumatic delirium
■ Vascular dementia

Cognitive disorders are caused by dysfunctions in brain anatomy or physiology. These disorders can cause marked change in intellectual functioning, judgment, and memory. Cognitive mental disorders also can result in a severe disruption of mental status called **psychosis.**

A psychosis is the most serious form of mental disorder. A person who is psychotic temporarily loses contact with reality. There are two main types of organic psychosis: delirium and dementia. Generally, **delirium** is an acute condition that develops rapidly and subsides spontaneously or when the underlying physical cause is treated. **Dementia** is caused by a chronic, irreversible physical deterioration of anatomic parts of the brain. Accordingly, dementia usually cannot be reversed. Delirium and dementia are discussed later in this chapter.

Psychoses caused by cognitive disorders with an organic or physiologic etiology are different from functional psychoses, such as those caused by schizophrenia. Functional psychoses are not associated with any known physical abnormality (although researchers in the field of neuropsychiatry believe that there is a basic defect in the biochemistry of the brain that causes functional psychoses). Cognitive psychotic conditions have a variety of causes or etiologies. The following **MEND A MIND** mnemonic aid can assist in recalling the various biologic causes of cognitive disorders:

**M** Metabolic disorder
**E** Electrical disorder
**N** Neoplastic disease
**D** Degenerative disease
**A** Arterial disease
**M** Mechanical disease
**I** Infectious disease
**N** Nutritional disease
**D** Drug toxicity

The types of physical conditions that belong to the various categories are outlined below.

| | |
|---|---|
| Metabolic | Endocrine gland disorders |
| | Electrolyte imbalances |
| Electrical | Epileptic disorders |
| Neoplastic | Benign or malignant tumors of the brain or elsewhere |
| Degenerative | Alzheimer's disease |
| | Huntington's chorea |
| Arterial | Cerebrovascular accident (CVA) |
| | Degenerative changes of cerebral arteries |
| | Vascular dementia (formerly multiple infarct dementia) |
| Mechanical | Head injury |
| Infectious | Encephalitis |
| | Meningitis |
| | Cerebral abscess |
| | General systemic infections |
| | AIDS |
| Nutritional | Nicotinic acid |
| | Vitamin B |
| | Thiamine |
| | Folic acid |
| Drugs | Alcohol |
| | Controlled substances |
| | Prescribed drugs |

The conditions listed above can produce a variety of acute psychiatric symptoms, including acute confusion, hallucinations, and delusions. Generally speaking, one of the differences between the psychotic episodes of people with cognitive disorders and those of people with functional psychiatric illness is that the hallucinations of the client with cognitive disorder tend to be primarily visual, whereas those of the functionally ill client are usually auditory. Some of the conditions (for example, epileptic disorders) do not routinely cause psychiatric disturbance. On occasion, depending on the types of neurologic dysfunction in the different parts of the brain, psychiatric symptoms of various types and severity may occur. In addition, the neurologic disorder can cause the basic personality tendencies of the person to be magnified. For example, a person who has always been mildly suspicious may become paranoid.

Table 17-1 presents the symptoms seen in delirium and dementia. Development of a nursing care plan for the client with a cognitive disorder includes nursing assessment of the mental status categories in this chart. The planning and intervention steps of the nursing process can be developed more easily when the specific types and symptoms of mental dysfunction are identified.

## TABLE 17-1. Symptoms of the Two Types of Cognitive Disorders

| Categories | Delirium | Dementia |
|---|---|---|
| Onset | Usually rapid: waxes and wanes abruptly | Usually slow: 1 month or more |
| Level of awareness | Increased or decreased | Normal or decreased |
| Orientation | Disoriented | Usually not affected until late in course |
| Appearance and behavior | May be semicomatose; agitated | Usually slowed responses |
| Speech and communication | Incoherent; degree of change based on severity of delirium | Usually slowed because of cognitive deficits |
| Mood | Labile; anxiety or panic common | Constricted affect or depression |
| Thinking process | Markedly altered | Mildly altered decreased intellectual ability |
| Memory | Partial or full loss of recent memory; remote memory intact | Partial loss of both recent and remote memory |
| Perception | Usually markedly altered | Usually intact or mildly affected |
| Abstract thinking and judgment | Markedly decreased | Mildly decreased |
| Sleep-wake cycle | Disrupted | Not affected |
| Treatment | Identify and remove underlying cause; symptomatic treatment | Symptomatic treatment |
| Prognosis | Reversible in most cases | Usually irreversible |

Adapted from Barry, P. (1996). The physical cause of cognitive mental disorders. In P. Barry (Ed.). *Psychosocial nursing: Care of physically ill patients and their families* (3rd ed.). Philadelphia: Lippincott Williams & Wilkins; Murray, G.B. (1997). Confusion, delirium, and dementia. In N.H. Cassem (Ed.). *Massachusetts General Hospital handbook of general hospital psychiatry* (4th ed.). St. Louis: Mosby–Year Book; Sadock, B., & Kaplan, H. (1998). *Synopsis of psychiatry: Behavioral sciences/clinical psychiatry.* Philadelphia: Lippincott Williams & Wilkins.

## ◆ DELIRIUM

Delirium is an acute cognitive disorder that produces a marked change in mental status. A toxic condition related to one of the categories described in the preceding mnemonic causes delirium. To determine its cause and prevent its occurrence, an immediate assessment of physiologic status is needed: a physical examination, diagnostic workup including laboratory tests and other tests as indicated, and review of all medications. Once the underlying cause is diagnosed and treated, the person usually returns to his or her previously existing mental status and personality style.

## NURSING CARE OF CLIENTS WITH DELIRIUM

A client who is developing a toxic cognitive disorder, whether he or she is on a psychiatric, medical, or surgical unit, often demonstrates symptoms of changing mental status before full-blown delirium occurs. Regardless of mental status on admission, the client becomes more restless and agitated. There may be physiologic changes such as increased temperature, blood pressure, and pulse, and facial flushing. Such changes indicate that the client's status is changing; good nursing care requires monitoring mental status changes frequently to determine how quickly the client's mental or physical state is deteriorating. Notify the physician as soon as specific changes are noted. Ideally, a delirious episode can be avoided if a diagnostic evaluation is performed with little delay and proper medication is ordered.

The drug of choice for many clients with cognitive disorder is haloperidol (Haldol). It is a major tranquilizer of the butyrophenone group, which is chosen over the major tranquilizers of the phenothiazine group because it has fewer anticholinergic effects on the other body systems. A client with an organic brain syndrome suffers from an illness in one or more of the many physiologic systems; therefore, it is important to avoid a medication with anticholinergic effects, because it likely will further disrupt the body's homeostasis. One of the side effects of haloperidol is the risk of tardive dyskinesia (see Chapter 28, Psychopharmacology and Electroconvulsive Treatment of Mental Disorders). Because of this risk, this medication should be discontinued as soon as the acute delirious episode has passed. If a client continues to be maintained on this medication, the charge nurse should be consulted to be sure that the need for the medication continues to be present. Generally speaking, once the underlying physical cause of the cognitive disorder is treated, and if the client has had no prior history of major psychiatric illness, the medication can be discontinued or replaced by a minor tranquilizer that has fewer toxic effects.

Caring for a client experiencing a delirious episode can be frightening. It is important for the nurse to maintain composure during the time with a delirious client. Although out of control, the client with cognitive disorder often remembers what happened. Avoid saying or doing anything that could further alarm the client or cause additional anxiety relating to the delirious period. Caring firmness and honesty are the most therapeutic behaviors that one can display.

### Restraints

The use of restraints is an area of nursing care that must conform to the hospital policy and procedure manual. Safeguard the client's safety during such an episode using hospital guidelines. If the client is totally out of control, there are hospital procedures that outline the policies regarding level of restraint and the manner in which restraint is applied and by whom. A review of Chapter 6, Professional, Legal, and Ethical Issues, describes the specific issues of the use of restraints in the mental health setting. These policies may include the roles of non-nursing personnel who may use stronger restraint than is allowed or is necessary to restrain and subdue the client. The nurse's composure and quiet directions can calm the situation and affect the restraint of the client. Physical restraint should not cause injury to the client unless lives are at risk.

The client should never be left alone during an acute psychotic episode. Restraints may or may not be used depending on the policies of the institution, the orders of the physician, and the circumstances of the client's cognitive disorder. Although medication decreases the acute state, it still may be necessary to restrain the client for his or her own safety.

Restraints are frightening to a client who is confused as the result of delirium. They should be used only after careful assessment of the client's problem. The need for restraints should be explained quietly to the client, even if he or she does not appear to be able to understand. It is important to obtain the order of a physician or to know what the *written* policy of the institution states about the use of restraints. The use of restraints and their abuse are important legal issues for nurses. Liability can result in lawsuits if the nurse using restraints is not legally covered by such a policy or if the guidelines are modified in any way.

The types of restraints available include wrist and ankle restraints and camisoles. Wrist and ankle restraints should be properly padded to safeguard the integrity of the skin. Restraints should be released following the policies of the nurse's institution or at least every 2 hours to allow for freedom of movement and to check the condition of the skin. Good body positioning is important when restraints are used.

Another important point to remember when caring for a client who has had a delirious episode is that the terror experienced during delirium remains repressed in his or her unconscious. The client may demonstrate increased levels of anxiety or experience frightening nightmares after the psychotic episode. If the client is gently asked what he or she remembers feeling and thinking while the delirium was occurring, he or she may be relieved to be able to describe it. As the painful thoughts and feelings are released, anxiety and nightmares should diminish. Attentive caring and knowledge in listening to the details of the experience can comfort and reassure the client.

## ◆ DEMENTIA

Dementia is a change in mental status caused by physical changes in the brain. It usually is a chronic condition that progresses slowly and is not reversible. Dementia is frequently associated with the elderly and is often incorrectly assumed to be a part of the aging process. Actually, many elderly people retain their intellectual functioning into their eighties and nineties. Important factors determining whether dementia occurs are genetic predisposition, family history, nutritional status, and general level of health.

## NURSING CARE OF CLIENTS WITH DEMENTIA

Often people who are hospitalized in nursing homes have varying levels of dementia, as do elderly people in the acute hospital setting. When dementia progresses to an advanced stage, psychosis can occur. When psychosis is present, the nursing care outlined earlier for the psychotic client with delirium should be followed. Most clients with early or moderate dementia require the nursing care described below. Table 17-1 identifies the various symptoms of dementia the client is experiencing. In developing the nursing care plan, it is crucial to record the severity of these symptoms and take them into consideration as nursing care approaches are considered. The participation of family members in planning and administering care is valuable because the client's altered mental status, including impaired memory, may result in an inaccurate or incomplete database. The following nursing approaches should be considered when administering care to a person with dementia:

- Give good basic physical care.
- Provide simple verbal directions in a calm voice.
- Avoid sensory overload.
- Provide a regular toileting schedule. Clients may forget to void and become embarrassed by their incontinence.
- Monitor and document bowel activity.
- Check and document nutritional intake.
- Maintain reality orientation by mentioning the day of the week and discussing seasonal and current events.
- Provide a night light. Clients with cognitive disorders are susceptible to **sundowning,** a decrease in orientation at night.
- Provide some type of enjoyable activity.
- Avoid using physical restraints unless indicated.
- Do not place intravenous lines in the lower arm. Confused clients often displace intravenous tubing.

Elderly people who are mildly confused, forgetful, and listless should not automatically be assumed to have dementia. Remember that elderly people have experienced a profound number of losses, and they may be acutely depressed. Nutritional deprivation, a possible cause of cognitive disorder, also can cause depression. The symptoms of acute depression and mild dementia can appear similar. If depression is suspected, psychiatric consultation can be requested if the client is in a nonpsychiatric institution.

## ◆ OTHER COGNITIVE DISORDERS

All of the following mental disorders have an organic etiology, which can be discovered in the client's history, physical exam, or laboratory tests, but they do not meet the specific criteria of delirium and dementia.

**Amnestic disorder** is a cognitive disorder in which the level of consciousness is not affected as it is in other organic brain disorders. Short-term and long-term memory are impaired, and the client is in an amnestic state. It is a rare condition.

### SUBSTANCE-INDUCED DELIRIUM

This section concentrates on the most frequently seen substance-related mental disorders in the clinical setting. In the event that there is a client whose condition is not described in this section, it is helpful to refer to the *Diagnostic and Statistical Manual of Mental Disorders,* fourth edition (DSM-IV), on the clinical unit or in the library. It describes the specific symptoms of the condition.

**Substance intoxication delirium** is a separate syndrome unlike those caused by other cognitive disorders. It is caused by recent intake of one or more psychoactive substances. The result is abnormal behavior, such as impairment of judgment, occupational functioning, or social functioning. These behavioral changes are due to the effects of the substance on the central nervous system. **Substance withdrawal delirium** is caused by the reduction or cessation of ingestion of a psychoactive substance following its regular use.

DSM-IV categories of substance-induced cognitive disorders include a large number of syndromes. These conditions present a wide variety of symptoms. The full presentation of symptoms for all conditions can be found in the DSM-IV. Here, the symptoms of intoxication and withdrawal are described for each of the major drug-induced cognitive disorders. In each case, none of the physical or mental symptoms is caused by any other type of medical condition. The names of other conditions that can develop with prolonged drug use appear under each major drug abuse group.

### ALCOHOL-INDUCED COGNITIVE DISORDERS

**Alcohol intoxication** is a condition in which recent ingestion of alcohol causes negative behavioral effects, including at least one of the following signs: slurred speech, lack of coordination, unsteady walking, nystagmus, or flushed face. In addition, at least one of the following psychological symptoms appears: mood change, irritability, excessive talking, or impaired attention.

## AMPHETAMINE (OR AMPHETAMINE-LIKE SUBSTANCE)-INDUCED COGNITIVE DISORDER

The drugs included in this category are those of the substituted phenethylamine: amphetamine, dextroamphetamine, and methamphetamine (speed). Other differing drugs such as methylphenidate or appetite suppressants (diet pills) are also included. Intoxication in this category includes the same physical and psychological symptoms as those of cocaine intoxication. **Abrupt or gradual withdrawal** from the drug induces depression and two or more of the following symptoms: increase in dreaming, disturbed sleep, and fatigue. Those who abuse these drugs can also develop delirium and delusional disorders.

## CANNABIS-INDUCED COGNITIVE DISORDER

The symptoms in **cannabis** (marijuana, hashish, or THC) **intoxication** are tachycardia and at least one of the following psychological symptoms that occur shortly after use: perception of slowed time, intensified subjective perceptions, apathy, and elation. In addition, one or more of the following physical symptoms appear: dry mouth, increase in appetite, and redness of the eyes. Disruption in social and occupational functioning and suspiciousness can result. A more severe form of cannabis-related mental disorder is **cannabis intoxication delirium.** There are no changes in level of consciousness and intellectual abilities, no major symptoms of depression, and no hallucinations or delusions.

## COCAINE-INDUCED COGNITIVE DISORDER

**Cocaine intoxication** occurs within 1 hour of using the drug and includes at least two of the following psychological symptoms: euphoria, grandiosity, excessive wordiness, excessive vigilance, and psychomotor agitation. In addition, at least two of the following physiologic conditions are present: dilated pupils, elevated blood pressure, tachycardia, nausea and vomiting, and chills or perspiration. There also are symptoms of antisocial behavior.

## HALLUCINOGEN-INDUCED COGNITIVE DISORDER

The drugs included in this category are substances related to 5-hydroxytryptamine (eg, LSD), dimethyltryptamine (DMT), and catecholamine (eg, mescaline). The hallucinogenic drugs are not categorized by intoxication or withdrawal. Rather, they markedly alter the mental status of those who use them and can cause hallucinosis, delusional disorder, and affective disorder.

## INHALANT-INDUCED COGNITIVE DISORDER

**Inhalant intoxication** follows the use of an inhalant that results in abnormal changes in behavior such as truculence, impaired judgment, belligerence, and impaired occupational or social functioning. At least two of the following signs must be present: dizziness, nystagmus, lack of coordination, slurred speech, unsteady gait, lethargy, depressed reflexes, psychomotor retardation, tremor, generalized muscle weakness, blurred vision, stupor or coma, and euphoria.

## OPIOID-INDUCED COGNITIVE DISORDER
The drugs included in this category are heroin, morphine, and the morphine-like drugs, such as meperidine (Demerol) and methadone. The diagnostic criteria for **opioid intoxication** are recent use of an opioid; constriction of pupils, or dilation if there is a major overdose; and the presence of one or more emotional or neurologic signs: euphoria, dysphoria, apathy, or psychomotor retardation.

Symptoms of **opioid withdrawal** include at least four of the following signs: tachycardia, mild hypertension, fever, lacrimation, dilated pupils, rhinorrhea (running nose), piloerection (hairs of skin standing on end), sweating, diarrhea, and yawning.

## PHENCYCLIDINE OR PHENCYCLIDINE-LIKE SUBSTANCE–INDUCED COGNITIVE DISORDER
The most common drugs in this category are known by the following names: Ketalar, TCP, PCP, angel dust, THC, crystal, and peace pill. These substances are usually ingested by inhaling or smoking. The symptoms of **phencyclidine (PCP) intoxication** shortly following ingestion include at least two of the following physiologic symptoms: decreased pain response, tachycardia and elevated blood pressure, dysarthria, decrease in voluntary muscle coordination, and horizontal or vertical nystagmus. In addition, there should be at least two of the following psychological symptoms: severe anxiety, mood swings, elation, grandiosity, psychomotor agitation, and sensation experienced in a different part of the body from where pressure is applied. Abuses of this class of drugs can also cause delirium and mixed mental disorder.

## SEDATIVE, HYPNOTIC, OR ANXIOLYTIC-INDUCED COGNITIVE DISORDER
Intoxication within this category can be caused by any of the following drugs: sedatives, including pentobarbital sodium (Nembutal), secobarbital (Seconal), and a combination of secobarbital sodium and amobarbital sodium (Tuinal); the minor tranquilizers; and benzodiazepines, including chlordiazepoxide (Librium), diazepam (Valium), and oxazepam (Serax). The common hypnotics are ethchlorvynol (Placidyl), flurazepam hydrochloride (Dalmane), glutethimide (Doriden), methyprylon (Noludar), chloral hydrate, and methaqualone. The symptoms of intoxication are the same as those for alcohol. Any distinctions are caused by differences in basic personality structures of diverse people.

Withdrawal symptoms following prolonged, heavy use of these drugs are also similar to alcohol withdrawal symptoms. At least three of the following physical symptoms are present in this brain syndrome:

Coarse tremors of the hands, eyelids, and tongue
Nausea and vomiting
Malaise or weakness
Autonomic hyperactivity
Anxiety
Depressed or irritable mood
Orthostatic hypotension

Other syndromes that can develop in abusers of this family of drugs are withdrawal delirium and amnestic disorder.

## ◈ PHYSICAL CONDITIONS THAT CAN CAUSE MENTAL DISORDERS

The physical conditions that can cause mental disorders follow the MEND A MIND mnemonic. A mnemonic is a word created to help people remember a list or some other type of information that may otherwise be difficult to classify. The purpose of this section is to provide knowledge of physical conditions that can disrupt the anatomy or physiology of the brain. Such disruption can cause changes in mental status.

### PSYCHOSIS ASSOCIATED WITH METABOLIC DISORDERS

This category of cognitive disorders includes those caused by endocrine disorders: complications of diabetes (other than cerebral arteriosclerosis) and disorders of the thyroid, pituitary, adrenals, and other endocrine glands.

Hyperactivity or hypoactivity of the thyroid gland often results in mental disturbances. If the secretion of the gland is insufficient, a condition known as **myxedema** develops. In addition to a well-known syndrome of physical symptoms (lowered blood pressure, temperature, pulse rate, and respiration rate; chilliness of the body, especially cold hands and feet; slowed physical activity; and dullness of facial expression), such clients become slow in their thinking and ability to grasp ideas. Their memory becomes impaired and their speech becomes slow and listless. Some are irritable, fretful, fault finding, or even paranoid in their ideas and attitudes. Congenital insufficiency of the thyroid gland results in a condition called **cretinism,** in which there are both mental and physical defects.

An overactive thyroid gives rise to a condition known as **exophthalmic goiter** or **Graves' disease.** The client's symptoms are the exact opposite of those seen in clients suffering from insufficient thyroxine. The client is nervous, high-strung, irritable, very active, anxious, and apprehensive. In acute thyroid intoxication, he or she may go into acute delirium, accompanied by incoherence, hallucinations, and great restlessness. This intoxication may lead to coma and death.

An undersecretion of the islands of Langerhans in the pancreas causes **diabetes mellitus.** Diabetes is characterized by hyperglycemia (or excessive amount of sugar in the blood) due to a deficiency of insulin that helps the cells burn up sugars. When the hyperglycemia mounts too high, the client goes into diabetic coma. He or she becomes irritable, anxious, and confused, hallucinates, and may even become delirious before reaching the convulsion state. Without treatment, coma usually results.

In addition to the disorders of the endocrine system, another type of metabolic disturbance is related to **electrolyte imbalance.** The brain is accustomed to functioning in homeostatic balance. Owing to illness or other factors, the body's electrolytes may be out of balance. Excessively high or low levels of electrolytes affect sensitive brain tissue that is bathed in the body fluids of blood and cerebrospinal fluid. Table 17-2 lists the electrolytes and their generally accepted normal ranges as a guideline for recognizing electrolyte imbalance as the cause for mental status changes in a general hospital client.

When clients have been chronically physically ill, their body tissues have had a period of time to allow for a gradual adjustment to altered electrolyte levels. Accordingly, their electrolyte levels may extend above or below the ranges shown in the table with no symptoms that reflect toxic effects on brain tissue.

TABLE 17-2. **Electrolytes That Can Alter Mental Status**

| Electrolyte | Normal Range | Abnormal Levels |
| --- | --- | --- |
| Calcium | 8.5–10.5 | Hypocalcemia, hypercalcemia |
| Sodium | 135–145 MEq/liter | Hyponatremia, hypernatremia |
| Phosphorus | 2.6–4.5 | Hypophosphatemia, hyperphosphatemia |
| Potassium | 3.5–5.0 MEq/liter | Hypokalemia, hyperkalemia |
| Base bicarbonate | Blood pH 7.38–7.42 Bicarb level 24 MEq/liter | Acidosis, alkalosis |

Adapted from Barry, P. (1996). The physical causes of cognitive mental disorders. In P. Barry (Ed.). *Psychosocial nursing: Care of physically ill patients and their families* (3rd ed.). Philadelphia: Lippincott Williams & Wilkins; Murray, G.B. (1997). Confusion, delirium, and dementia. In N.H. Cassem (Ed.). *Massachusetts General Hospital handbook of general hospital psychiatry* (4th ed.). St. Louis: Mosby–Year Book; Sadock, B., & Kaplan, H. (1998). *Synopsis of psychiatry: Behavioral sciences/clinical psychiatry.* Philadelphia: Lippincott Williams & Wilkins.

## PSYCHOSIS ASSOCIATED WITH ELECTRICAL DISORDERS

In certain clients with idiopathic epilepsy, the epileptic attack may take the form of an episode of excitement with hallucinations, fears, and violent outbreaks. Most commonly, clouding of consciousness occurs before or after a convulsive attack or, instead of a convulsion, the client may show only a dazed reaction with deep confusion, bewilderment, and anxiety. There are no psychiatric disorders directly related to epilepsy, however, and this type of occurrence is relatively rare.

## PSYCHOSIS ASSOCIATED WITH NEOPLASTIC DISORDERS

Tumors that develop in the brain can produce psychotic reactions. Such tumors may be benign or malignant. The benign tumors are usually encapsulated. If diagnosed before their growing pressure has done much damage and if located in an area where surgery is feasible, they are often successfully removed. Angiomas, or blood tumors, although benign, do not lend themselves well to surgical removal. Malignant tumors spread rapidly and usually result in severe mental imbalance. Surgery is of little avail, and although radiation therapy is usually tried, it merely slows down the spreading of the tumor. Chemotherapy may or may not help. An additional type of neoplasm that frequently results in acute depression is carcinoma of the pancreas. The cause of this acute change in mental state is not known.

## PSYCHOSIS ASSOCIATED WITH DEGENERATIVE DISORDERS

Alzheimer's disease is the most common degenerative condition that results in significant dementia, which is now categorized as **dementia of the Alzheimer's type.** It is a condition that begins with gradual decrease in memory, emotional stability, and general functioning. The initial symptoms usually appear between the ages of 40 and 60. Intellectual ability and personality functioning gradually decrease. Memory fails markedly. There are muscular and gait changes. Within a year, profound dementia accompanied by hallucinations and delusions usually occurs. Complete nursing care is required.

Another example of this type of disorder is **Huntington's chorea,** a hereditary, sex-linked form of psychosis. It appears chiefly in men, usually in their early thirties, and progresses rapidly so that the client ages mentally in a very short time and becomes helplessly psychotic in a few years.

## PSYCHOSIS ASSOCIATED WITH ARTERIAL DISORDERS

The brain must receive a rich supply of oxygen in order to function normally. Anoxia, from whatever cause, can seriously affect the nervous tissue and result in brain damage. **Cerebral arteriosclerosis** (hardening of the arteries of the brain) is a frequent cognitive disorder. The number of clients admitted to public mental hospitals with this disorder is exceeded only by schizophrenics. The onset of arteriosclerotic mental disorder varies widely but, in general, may appear between the years of 50 and 65. Among the early symptoms are headaches, dizziness, inability to sustain concentration, short attention span, emotional instability, memory impairment, and episodes of confusion. Some clients develop paranoid delusions; some develop epileptiform convulsions; others show fluctuations in orientation and memory.

When this disease becomes advanced, small thromboses may form in small intracranial blood vessels, and the client has a series of minor strokes. Following the rupture of such a vessel and until the small blood clot is absorbed again, the client will be confused and have difficulties in speech, memory will ramble back into youth, and he or she will, perhaps, show some small degree of muscular paralysis. This is called **vascular dementia.**

Also included in this category are circulatory disturbances such as cerebral thrombosis, cerebral embolism, arterial hypertension, cardiorenal disease, and cardiac disease (particularly in decompensation). When a large blood vessel becomes occluded by a large clot or ruptures, the symptoms are much more severe, and we say the client has had a stroke, also known as a **cerebrovascular accident** (CVA).

In about half of these vascular accidents, consciousness is either lost or greatly disturbed. If a coma develops, it may be only a brief episode or it may terminate in death. Paralysis of the muscles on the opposite side of the body from the site of the cerebral hemorrhage usually results (*hemiplegia*), or there may be *monoplegia* (paralysis of just one extremity), *paraplegia* (paralysis of both legs), or *quadriplegia* (paralysis of all four extremities or the entire body). **Aphasia** (the inability to correctly say the words one is thinking) is frequently present, swallowing may be difficult or impossible, and bladder and bowel control may be lost.

## PSYCHOSIS ASSOCIATED WITH MECHANICAL DISORDERS

These disorders include injury or trauma to the brain from an external force. Oddly enough, relatively few head injuries result in permanent brain damage. The brain tissue, although extremely delicate, is very well protected by its meningeal coverings and the bony case of the cranium; however, some injuries *do* result in extensive brain damage. In this event, scar tissue usually develops in the injured area.

Three types of acute psychoses owing to trauma are **concussion, traumatic coma,** and **traumatic delirium.** Concussion very commonly results from a head injury. Its symptoms are amnesia (the client has a memory loss from just before the time of the accident up until awakening from unconsciousness), unconsciousness (which may be momentary or continue for several hours), and nausea (the client may vomit while regaining consciousness). He or she may regain consciousness suddenly or pass through a variable period of clouded consciousness and confusion. The client usually recovers fully in a short time, but if the brain damage is more pronounced, coma may develop or the concussion may be followed by a chronic state of deterioration, personality change, or chronic emotional invalidism.

Traumatic delirium may follow emergence from a traumatic coma or stupor. If the delirium is mild, the client acts more or less bewildered, irritable, and restless. If it is severe, he or she may be noisy, belligerent, demanding, and verbally abusive. Delirium or coma of more than 1 month's duration usually indicates severe brain damage.

In the event the client does not recover from the concussion (ie, the brain damage becomes chronic), he or she may show mental enfeeblement accompanied by epileptic seizures, paralysis, and other neurologic disturbances. The client may develop a definite personality change, becoming unstable, aggressive, quarrelsome, and destructive, or he or she may become depressed, apprehensive, and easily fatigued—in short, a chronic, complaining invalid.

## DEMENTIA ASSOCIATED WITH INFECTIOUS DISORDERS

AIDS dementia complex is a mental state that can occur in the advanced stage of HIV-1 infection. The symptoms that appear in this condition are a decrease in cognitive, emotional, behavior, and motor abilities. Three stages of progression are associated with this condition:

1. Symptom occurrence related to disease development
2. Concurrent involvement of different levels of the neurologic system
3. Development of multiple pathologic processes within one part of the nervous system

The nursing care of AIDS complex is symptom specific. Emotional distress is addressed by supporting effective coping. As the neuropathology progresses, issues of safety may become the most important problem to address. Delirium may occur as an outcome of the acute neurologic deterioration. The management of delirium associated with AIDS is described in the next section.

## PSYCHOSIS ASSOCIATED WITH INFECTIOUS DISORDERS

AIDS and intracranial infections such as encephalitis, meningitis, and cerebral abscess can result in hallucinations, delusions, and other psychotic symptoms. Once the acute episode has passed, there usually are no ongoing psychiatric side effects. On occasion, there can be some ongoing changes in personality traits, such as increased stubbornness, that become part of a person's permanent personality style.

In addition, systemic infections (eg, pneumonia, typhoid, malaria, acute rheumatic fever) are very often associated with acute mental disturbances. Toxins produced by viral and bacterial invasion of the bloodstream may involve the central nervous system, and delirium is frequently seen. The higher the fever, usually the more intense is the delirium.

## PSYCHOSIS ASSOCIATED WITH NUTRITIONAL DISORDERS

Certain vitamins are essential to a well-functioning neurologic system. Often, inadequate nutrition can result in deterioration of neurologic functioning within the tissues of the brain. When this occurs, psychiatric symptoms may develop. Deficiencies in several B vitamins can cause these changes in mental status. The vitamins are nicotinic acid, $B_{12}$, thiamine, and folic acid.

Although **pellagra** is not common today, it may occur in the chronic alcoholic whose diet has consisted chiefly of alcohol over a period of several months, in poverty-stricken areas where residents are very restricted in their choice of foods, and in people suffering from intestinal diseases that prevent the absorption of food. Clients with advanced pellagra exhibit symptoms of mental confusion and delirious states. Irritability, distrust, anxiety, and depression are also common. The disorder is caused by a lack of vitamin B (especially the nicotinic acid factor).

**Pernicious anemia,** although seldom reaching the frank psychotic state, does exhibit the milder symptoms of mental fatigue, memory loss, irritability, depression, and apprehension.

Thiamine deficiency can result in Wernicke's encephalopathy, most commonly seen in chronic alcoholic clients. It also may be present in clients with carcinomas of the digestive tract, tuberculosis, or toxemia.

Folic acid deficiency is an important *and* reversible cause of dementia symptoms in the elderly. The symptoms are progressive dementia, depression, and, in some cases, epilepsy. When given therapeutic doses of folic acid, the client's mental status improves in many cases. It can take several months, however, for improvement to occur.

## PSYCHOSIS ASSOCIATED WITH DRUG SIDE EFFECTS

A significant cause of drug-related cognitive disorders is the side effects of medications used in physical illness. Many cardiac drugs cause psychiatric symptoms, such as anxiety, depression, short-term memory loss, disorientation, emotional lability, and hallucinations. In addition, synergistic effects of two or more medications may result in a toxic level of medication that affects neurophysiologic functioning. **Synergism** is the effect of separate entities that, when combined, have a greater effect than the sum of their individual actions. It is similar to a $1 + 1 = 3$ result. Any good drug reference lists the reported psychiatric side effects that can occur with use of specific medications.

## KEY POINTS

---

- Possible causes of cognitive disorders include the following:
  —**Metabolic disorder:** endocrine gland disorder, electrolyte imbalance
  —**Electrical disorder:** epileptic disorders
  —**Neoplastic disease:** tumors
  —**Degenerative disease:** Alzheimer's disease, Huntington's chorea
  —**Arterial disease:** CVA, vascular dementia
  —**Mechanical disease:** head injury
  —**Infectious disease:** meningitis, encephalitis, abscess, systemic infections
  —**Nutritional disease:** vitamin deficiency or toxicity
  —**Drug toxicity:** alcohol, prescribed medications
- Delirium is an acute cognitive disorder that produces a marked change in mental status. Once its cause is determined and treated, mental status usually returns to its previous state.
- Dementia is a change in mental status caused by physical changes in the brain. It progresses slowly and usually is not reversible.
- Intoxication is caused by the intake of one or more psychoactive substances.

---

### BOX 17-1. Web Resources

*http://www.alzheimers.com*
Provides general information about Alzheimer's disease, coping, treatment and resources for the client and caregiver.

*http://www.mentalhealth.com/fr20.html*
Provides overviews of diagnoses and treatment for numerous psychiatric illnesses. American descriptions based on DSM-IV.

*http://www.healthfinder.gov/hottopics.htm*
Sponsored by the government. Provides general information about a variety of disorders as well as links to additional resources.

- Withdrawal is a syndrome that results when a person reduces or stops ingesting a psychoactive substance that he or she has been using regularly.
- Both alcohol intoxication and alcohol withdrawal can cause delirium.
- Other substances that can cause substance-induced cognitive disorders include amphetamines, cannabis, cocaine, hallucinogens, inhalants, opioids, phencyclidines, sedatives, and hypnotics.
- Some medications for physical conditions can create psychiatric symptoms. In addition, the combined effects of medications may create more symptoms than the two medicines would if taken separately. This is called synergism.

## SELF-AWARENESS ACTIVITY

- Have you known elderly people who were forgetful or had other symptoms of dementia?
- What was your opinion of these people?
- Did you attempt to communicate with them?
- What happened as you were talking with them?
- How did you feel?
- Are you surprised at the many different types of contributing causes that result in changes in brain functioning?
- Were you aware that most types of dementia are irreversible and that most types of delirium can be treated and the person can return to normal?

## QUESTIONS

1. When teaching a family member about dementia, the nurse should teach that:
   a. Dementia is reversible and therapy is aimed at treating the underlying cause of the dementia.
   b. Dementia and delirium are interchangeable diagnostic labels.
   c. Clients with dementia cannot benefit from health care interventions.
   d. Dementia is usually a progressive disorder and is not a part of the normal aging process.
2. Which of the following is an example of an appropriate nursing intervention for the client with dementia?

a. Assigning the client the responsibility of orienting new clients to the unit.
b. Turning off all unit lights at night to facilitate sleep.
c. Providing frequent visual and verbal cues regarding the time of day and unit routine.
d. All of the above.

3. Examples of metabolic disorders that may be implicated in the development of cognitive disorders include
a. endocrine gland disorders and electrolyte imbalances.
b. cerebral abscess and encephalitis.
c. cerebrovascular accident and degenerative changes of cerebral arteries.
d. Alzheimer's disease and Huntington's chorea.

4. When a nurse suspects that a client is experiencing an episode of delirium, he or she should first
a. notify the client's family of this change in condition.
b. assess the client's physiologic status.
c. give a medication to help the client sleep.
d. document the client's change in condition.

---

### BOX 17–2. **Clinical Vignette**

Thomas Bergin is 86 years old. He is a retired electrician and lives alone. He has been socially isolated since the death of his wife 7 years ago. His daughter, Alice, lives 30 miles away and does not see him frequently. Recently Alice visited her father. She was surprised to see that he had not shaved for several days. Mr. Bergin was reluctant to let her enter his apartment. Even after she told him who she was, he continued to be suspicious of her. When she entered his apartment it was much messier than usual. Several unread newspapers littered the entry hall. When she looked in the refrigerator, there was no food. As she was standing at the refrigerator, Mr. Bergin's cat began to meow loudly, as though seeking to be fed. Mr. Bergin has a chronic heart ailment for which he takes daily medication. When Alice asked her father to show her his medicine bottle, he didn't know where to find the bottle.

What is your initial impression of what is happening here? What are the first questions you would ask to begin to gather more information?

---

BOX 17–3. **Nursing Diagnoses Associated With Clinical Vignette**

**CONFUSION, ACUTE**
**Definition:** A state in which there is an abrupt onset of a cluster of global, fluctuating disturbances in consciousness, attention, perception, memory, orientation, thinking, sleep–wake cycle, and psychomotor behavior (American Psychiatric Association [APA], 1994).

Related Nursing Diagnosis: Acute confusion related to possible dementia as evidenced by increased suspiciousness and forgetfulness about feeding pet.

**INSTRUMENTAL SELF CARE DEFICIT**
**Definition:** The state in which the individual experiences an impaired ability to perform certain activities or access services essential for managing a household.

Related Nursing Diagnosis: Instrumental Self-Care Deficit related to inability to take prescribed medications as directed.

**IMPAIRED HOME MAINTENANCE MANAGEMENT**
**Definition:** The state in which an individual or family experiences or is at risk to experience a difficulty in maintaining a safe, hygienic, growth-producing home or environment.

Related Nursing Diagnosis: Impaired home maintenance management as evidenced by decreased home cleanliness and lack of adequate food supply.

---

## BIBLIOGRAPHY

Barry, P. (1996). The physical causes of cognitive mental disorders. In P. Barry (Ed.). *Psychosocial nursing: Care of physically ill patients and their families* (3rd ed.). Philadelphia: Lippincott Williams & Wilkins.

Boyd, M., & Nihart, M. (1998). *Psychiatric nursing: Contemporary practice.* Philadelphia: Lippincott Williams & Wilkins.

Carpenito, L. (1999). *Handbook of nursing diagnosis* (8th ed.). Philadelphia: Lippincott Williams & Wilkins.

Carpenito, L. (2000). *Nursing diagnosis: Application to clinical practice* (8th ed.). Philadelphia: Lippincott Williams & Wilkins.

*Diagnostic and statistical manual of mental disorders* (4th ed.). (1994). Washington, D.C.: American Psychiatric Press.

Murray, G.B. (1997). Confusion, delirium, and dementia. In N.H. Cassem (Ed.). *Massachusetts General Hospital handbook of general hospital psychiatry* (4th ed.). St. Louis: Mosby–Year Book.

Nettina, S.M. (1996). *The Lippincott manual of nursing practice* (6th ed.). Philadelphia: Lippincott Williams & Wilkins.

Sadock, B., & Kaplan, H. (1998). *Synopsis of psychiatry: Behavioral sciences/clinical psychiatry.* Philadelphia: Lippincott Williams & Wilkins.

## BOX 17–4. Family Teaching When a Client Has Delirium, Dementia, or Other Cognitive Disorder

When a family member has delirium, dementia, or other cognitive disorder, the following recommendations can provide support for the client and give the family more confidence in knowing how to support their family member. Family members should be encouraged to call the client's mental health caregiver whenever the client appears to be at risk for harm.

The family responses that will be therapeutic to this client include:

- Provide safe environment for client, including assessment of all environmental conditions that may cause or create potential harm to client
- Maintain adequate nutritional support
- Provide sanitary conditions in environment
- Support personal hygiene
- Encourage client to plan with family around his or her needs and expectations
- Support client in seeing mental health care provider and attending groups if he or she is able to do so
- Assess client's judgment frequently when there is fluctuating mental status
- Provide collaborative problem solving
- When anxiety, depression, suicidality, or other mental disorder is suspected or is present, follow the family teaching recommendations in the pertinent chapters in this book
- Review medication compliance

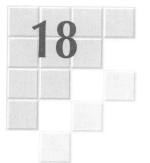

# 18

# The Client With Schizophrenia and Other Psychotic Disorders

---

## Behavioral Objectives

*After reading this chapter the student will be able to:*

- List five major criteria necessary for a diagnosis of schizophrenia and describe them.
- Name the five types of schizophrenia and explain the main characteristic of each.
- Describe the possible causes of schizophrenia using the psychoanalytic theory and the physiologic theory.
- Describe the four components of nursing care for the client with schizophrenia.
- Name the seven types of delusional disorders and explain the main characteristics of each.

---

## Key Terms

- Blunting
- Brief psychotic disorder
- Catatonia
- Catatonic excitement
- Catatonic negativism
- Catatonic rigidity
- Delusion
- Disintegration
- Echolalia
- Echopraxia
- Erotomanic
- Fragmentation
- Grandiose
- Hallucination
- Loosening of associations
- Neologism
- Persecutory
- Regression
- Schizoaffective disorder
- Schizophreniform disorder

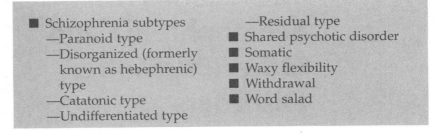

- Schizophrenia subtypes
  —Paranoid type
  —Disorganized (formerly known as hebephrenic) type
  —Catatonic type
  —Undifferentiated type
  —Residual type
- Shared psychotic disorder
- Somatic
- Waxy flexibility
- Withdrawal
- Word salad

The functional group of psychoses, of which schizophrenia is the most prevalent, is divided into five types: schizophrenia, major mood disorders, paranoid states, other nonorganic psychoses (primarily psychotic depressive reaction), and psychoses with origin specific to childhood. Each of the psychotic mental states has its own specific type of disordered mental state with related symptoms of changes in mental status.

A person's basic type of personality is the predisposing factor as to which form of psychosis he or she will develop. It occasionally happens that a person with recurrent psychosis *may* show a different form than the one evidenced earlier. As a rule, however, if psychosis occurs several times in the life of a person, it tends to follow the same behavioral pattern each time.

## ◆ SCHIZOPHRENIC DISORDERS

The behavioral patterns of schizophrenic clients are characterized by much disorganization and discord of the personality. Schizophrenia comes from two Greek words—*schizo,* meaning *to split,* and *phrenia,* meaning *mind.* Schizophrenia includes a large group of disorders characterized by disturbances of thinking, mood, and behavior. Disturbances of thinking are shown by changes in concept formation that often lead to misinterpretation of reality and, on occasion, delusions and hallucinations. These delusions and hallucinations often appear to be psychologically self-protective.

Accompanying mood changes may include ambivalent, constricted, and inappropriate emotional responsiveness and loss of empathy with others. Behavior may be withdrawn, regressive, and bizarre. In the schizophrenias, the mental status is primarily due to a thought disorder. These states must be distinguished from the major affective disorders, which are disorders of mood. In paranoid states, psychotic symptoms are absent, other than a narrow but deep distortion of reality.

### THEORIES OF CAUSES OF SCHIZOPHRENIA
Today's researchers are probing into body and brain chemistry to determine which chemical substances affect the nervous tissues of per-

sons with schizophrenia. The biochemical substances released in the brain are known as neurotransmitters. The purpose of the neurotransmitters, as their name implies, is to transmit or send messages within the brain or between the brain and various parts of the body. There are many known neurotransmitter substances in the brain, and perhaps others that have not yet been identified by neurobiologists. Dopamine is the neurotransmitter most frequently viewed as a factor in the development of schizophrenia and its ongoing course. Research has demonstrated that there is an association between the behavioral symptoms of schizophrenia and the presence of elevated levels of dopamine in schizophrenic clients. Figure 18-1 shows the multiple causative factors that are believed to contribute to the development of schizophrenia.

One of the factors that contributed to the research into the relationship between neurotransmitters and schizophrenia was the recognition that the mental status that resulted from the use of lysergic acid

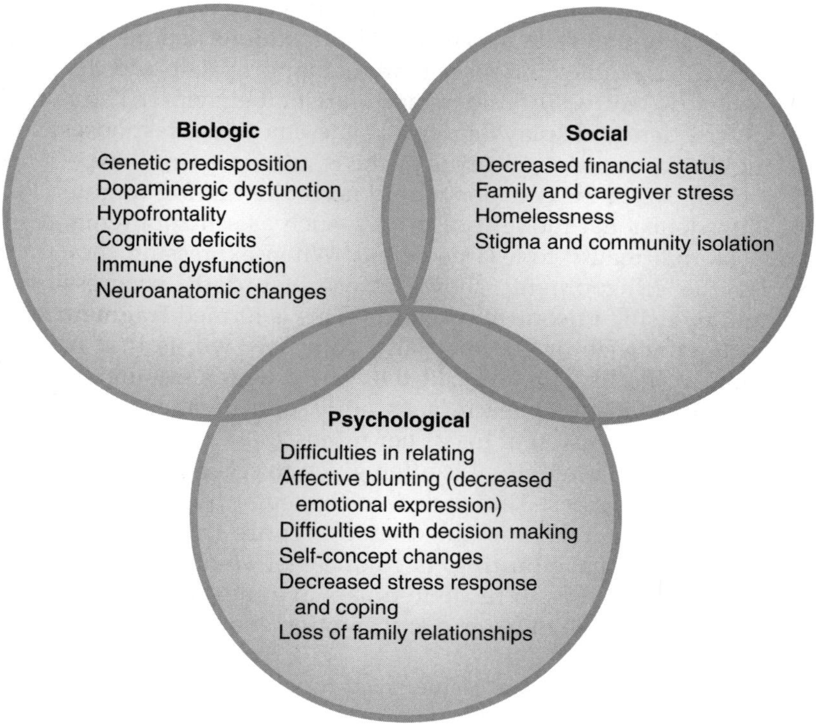

**Biologic**

Genetic predisposition
Dopaminergic dysfunction
Hypofrontality
Cognitive deficits
Immune dysfunction
Neuroanatomic changes

**Social**

Decreased financial status
Family and caregiver stress
Homelessness
Stigma and community isolation

**Psychological**

Difficulties in relating
Affective blunting (decreased
    emotional expression)
Difficulties with decision making
Self-concept changes
Decreased stress response
    and coping
Loss of family relationships

FIGURE 18–1. Biopsychosocial etiologies for patients with schizophrenia. (Boyd, M. A. & Nihart, M. A. [1998]. *Psychiatric nursing: Contemporary practice*. Philadelphia: Lippincott Williams & Wilkins.)

diethylamine (LSD) was similar in many ways to the mental status changes experienced by people with schizophrenic illness.

Should research bear out the theory that the schizophrenic has a chemical or physiologic basis of psychosis, we shall have to classify this large group of psychoses as organic rather than functional. An alternative finding may be that the schizophrenic person has both a physiologic and psychological cause for his or her psychotic state.

According to general mental health theory, many schizophrenic clients appear to have childhoods deprived of meaningful relationships with the important people in their family circles. An outstanding fact is that most of these people have felt that as children they were unloved, unwanted, and unimportant to their families. This lack of good, firm interpersonal relationships at an early age results in immature adult personalities that find it difficult to adjust socially or relate with other people intimately.

## SYMPTOMS OF SCHIZOPHRENIA

Thought disorder is evidenced by behavior or spoken thoughts that are disorderly, unrealistic, and often irrational. Autism is common. Autism is a mental state in which a client exhibits actions, thoughts, feelings, ideas, and experiences that are inappropriate and distorted. Observers do not easily understand autistic behaviors. The autistic person frequently displays inappropriate emotional responses, such as laughing or showing pleasure as the result of a painful experience, or weeping when the occasion would normally call for laughter. People with delusional thought disorders, such as schizophrenia, disregard external reality to a large extent. When expressing thought in words, the schizophrenic shows a loss of orderly progression of thought by using unconnected words. This is termed **fragmentation,** or **word salad.** He or she may also coin new words that have no meaning to the listener. We call these new words **neologisms.** The schizophrenic client's speech lacks unity, clearness, and coherence, reflecting the confusion of his or her mind.

The schizophrenic client is often given to eccentric, unexplained, and sudden activities. Undirected restlessness, fitful behavior, and impulsive, apparently unpremeditated acts are frequent. A **lack of affect,** or emotional **blunting,** is coldness of emotional response to others. The client fails to relate to others in a meaningful way. He or she is emotionally shallow, and any emotion shown is often inappropriate.

**Withdrawal** is a progressive shutting out of the world. There is reduction in interest, initiative, and spontaneity. Many clients seem to have withdrawn behind barriers, which would reveal loneliness, hopelessness, hatred, and fear if they could be penetrated. The client may build a shell of indifference in self-defense. The withdrawal may vary from a mild degree of isolation to one so profound that the client seems to be completely unaware of his or her surroundings. However, these severely withdrawn people, in spite of appearances, are sometimes acutely aware of all that goes on in the environment.

**Regression** varies in degree from slight to profound. There is a tendency for the schizophrenic client to retreat to a more primitive and infantile level of thinking and behaving.

A **delusion** is a fixed, false belief based on a misinterpretation of fact. Because the ideas, or mental content, of the schizophrenic client are so often delusional, and because the client's needs are so often disguised by symbolism, his or her thought content often appears complicated and difficult to understand. Delusions tend to center around themes of persecution, grandiosity, sex, and religion. The client dramatizes problems, strivings, and conflicts in fantastic delusional beliefs.

**Hallucinations** are another common symptom of schizophrenia. Hallucinations are sensory perceptions that have no basis in fact. They come, instead, from troublesome material from the client's inner life. They are very real to the client. Sometimes they are terrifying, sometimes accusing, and sometimes pleasurable.

## DIAGNOSTIC CRITERIA OF SCHIZOPHRENIA

When unresolved anxiety mounts too high, the schizophrenic person tends to meet problems by turning away from the real world and withdrawing into a dream world produced through fantasy, projection, delusions, and hallucinations. In other words, he or she becomes psychotic.

Although there are five major subdivisions of schizophrenia, each with distinguishing characteristics, there are several overall characteristics common to all subgroups.

## ◆ SCHIZOPHRENIA

Characteristic symptoms include two (or more) of the following, each of which is present for a significant portion of time during a 1-month period (or less if successfully treated):

1. Delusions
2. Hallucinations
3. Disorganized or incoherent speech
4. Grossly disorganized or catatonic behavior. **Catatonia** is a type of motor activity observed in some persons with schizophrenia in which there is either violent physical activity or inhibited or "paralyzed" physical activity.
5. Other types of negative symptoms, such as blunted affect, inability to speak, and inability to carry out one's will

## MAJOR SUBTYPES OF SCHIZOPHRENIA

The subtypes of schizophrenia are defined by the prominent symptoms at the time of evaluation. They are as follows:

Paranoid type
Disorganized type
Catatonic type
Undifferentiated type
Residual type

### Paranoid Type

The **paranoid schizophrenic** adds suspiciousness, projection, and delusions of persecution to his or her other basic schizophrenic traits. Delusions occupy a prominent place in his or her mental concepts, and hallucinations are tied in with these delusions.

Voices issue commands to the client from the air or out of the walls; he or she may refuse medications or food for fear of being poisoned. The paranoid schizophrenic client is usually highly verbal and will tell the nurse about the detectives who are following him or her everywhere or about unseen instruments that are reading his or her mind. At times, the paranoid schizophrenic client may become quite aggressive and even combative, and utterances may become disconnected and fragmentary.

The paranoid schizophrenic does *not* demonstrate the following traits normally associated with other forms of schizophrenia: incoherence, marked loosening of associations, catatonic behavior, grossly disorganized behavior, or flat or very inappropriate affect.

### Disorganized Type

The **disorganized type,** formerly known as the **hebephrenic type,** has an insidious onset that usually begins in adolescence. The client's emotions become shallow and inappropriate. He or she withdraws from social contacts, appears preoccupied, and smiles and giggles frequently in a silly manner. The client's speech becomes badly fragmented, often to the point of incoherence. Bizarre delusions and hallucinations, often of a pleasant type, if present, are transient and not well organized. Hypochondriacal complaints are frequent. There is more disorganization of personality and habits in the disorganized type than in any of the other types of schizophrenia, but it is rarely seen today because of early intervention, the use of the powerful phenothiazine drugs, and the end of the era of long-term institutionalization of clients.

### Catatonic Type

The **catatonic type** appears primarily in two major forms. One form is characterized by apparent stupor, immobility, mutism, and negativism;

the other phase is characterized by unorganized, excessive, impulsive, and sometimes destructive behavior. The diagnosis can be made if any of the symptoms described in the following are present.

In catatonic stupor, or withdrawal, the client shows no interest in the environment. The client's facial expression is vacant; he or she may stare into space, frequently with head bowed, and may lie, sit, or stand very still for long periods of time. The client often must be tube fed and given complete physical care when in this state. Although apparently unheeding and insensible, the client's consciousness is actually very clear, and after recovery he or she will often relate minute details of what went on. The client lives in an unreal world and seems oblivious to the external environment. Occasionally, the client may be seen whispering and smiling slightly; at other times, he or she may exhibit odd mannerisms and strange positioning of the head and extremities.

If someone raises the client's arm into an upright position, he or she will maintain this position for an amazingly long time. The term **waxy flexibility** is used to describe this phenomenon. Two other peculiar mannerisms occasionally are seen: **echolalia,** in which the client repeats the words or phrases of others but offers no conversation of his or her own, and **echopraxia,** in which the client mimics all actions of the person who is addressing him or her, but makes no answer at all.

**Catatonic negativism** is marked by resistance to instructions of others or to purposeful action. **Catatonic rigidity** is the holding of a particular posture for long periods of time and resistance to being moved.

In **catatonic excitement,** the client's behavior is characterized by impulsive and stereotyped activities, poorly coordinated and often lacking apparent purpose. Hostility and feelings of resentment are common; unprovoked outbursts of violence and destructiveness may occur; hallucinations are frequent. The flow of speech may vary from mutism to a rapid speech, also known as pressured speech, suggesting flight of ideas. Some excitements are in the form of short panic reactions.

The characteristic symptoms of catatonia are withdrawal, regression, repetitive stereotyped actions, odd mannerisms, strange positioning of parts of the body, waxy flexibility, mutism, and hallucinations.

### Undifferentiated and Residual Types
**Schizophrenia, undifferentiated type** refers to less severe psychotic symptoms that cannot be classified in the types described previously or to symptoms that meet the criteria for more than one of the other schizophrenia categories.

**Schizophrenia, residual type** is a classification used when the client has had at least one episode of schizophrenia but does not display acute psychotic symptoms. Other symptoms of schizophrenia are present, however. They include the following:

Eccentric behavior
Emotional blunting or blunted affect
Social withdrawal
Disordered thinking
Loosening of associations

**Loosening of associations** is a type of thinking in which the normal connectedness between ideas or thoughts seems haphazard. The thinking process does not flow in a normal pattern.

## PROGNOSIS

Over the 5- to 10-year period following the first psychiatric hospitalization for schizophrenia, approximately 10% to 20% of clients are viewed as having a good outcome. More than 50% of clients are viewed as having a poor outcome. It should be noted, however, that new antipsychotic medications recently released from pharmaceutical companies indicate that the prognosis for schizophrenia can be much improved, provided that the person with schizophrenia takes medication on a regular basis. The more recent medications also are available in long-term timed-release forms that are more likely to promote medication compliance. Table 18-1 shows the types of factors that may be predictive of the prognosis for individuals with schizophrenia.

### TABLE 18–1. Features Weighting Toward Good to Poor Prognosis in Schizophrenia

| Good Prognosis | Poor Prognosis |
|---|---|
| Late onset | Young onset |
| Obvious precipitating factors | No precipitating factors |
| Acute onset | Insidious onset |
| Good premorbid social, sexual, and work histories | Poor premorbid social, sexual, and work histories |
| Mood disorder symptoms (especially depressive disorders) | Withdrawn, autistic behavior |
| Married | Single, divorced, or widowed |
| Family history of mood disorders | Family history of schizophrenia |
| Good support systems | Poor support systems |
| Positive symptoms | Negative symptoms |
| | Neurological signs and symptoms |
| | History of perinatal trauma |
| | No remission in 3 years |
| | Many relapses |
| | History of assaultiveness |

## NURSING CARE OF CLIENTS WITH
## SCHIZOPHRENIC DISORDERS

The schizophrenic client admitted to a psychiatric institution is out of control. His or her thoughts and feelings are bizarre. The schizophrenic client may be terrified or overwhelmed with grief or rage, or may seem to be falling apart psychologically (also known as disintegrating). **Disintegration** is the disruption of the normal influence of the mind on combining thoughts, feelings, memories, and perceptions into a realistic view of oneself and one's environment. When the mind loses its ability to maintain these psychological functions in balance, the client feels as though he or she really is falling apart.

The client who is experiencing an acute schizophrenic episode appears to have indeed lost the ability to function psychologically. For nurses new to the psychiatric setting, observing this can be a frightening experience. Seeing a fellow human in the rawest emotional state touches the caregiver's vulnerability as a human being. The safety of caregivers can be at risk. In addition, it is common for new professionals in the mental health setting to wonder whether such a loss of mental control could happen to them.

Sometimes a mental health professional may have a family member or friend who has experienced a psychotic disorder. Memories associated with their psychotic episodes may create fear, anxiety, or sadness. It is important to realize that these feelings are common to all people new to the psychiatric unit, regardless of their caregiving discipline: nursing, medicine, social work, and so on. As a nurse learns more about the nature of the illness, its treatment, and prognosis and discusses his or her feelings with peers, supervisors, or instructors, these feelings can gradually diminish.

### Assessment

A basic rule governs those who work with psychiatric clients: ideally, a consistent nurse should be assigned to the care of each client. This is essential, especially for the psychotic client whose level of functioning is, in some way, severely regressed. As a young child benefits from the security of a consistent caregiver and is disturbed by frequent changes in caregivers, so too is the client with a psychotic disorder.

The assessment of the newly admitted schizophrenic client is a slow process that requires obtaining information from many people, including the client. Despite the psychotic episodes the client is experiencing, he or she may be able to give reliable information at certain times. The family or friends of the client are important because they can often give facts that validate the client's statements or fill in the many gaps of knowledge that are important in understanding the client's current illness. It is also possible to discern maladaptive family relationship patterns that may have contributed to the person's current disorder. In addition, if these dynamics are not addressed in the treatment setting, they can undermine the client's ability to function independently once he or she is discharged from the hospital.

When talking with the client early in the admission process, it is helpful for the nurse to remember his or her own personal need for safety. Accordingly, it is important to maintain a nonthreatening, calm communication style, observing for signs of increasing anxiety and agitation in the client. Rather than continue an interview with an increasingly anxious psychotic client, the nurse should tell the client that he or she will return later. The types of questions that assist in developing the therapeutic relationship and gathering information for the nursing process appear in Chapter 7, Communicating in the Therapeutic Relationship. These concepts can be modified to accommodate the client's level of functioning.

The assessment of the psychotic client includes the data obtained by members of other disciplines on the treatment team. Depending on the particular treatment philosophy of the institution in which a nurse is working, this information may be pooled and used in a unified team approach to provide a comprehensive and therapeutic care plan. The nursing diagnoses that are determined in reviewing the data form the basis of the planning step. In order to meet the evaluation criteria, the symptoms or problems the client demonstrates should diminish during the treatment process.

### Planning

The planning step of the nursing process should be integrated with the overall plan of the multidisciplinary treatment team as developed by the client's primary therapist. The recommendations in Chapter 10, Nursing Process in the Mental Health Setting, can be used in developing the care plan according to the nursing process model. The discussion about the nursing care of the psychotic client is limited to specific recommendations for interventions with this type of client. One is wise to remember that the treatment process of the psychotic client may be lengthy. Accordingly, planning includes both short- and long-term goals. In this way, the client and caregivers set realistic, achievable goals that minimize discouragement if progress is slow.

### Implementation

The most important concern for all clients is the client's safety and physical well being. The psychotic client who experiences loss of contact with reality is at particular risk of inflicting harm to self and others. The assessment process should include this major consideration. Intervention includes active steps to ensure the safety of the client and all others with whom he or she comes in contact. This includes careful monitoring of the environment by the nurse. It may be necessary for the high-risk client to be secluded until medication reduces the level of risk. Limits and controls carried out in a therapeutic and supportive manner promote the client's sense of control and security. These should be outlined carefully in the nursing care plan so that other nurses carry them out in a consistent manner.

The psychotic client is often unable to care for him or herself. Nursing intervention includes ensuring that bathing, dressing, eating, and toileting are adequately maintained. If it is necessary for the nurse to encourage the client to undertake self-care, or if assistance in self-care becomes necessary, then the nurse's attitude and actions will preserve the client's self-esteem and dignity.

It is important for a nurse who begins working on a unit with psychotic clients to know the procedures and safety precautions used on the unit when there is a clinical crisis. Knowing how to intervene therapeutically when the client is experiencing hallucinations or delusions is essential information. These periods can be very frightening to the client. The client becomes highly anxious because one aspect of his or her mind is aware of the loss of contact with reality. When a nurse sits quietly, accepting and understanding the client's distress, the client's sense of trust can slowly develop. The nurse will gradually come to understand the cause of the client's emotional distress and can respond to the client's statements about his or her perceptions, thoughts, or feelings in ways that can gently restore a stronger sense of reality.

When caring for a person with psychotic beliefs, it is important not to agree with or in any way enter into the client's misperceptions. Rather, the nurse can repeat the client's statements to show that he or she is being heard. Then, the nurse can clarify reality by telling the client that he or she does not hear the same voices. Reality-based statements by the client can be validated, and the nurse can encourage reality orientation by the nature of questioning used in discussion with the client.

It is especially important to use a family therapy approach with the families of schizophrenic clients. Nurses can sometimes actively participate in this process. The nurse can attend treatment team meetings in which the family patterns are discussed. Regardless of his or her level of involvement, the nurse can become aware of the issues that the client has faced and will continue to face in his or her family. The nurse's interventions should be supportive to the overall family system of which the client is an integral member.

### Evaluation
Evaluation of the nursing intervention should be based on whether there is a decrease in the original symptoms observed in the assessment

process. Evaluation of both short- and long-term goals should be an ongoing process. When revision is indicated, the nursing process should be reinstituted.

### Outpatient Nursing Care

Over the past several years, there has been a trend toward "deinstitutionalization" and increased community-based outpatient care of people with psychiatric disorders, including people with schizophrenia and other psychotic disorders. People with these disorders may be hospitalized for a time. After being stabilized, schizophrenic clients are often released and treated primarily in an outpatient setting.

The basic needs of the outpatient client with schizophrenia—medication, physical safety, and general well being—remain the same as for the inpatient client. However, the very nature of these disorders may make consistent client care difficult to attain, and a client most in need of medication or other care may "fall through the cracks." This reality is reflected in the increasing incidence of people with schizophrenia among the homeless population. Responding to the needs of these clients is an ongoing challenge for the community-based psychiatric nurse (Box 18-1).

## ◆ DELUSIONAL DISORDERS

A firm, fixed system of delusion in an otherwise well-balanced personality characterizes the behavioral pattern in these disorders. This delusional system centers on feelings of persecution and grandiosity. The major areas of activity most frequently involved are those of religion, politics, or another person. The delusional system slowly develops after a false interpretation of an actual occurrence. There are no hallucinations. The client simply becomes convinced that a certain thing or situation is true and will accept no proof, regardless of how convincing it is, that he or she has a wrong concept of the thing or situation.

The types of delusional disorders are as follows:

Erotomanic
Grandiose
Jealous
Persecutory
Somatic
Mixed
Unspecified

In the **erotomanic** disorder, the individual believes that someone, usually of higher status, is in love with him or her. In the **grandiose** type, the person has an inflated sense of self-worth, power, identity, knowledge, or special relationship to a famous person or to God. In the

> ## BOX 18–1.   Family Teaching When a Client Has Schizophrenia
>
> When a family member has schizophrenia, the following recommenda-tions can provide support for the client and give them more confidence in knowing how to support their family member. Family members should be encouraged to call the client's mental health caregiver whenever the client appears to be at risk for harm.
> The family responses that are therapeutic to this client include:
>
> - Assess needs regarding safety, nutrition, hygiene, and other activities of daily living that may change with altered mental state.
> - Review medication compliance.
> - Avoid direct challenge of client's disturbed thoughts.
> - Communicate clearly, simply, and truthfully with client using reality-based language.
> - Avoid statements or behavior that increase agitation in client or provoke potential for violence.
> - Identify disturbed thoughts that family member cannot understand and provide feedback that restores reality and control to client.
> - Identify disturbed behavior and gently clarify expectations.
> - Support change in client's behavior by setting reasonable expectations.
> - Avoid rapid gestures.
> - Use careful judgment in touching the client when he or she is demon-strating disturbed thinking.
> - Encourage client to plan with family around his or her needs and expec-tations during recovery.
> - Support client in seeing mental health care provider and attending groups.
> - Ask client to describe situations that create disturbed thinking.

jealous form, the individual believes incorrectly that his or her sexual partner is unfaithful.

In the **persecutory** type, the person becomes increasingly suspi-cious of people and situations and feels that people are spying on him or her with harmful intentions. The client with a persecutory disorder assumes anything other people are talking about concerns him or her. As this persecution complex enlarges, the client becomes grandiose. This increased sense of self-importance is reflected in statements such as "a foreign government is after me" or "an international ring is pur-suing me."

In the **somatic** type, the individual believes he or she has some physical disease, disorder, or defect. In the mixed type, delusions of the preceding types appear but no one theme predominates. The unspeci-fied type does not fit any of the previous categories, but does have a general delusion that is not grounded in reality.

## NURSING CARE OF CLIENTS WITH DELUSIONAL DISORDERS

The general principles for nursing care of the client with schizophrenia should be employed with the delusional client. Depending on the level and type of delusion, the client can be a risk to himself or herself and to others. The delusions continue until the effects of medication and hospitalization gradually diminish the level of psychosis. Until that time, one of the primary roles of the nurse is to frequently monitor the client and, if indicated, use physical and pharmacologic restraints to ensure his or her safety and that of others.

When institutionalized, a client's suspiciousness often involves food and medications, and persuading him or her to eat or take medications often poses a real problem. The paranoid person is well oriented to person, place, and time, and speaks and acts rationally outside of his or her special delusional system. Thus, the paranoid client is frequently able to convince acquaintances that his or her "idea" is true and may be able to convince a group that he or she is a great reformer, leader, or prophet, until finally the fallacy of the client's claims becomes clearly evident to them and they turn away in disillusionment.

The outstanding symptoms of paranoia are a well-developed delusional system involving feelings of persecution and grandiosity, strong projection, and suspiciousness; there are no hallucinations. These people may become dangerous. So great is their fear of being harmed by others that they may strike out first in self-defense. Therapy has not been especially effective in changing these delusional concepts. Phenothiazine medication, electroconvulsive therapy (ECT), or a combination of the two may be helpful.

## ◆ OTHER PSYCHOTIC DISORDERS

This category includes the following disorders:

Brief psychotic disorder
Schizophreniform disorder
Schizoaffective disorder
Shared-induced psychotic disorder
Atypical psychosis

**Brief psychotic disorder** is a condition that can occur as the result of an acutely stressful episode before which the person functioned normally and had no other type of physical or mental disorder. The person experiences severe emotional distress and one or more of the following signs of psychosis: delusions, hallucinations, loose associations or incoherence, and severely catatonic or disorganized behavior. The symptoms disappear within 1 month, and the individual returns to his or her previous level of functioning.

**Schizophreniform disorder** meets some of the criteria of schizophrenia; however, the condition lasts less than 6 months, disallowing the schizophrenia diagnosis. There are two subclassifications of this type: the first is labeled *with good prognostic features*. These features include no flat affect, good pre-illness social and work role functioning, confusion or perplexity at the height of the psychotic episode, and onset of psychotic symptoms within 4 weeks of the first noted changes in normal behavior or functioning. The second subcategory is *without good prognostic features*. It includes the classic schizophrenia symptoms.

**Schizoaffective disorder** is a condition that manifests a mixture of symptoms of a major depressive episode or a manic episode of bipolar disorder, as well as some of the symptoms that meet the criteria of schizophrenia. There is a history of delusions or hallucinations during the period of the disturbance, but no permanent mood symptoms. The disorder does not meet all the criteria for schizophrenia. It is unknown whether there is an underlying organic cause.

**Shared psychotic disorder** (formerly induced psychotic disorder) is a condition in which a second person takes on a delusion similar to that of another who has a delusional (paranoid) disorder. The affected individual has no prior history of psychosis or schizophrenia.

Psychotic disorder not otherwise specified is a category for those conditions that involve the symptoms of psychosis but do not meet the full range of criteria of the other categories of functional psychotic mental disorders (Boxes 18-2 and 18-3).

## KEY CONCEPTS

■ Schizophrenia, the most prevalent of the functional group of psychoses, is characterized by disturbances of thinking, mood, and behavior.

---

### BOX 18–2. Clinical Vignette

Marissa is a 24-year-old single woman who is homeless. She stays occasionally at a shelter when the weather is bad. One day while walking down the street, Marissa falls down. You are the first person to find her. She is incoherent and tells you in garbled speech that God is going to strike you dead for talking to her. She does not appear to have bathed or washed her hair in several days. There is an odor of acetone on her breath, indicating that she has not had proper nutrition for several days. Her eyes are looking wildly about and her manner is threatening.

Before taking action, what are your initial considerations?

---

BOX 18–3. **Nursing Diagnoses Associated With Clinical Vignette**

**THOUGHT PROCESSES, ALTERED**
**Definition:** A state in which an individual experiences a disruption in such mental activities as conscious thought, reality orientation, problem solving, judgment, and comprehension related to coping, personality, and/or mental disorder.

Related Nursing Diagnosis: Altered thought processes as evidenced by disorientation and confusion related to statement "God will strike you dead if you talk to me."

**INSTRUMENTAL SELF-CARE DEFICIT**
**Definition:** The state in which the individual experiences an impaired ability to perform certain activities or access services essential for managing a household.

Related Nursing Diagnosis: Instrumental Self-Care Deficit related to inability to provide personal hygiene and nutrition to self as evidenced by personal hygiene, neglect, and odor of acetone on breath.

**VIOLENCE, RISK FOR**
**Definition:** A state in which an individual has been, or is at risk to be, assaultive toward others in environment.

Related Nursing Diagnosis: Risk for Violence related to mental confusion as evidenced by wild look in eye and threatening manner.

---

■ A person's basic personality is the predisposing factor as to which form of psychosis he or she will develop. Repeated incidences of psychosis in a person's life tend to follow the same behavioral pattern each time.

■ Current biomedical research links brain chemistry (especially the neurotransmitter dopamine) and the development of schizophrenia. According to current psychoanalytic theory, persons with schizophrenia were deprived of meaningful relationships with important members of the family circle in childhood.

■ The main symptoms of schizophrenia are thought disorder, fragmented speech, autism, inappropriate or absent emotional affect, withdrawal, regression, delusion, and hallucination.

■ Major subtypes of schizophrenia and their characteristics are as follows: catatonic (stupor, rigidity, unorganized or impulsive behavior); disorganized (inappropriate emotions, withdrawal, delusions); and paranoid (suspiciousness, projection, delusions of persecution).

■ Effective nursing care of clients with schizophrenia includes consistency of caregiver; a calm, nonthreatening communication style;

intervention to ensure client safety; listening to client's statements without validating misperceptions; and basing evaluation on the observable decrease in symptoms.

■ Delusional disorders are characterized by a firm, fixed system of delusion in an otherwise well-balanced personality. Major types of delusional disorders are erotomanic, grandiose, jealous, persecutory, and somatic.

■ Shared psychotic disorder is when a second person takes on a delusion similar to that of another person who has a delusional disorder.

## SELF-AWARENESS ACTIVITY

Schizophrenia and other types of psychotic disorders are often the image we have of "mental illness." In reality, only a small percentage of individuals—less that one half of 1% of the population—actually experience the symptoms of schizophrenia at any given time. These symptoms are manageable in a large majority of clients, provided that they take their medications. The individuals you see with symptoms of schizophrenia may not be taking medication.

- Have you ever thought about which aspect of mental illness behavior in a schizophrenic client feels most threatening to you?

- Is it possible that increasing your knowledge of this mental disorder can diminish your fear?

- What can you do to increase your own sense of safety and control in the following situations?

    —Working on a mental health unit where schizophrenic clients are present

    —Working in an outpatient setting where the individual has a history of schizophrenia, is compliant in taking medications, and currently has a physical illness that requires home care nursing

    —Walking on the street where there is a person who appears to be suffering from delusions

## QUESTIONS

1. The client tells the nurse that all women are "ridioxites." This is most likely an example of
   a. word salad.
   b. a neologism.
   c. a delusion.
   d. a hallucination.

2. When teaching about schizophrenia, the best description of delusions the nurse could give is that they are
   a. altered sensory perceptions.
   b. fixed false beliefs.
   c. a lack of orderly thought processes.
   d. inappropriate responses to situations.
3. Sharon, a client with schizophrenia, reports to the nurse that she is unable to sleep because she heard someone yelling her name. The best response by the nurse is:
   a. "That's not possible, I've been here all night and not heard anything."
   b. "Was it a man or a woman calling your name?"
   c. "That must be frightening, but I've not heard anything tonight."
   d. "You need to take this sleeping pill to help you sleep."
4. The client with paranoid schizophrenia would likely demonstrate which of the following traits?
   a. Loose associations.
   b. Grossly disorganized behavior.
   c. Describing unconfirmed harassment.
   d. Inappropriate affect.

---

**BOX 18–4. Web Resources**

*http://www.nami.org*
Sponsored by the National Alliance for the Mentally Ill, a nonprofit organization. Provides education and information on mental illness and treatment, as well as resources and advocacy support for the client or significant others.

*http://www.nimh.nih.gov/publicat/schizmenu.cfm*
Sponsored by the National Institutes of Health. Provides general information, publications, and links to other government agencies and programs.

*http://www.mentalhelp.net*
Provides information about common psychiatric disorders and treatments, as well as professional resources. Offers links to support groups and other online resources.

## BIBLIOGRAPHY

Barry, P.D. (1996). *Psychosocial nursing: Care of physically ill patients and their families* (3rd ed.). Philadelphia: Lippincott-Raven.

Boyd, M., & Nihart, M. (1998). *Psychiatric nursing: Contemporary practice.* Philadelphia: Lippincott Williams & Wilkins.

Carpenito, L.J. (2000). *Nursing diagnosis: Application to clinical practice* (8th ed.). Philadelphia: Lippincott Williams & Wilkins.

*Diagnostic and statistical manual of mental disorders* (4th ed.). (1994). Washington, D.C.: American Psychiatric Press.

Goff, D., Henderson, D., & Manschreck, T. (1997). Psychotic patients. In N.H. Cassem (Ed.). *Massachusetts General Hospital handbook of general hospital psychiatry* (4th ed.). St. Louis: Mosby–Year Book.

Sadock, B., & Kaplan, H. (1998). *Synopsis of psychiatry: Behavioral sciences/clinical psychiatry.* Philadelphia: Lippincott Williams & Wilkins.

Tomb, D. (1998). *Psychiatry.* Philadelphia: Lippincott Williams & Wilkins.

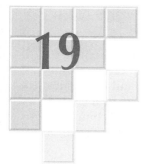

# 19

# The Client Who Is Contemplating Suicide

---

## B e h a v i o r a l    O b j e c t i v e s

*After reading*
*this chapter*
*the student*
*will be able to:*

■ Define suicide.
■ Describe the relationship between a no-suicide contract and the least restrictive environment for a client contemplating suicide.
■ Identify the risk factors for suicide.
■ Identify therapeutic services available in the hospital setting to a client contemplating suicide.
■ Name four nursing diagnoses related to clients contemplating suicide.

---

## K e y    T e r m s

■ Dysphoria
■ Informed consent
■ Involuntary hospitalization
■ Least restrictive environment
■ No-suicide contract

■ Suicidal ideation
■ Suicidal plan
■ Suicide
■ Suicide prevention
■ Suicide risk
■ Voluntary hospitalization

The client who is contemplating suicide presents a psychiatric emergency. **Suicide** is the conscious choice of a personal action to kill oneself. Approximately 30,000 people die each year because of suicide. It is estimated that nearly 8 to 10 times that number attempt suicide and do not complete their attempts. These statistics do not include several groups of individuals, such as those who are the victims of accidental deaths that were premeditated suicides. Another group of people are those who die because of the chronic effects of alcohol and other substances of abuse. Yet another group of individuals who can be included in this group are persons with chronic illness who are noncompliant with their medical care. These persons have medical conditions such as diabetes, obesity, and hypertension.

## ◆ CLINICAL ISSUES ASSOCIATED WITH RISK OF COMPLETED SUICIDE

**Suicide risk** is the assessment of the presence of specific factors that make a person more vulnerable to death by suicide. These factors have been identified in research on the lives and life circumstances of individuals who have completed suicides. The factors that increase the possibility of suicide are shown in Box 19-1.

These factors have been found to be associated with individuals who have completed suicide. They provide important assessment cues to evaluate suicide risk. If the nurse is working with a person who is contemplating suicide, this observation should be reported immediately to the nursing supervisor. If in the inpatient setting, the client's therapist should be called to meet with the client. If the nurse is in the outpatient setting, it is important to ask a series of questions that indicate the suicidal risk of the client. The questions are shown in Box 19-2.

Many times the nurse fears that by asking these types of questions, he or she may put the idea of suicide into someone's head. When the questions are asked sensitively, it can be a relief for a client to talk about his or her discouragement. If the client acknowledges that suicide is an option he or she is considering, then questions should be developed based on the following risk factors to determine how at risk the client is for committing suicide. **Suicide prevention** is the therapeutic process initiated when a client indicates one or more of the risk factors outlined above that indicate a risk for suicide.

---

BOX 19-1. **Factors That Contribute to Incidence of Suicide**

| | |
|---|---|
| Sex | Children |
| Type of method | Occupation |
| Age | Climate |
| Race | Physical health |
| Religion | Mental health |
| Marital status | History of prior suicide attempt |

BOX 19-2. **Assessment of Suicidal Episode**

**INTENT TO DIE**
1. Have you been thinking about hurting or killing yourself?
2. How seriously do you want to die?
3. Are there people or things in your life that might keep you from killing yourself?

**SEVERITY OF IDEATION**
1. How often do you have these thoughts?
2. How long do they last?
3. Can you dismiss them or do they tend to come back over and over?
4. How much do the thoughts distress you?

**DEGREE OF PLANNING**
1. Have you made any plans to kill yourself. If yes, what are they?
2. How likely is it that you could actually carry out the plan?
3. Have you done anything to put the plan into action?
4. Could you stop yourself from killing yourself?

From Boyd, M., & Nihart, M. (1998). *Psychiatric nursing: Contemporary practice.* Philadelphia: Lippincott-Raven.

**Suicidal ideation** is the experience of having unwanted, fleeting, and intrusive thoughts of being dead or wanting to be dead. Suicidal ideation may or may not be accompanied by a suicidal plan. A **suicidal plan** is a vision of how one would attempt suicide, that is, what means would be used to kill oneself, such as with pills, a gun, and so on. Individuals with suicidal ideation without a plan can be at high risk for suicide. A person with a suicidal plan is considered to be at very high risk. In either instance, a mental health professional should be consulted whenever an individual is at risk for suicide.

It is important that the nurse's supervisor be told immediately about the results of the nursing assessment of suicidal risk. Depending on the clinical judgment of the nursing supervisor, hospital admission may be recommended in order to safeguard the client's life. Obtaining a no-suicide contract helps to determine the least-restrictive environment for the client. A **no-suicide contract** is a written or verbal agreement between a mental health professional and a client in which the client agrees that he or she will not engage in suicidal behavior for a specified period of time. The **least restrictive environment** is the health care setting that provides the most therapeutic and safe environment for the client.

If hospitalization is recommended, then the client is told about his or her voluntary choice to be admitted to the hospital. This discussion supports the client's civil rights. **Informed consent** occurs when the client hears about his or her choices for treatment and decides to be admitted to the hospital. A client's decision to enter the hospital for treatment is called **voluntary hospitalization.** A client may resist hospitalization, yet caregivers believe that the client's safety and ultimate survival is dependent on being admitted to an inpatient hospital unit. In this situation health care professionals may seek a legal order for **involuntary hospitalization.**

## ◆ RISK FACTORS FOR SUICIDE

One of the factors that is very important to assess and is not included in this list of assessment factors is the *history of a recent significant loss.* This loss can be the loss of a partner or job, a professional failure, and so on. It is important to ask whether the individual has experienced a significant loss. If the answer is yes, the nurse should take the time to examine the meaning of this loss to the client.

### SEX
Men are three times more likely than women to commit suicide. Women are four times more likely than men to attempt suicide.

### TYPES OF METHODS
The type of method a person chooses and uses in a suicide attempt is an important indication of the seriousness of the intention of the suicidal person. Men are more likely to complete suicide because of the methods they choose, including firearms, hanging, and jumping from high places. Other methods, although less lethal, are effective. The intention of the person to complete his or her suicide attempt is the most critical factor.

### AGE
The most rapidly increasing age range of suicides is in men aged 15 to 24. Suicide is the third leading cause of deaths in men of this age group, following accidents and homicides. It is estimated that the number of attempted suicides in men aged 15 to 24 is 1 to 2 million annually. The suicide rates in women of the same age are also increasing, but less rapidly than in men. The suicide rates of men aged 25 to 34 increased almost 30% in the past decade. In men, the peak of suicide rates occurs after age 45. In women, suicide rates increase after age 55. The highest incidence of suicides is in men older than 65. Older people attempt suicide less often than younger people, but are more likely to complete the suicide. The completed suicide rate for people older than 75 is three times higher than all other age groups. Although people older than 65 encompass only 10% of the population, they comprise 25% of all suicides.

## RACE

White men constitute two of every three suicides. White men commit suicide at a rate that is 1.6 times that of black men. The incidence of suicide in black men is rising, however. The suicide rate of white men is four times that of white women and eight times that of black women. Young people who live in the inner city are far more likely to commit suicide. Young Native Americans and Inuit Eskimos are also at higher risk for suicide. Suicide rates for immigrants are also significantly higher than for native-born individuals.

## RELIGION

It is important to obtain answers about the meaning and integration of religion into a person's life in order to assess the impact of religion on suicidal risk. These factors can be more important in deterring suicide than religious affiliation. Roman Catholics have traditionally had lower rates of suicides compared with Protestants and Jews.

## MARITAL STATUS

Marriage and the presence of children are important suicide deterrents. The incidence of suicide in married persons is 11 per 100,000, significantly less than for those who are single, widowed, or divorced. Single people who have never married have a rate that is nearly double that of married persons. Socially isolated people also have a higher incidence of suicide than those who are more socially involved with others. Widowed persons have a rate that is slightly more than double that of married persons. Divorced persons have a rate that is nearly four times higher than married persons. The incidence of divorced men who commit suicide is 69 per 100,000 compared with 18 per 100,000 for divorced women.

## HISTORY OF SUICIDE IN FAMILY

The person who has a history of suicide in his or her family has a significantly higher risk of suicide than a person without such a history. Another risk factor to be assessed in a person contemplating suicide is the anniversary date or dates of family members who have committed suicide.

## OCCUPATION

Professional persons and individuals with above-average social status and incomes are at higher risk than others. The presence of full-time work is a deterrent to suicide. Unemployment presents a higher suicide risk. At-risk occupational groups include physicians, with psychiatrists carrying the highest risk; musicians, dentists, law enforcement officers, lawyers, and insurance agents. Times of economic recession and depression show higher rates of suicide.

## CLIMATE

Suicide rates are higher in temperate climates. It is theorized that these climates have fewer hours of sunlight in the fall and winter months and may have a higher incidence of seasonal affective disorder (SAD), a condition that results in increased levels of depression and **dysphoria,** defined as a depressed, disquieted, and restless mood.

## PHYSICAL HEALTH

The presence of a chronic health condition has been found to be a factor in people who commit suicide. Persons with a history of alcohol dependence and concurrent physical health problems related to alcoholism have a higher rate of suicide. Persons, both men and women, with cancer of the genitals, as well as women with breast cancer, have higher rates of suicide. Health-related factors in suicide risk include loss of mobility, especially when related to occupation or recreation; disfigurement, especially among women; and chronic, intractable pain.

## MENTAL HEALTH

Close to 95% of individuals who commit suicide have a psychiatric disorder at the time they commit suicide. Eighty percent of these persons have a depressive disorder. Ten percent of persons with a psychiatric disorder who commit suicide are schizophrenic.

## PRIOR SUICIDE ATTEMPT

Nearly 40% of all individuals who attempt suicide have attempted suicide previously. The risk of a second attempt is highest within 3 months of the initial attempt.

The following boxes provide additional information regarding assessment of suicidal risk factors. Box 19-3 shows the risk groups for completed suicides, and Box 19-4 describes the questions to be asked in assessing the warning signs of suicide.

## ◆ TREATMENT FOR SUICIDAL IDEATION, PLAN, OR ATTEMPT

Ideally, a person with suicidal ideation or a suicidal plan will make a no-suicide contract with his or her mental health professional. When such a contract is made and the client is viewed as reliable, then the person can remain at home, provided that 24-hour social support is available in the home and the health professional is available on a 24-hour basis (see Boxes 19-5 and 19-6). If client assessment indicates a necessity for inpatient hospitalization, then the following therapeutic services will be available:

- Overview of antidepressant and/or antipsychotic medication effectiveness

BOX 19-3. **Risk Groups for Completed Suicide**

Older, single, divorced, or widowed males
Caucasians
Protestants
Unemployed people
People in poor physical health
People living alone
People with an anniversary of death or loss
People with sudden changes in life situation
People who leave suicide notes
Older homosexual men

BOX 19-4. **Questions That Determine the Warning Signs of Suicide**

**THE FOLLOWING MUST BE LEARNED ABOUT *ALL*
SUICIDAL PATIENTS:**
1. The patient's intention—Why does he or she want to die?
2. Is a suicide plan made?—The more specific plan, the more likely the act.
3. Method—The more lethal the technique, the more serious the plan.
4. Presence of psychiatric or organic factors, e.g., psychotic depression, thought disorder, sedative self-medication, organicity.
5. Determine the role of impulsivity versus premeditation.
6. Is the precipitating crisis resolving?
7. Take an "inventory of loss."
8. Does the patient have plans for the future?
9. Does the patient have caring family or other supports?
10. Does the patient think he or she is going to commit suicide?

- 24-hour observation
- Individual psychotherapy
- Group therapy
- Family therapy

## ◆ NURSING DIAGNOSIS CATEGORIES RELATED TO CLIENT WHO IS CONTEMPLATING SUICIDE

Risk for Self-Harm
Risk for Self-Abuse
Risk for Self-Mutilation
Risk for Suicide

## BOX 19-5. Nursing Interventions With the Person Who Is Contemplating Suicide

- Immediately inform the patient's primary health care provider about the patient's risk for suicide.
- Psychiatric consultation is recommended to confirm lethality and plan for safety and therapeutic intervention.
- A patient with an immediate, lethal, and precise suicide plan needs strict safety precautions such as hospitalization or continuous or close supervision.
- If in the home care setting, call 911 if there is no other assistance available and the person appears to be at high risk for suicide.
- The patient in the general hospital or outpatient setting should be observed constantly, one-to-one, with eye contact, and not allowed to leave the room without constant supervision until the patient's therapist, the mental health consultant, or the nursing supervisor arrives.
- The low-suicide-risk patient should not be underestimated. If circumstances change, risk could change.
- Document the patient's behavior and verbatim statements as well as the time and date the provider was notified. If the provider is not responsive to the nurse's report of the patient's suicidal ideation, it is important to maintain observation and continue to pursue psychiatric consultation.
- The legal responsibility for an attempted or completed suicide, at least partially, belongs to the nurse on duty at the time.
- A written and signed no-suicide contract, ensuring a safe environment, reducing symptoms, increasing social support, encouraging a plan for living, and providing referrals are important nursing interventions. A no-suicide (or no-harm) contract may be ineffective with impulsive people or manipulative and/or angry patients who lack a therapeutic relationship with the provider.
- Members of some cultural groups may be uncomfortable with the formality of signing a contract with a health care provider.
- Transfer to a psychiatric unit can best ensure safety.
- Issues around voluntary or involuntary hospital admission are the responsibility of the nursing or psychiatric supervisor.
- If the patient must remain on a medical or surgical unit, specific nursing care recommendations should be obtained from the psychiatric or psychiatric nursing consultant.
- It is necessary to assess suicide potential continuously by observing impulse control, suicidal ideation and intent, behavior changes, emotional state, physical complaints, the patient's response to observation, and safety needs. These observations should be documented on a regularly scheduled basis.

> ## BOX 19-6. Family Teaching When a Client Is Contemplating Suicide
>
> When a family member is contemplating suicide, the following recommendations can provide support for the client and give the family more confidence in knowing how to support their family member. Family members should be encouraged to call the client's mental health caregiver whenever the client appears to be at risk for harm.
> The family responses that are therapeutic to this client include:
>
> * Obtaining recommendations from nursing staff during discharge planning about:
>   —Current lethality of client's suicidal thinking at time of discharge
>   —Immediate community resources and options if family member becomes concerned that suicidal risk increases and becomes acute when client is at home
> * In immediate postdischarge period:
>   —Providing environment that includes the presence of a family member or other companion for the first few post-discharge days
>   —Asking client to identify triggers for suicidal thoughts
>   —Asking client how he or she is feeling at intervals during the day
>   —Inquiring if client is having current thoughts of self-harm at intervals during the day
>   —If answer is yes, assessing if the client believes that he or she is prepared to follow through with the plan
>   —If answer is yes, preparing to implement the plans recommended by the staff during discharge planning
> * Providing therapeutic environment, following recommendations in Chapter 15, The Client with a Mood Disorder
> * Encouraging client to plan with family around his or her needs and expectations during recovery
> * Supporting client in seeing mental health care provider and attending groups
> * Reviewing medication compliance

Other nursing diagnoses may be applicable following assessment (see Boxes 19-7, 19-8, and 19-9). These nursing diagnoses and their related diagnostic information are available in Carpenito, L. (2000). *Nursing diagnosis: Application to clinical practice* (8th ed.). Philadelphia: Lippincott Williams & Wilkins.

## KEY POINTS

■ A client contemplating suicide is a psychiatric emergency.

BOX 19-7. **Clinical Vignette**

Ana is a 19-year-old college student from Malaysia. Before arriving in the United States to attend college, she had never been away from home. Ana's younger brother was seriously injured in a fire 2 months ago. Ana has been preoccupied with thoughts of him and his physical pain. Ana's roommate has been increasingly concerned about her because she has recently been withdrawn, missing about half of her classes, not eating, and appearing thin. She spends much of her time in her room and is sleeping 14 or 15 hours per day. When her roommate expresses concern about her lack of eating, excessive sleeping, and missing classes, Ana says that nothing matters. When registration occurred for the upcoming semester, Ana said that she wouldn't be around to go to classes.

If you were Ana's roommate, what would you do?

■ Suicide risk is the assessment of the presence of specific factors that make a person more vulnerable to death by suicide.
■ Signing a no-suicide contract can allow a client to stay in the least restrictive environment and still be safe from a suicide attempt.
■ Risk factors for suicide include history of recent significant loss, sex, types of methods, age, race, religion, marital status, history of suicide in family, occupation, climate, physical health, mental health, and prior suicide attempt.
■ Treatment available in the hospital setting to a client contemplating suicide includes overview of medications and effectiveness, 24-hour observation, individual psychotherapy, and group and family therapy.
■ Possible nursing diagnoses for clients contemplating suicide are Risk for Self-Harm, Risk for Self-Abuse, Risk for Self-Mutilation, and Risk for Suicide.

## SELF-AWARENESS ACTIVITY

• Suicide is a serious subject. Many people are uncomfortable talking about suicide. What was it like to read this chapter?
• What feelings did you experience as you read this chapter?
• Over the course of their lives, many people experience occasional periods of thought about death. Has this ever happened to you? What triggered these thoughts? Did you tell anyone about your experience?

BOX 19-8. **Nursing Diagnoses Associated with Clinical Vignette**

**RISK FOR SELF-HARM**

**Definition**
A state in which an individual is at risk for inflicting direct harm on one-self. This may include one or more of the following: self-abuse, self-mutilation, and suicide.

**Related Nursing Diagnosis**
Risk for Self-Harm related to feelings of helplessness about brother's injury as evidenced by statement "I won't be around to take courses next semester."

**INSTRUMENTAL SELF-CARE DEFICIT**

**Definition**
The state in which the individual experiences an impaired ability to perform certain activities or access services essential for managing a household.

**Related Nursing Diagnosis**
Instrumental Self-Care Deficit related to altered nutritional status as evidenced by lack of eating and loss of weight.

**COPING, INEFFECTIVE INDIVIDUAL**

**Definition**
A state in which the individual experiences, or is at risk to experience, an inability to manage internal or environmental stressors adequately because of inadequate resources (physical, psychological, behavioral, and/or cognitive).

**Related Nursing Diagnosis**
Ineffective Individual Coping related to separation from home and family and recent serious injury of brother as evidenced by statement "I won't be around to take courses next semester," social isolation, and lack of adequate nutrition.

- As you were reading the recommendations about questions to ask a client who may be at suicidal risk if you are working by yourself with no other health professional available, were you able to imagine yourself asking these questions? How would you feel if you found that a person was actively thinking about suicide?

## QUESTIONS

1. Which of the following clients would likely present the highest suicide potential?

> BOX 19-9. **Web Resources**
>
> *http://www.cdc.gov/safeusa/suicide.htm*
> Sponsored by the Centers for Disease Control. Provides general information about suicide and links to additional resources.
> *http://www.mentalhelp.net*
> Provides information about common psychiatric disorders and treatments, as well as professional resources. Offers links to support groups and other online resources.
> *http://www.nimh.nih.gov/research/suicide.htm*
> Sponsored by the National Institutes of Health. Provides general information, publications, and links to other government agencies and programs.

    a. A 55-year-old never-married woman, with poorly controlled diabetes and few friends

    b. A 60-year-old man, healthy and married with children and grandchildren nearby

    c. A 27-year-old woman, married with two children, employed part-time

    d. A 40-year-old woman, never married, with several friends and close relationships

2. The nurse is conversing with a client who says, "Sometimes I think it would be nice just to go to sleep and never wake up." The best initial response by the nurse would be to

    a. ignore the comment and divert the client's attention to another topic.

    b. say to the client, "Some days are like that, aren't they?"

    c. ask the client if he or she has thoughts about suicide.

    d. ask the client, "Why do you think that way?"

3. The nurse asks a depressed client the following questions. Which question, if answered in the affirmative, would lead the nurse to further evaluate the client for suicidal ideations?

    a. "Are you actively involved in a religious organization?"

    b. "Have you recently experienced any personal or professional losses?'"

    c. "Do you have children?"

    d. "Do you have close friends with whom you spend time?"

4. If an outpatient client admits to having suicidal ideations, the best initial action of the nurse is to

    a. notify the police, so the client can be placed in protective custody.

    b. obtain a no-harm contract from the client and notify a nursing supervisor.

c. tell the client not to do anything dangerous and notify the psychiatrist.

d. tell the client that if he or she promises not to do anything harmful, no hospitalization will be necessary.

## BIBLIOGRAPHY

Boyd, M., & Nihart, M. (1998). *Psychiatric nursing: Contemporary practice.* Philadelphia: Lippincott-Raven.

Carpenito, L.J. (2000). *Nursing diagnosis: Application to clinical practice* (8th ed.). Philadelphia: Lippincott Williams & Wilkins.

Conwell, Y., Duberstein, P., & Cox, C., et al. (1996). Relationship of age and Axis I diagnoses in victims of completed suicides: A psychological autopsy study. *American Journal of Psychiatry, 153*(8), 1001–1008.

*Diagnostic and statistical manual of mental disorders* (4th ed.). (1994). Washington, D.C.: American Psychiatric Press.

Sadock, B., & Kaplan, H. (1998). *Synopsis of psychiatry: Behavioral sciences/clinical psychiatry.* Philadelphia: Lippincott-Raven.

Valente, S. (1993). Evaluating suicide risk in the medically ill patient. *Nurse Practitioner, 18,* 42–43.

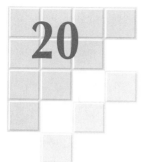

# The Client With a Substance-Related Mental Disorder

## 20

—Hallucinogen        —Sedative, hypnotic, or
—Inhalant            anxiolytic
—Nicotine          —Polysubstance abuse
—Opioid              ■ Substance abuse
—Phencyclidine (PCP) or   ■ Substance dependence
    similarly acting        ■ Substance-related disorder
    arylcyclohexylamine    ■ Withdrawal sickness

The diagnosis **substance-related disorder** is now used in place of psychoactive substance-use disorder and the term *drug addiction*. It is used for clients whose mental states are altered by alcohol, drugs, tobacco, and ordinary caffeine-containing beverages. Included are changes in mental status caused by the side effects of medically prescribed drugs taken as medically indicated.

This chapter includes information on the behavioral aspects of the maladaptive use of substances. The changes in mental status caused by such use are described in Chapter 17: The Client With Delirium, Dementia, Alzheimer's, and Other Cognitive Disorders.

There are 12 major categories of substances that are abused under this classification:

Alcohol
Amphetamine or similarly acting sympathomimetic
Caffeine
Cannabis
Cocaine
Hallucinogen
Inhalant
Nicotine
Opioid
Phencyclidine (PCP) or similarly acting arylcyclohexylamine
Sedative, hypnotic, or anxiolytic
Polysubstance abuse

The classification also includes other substance-related disorders, such as changes in mental state caused by side effects of medications prescribed for medical conditions.

## ◆ ETIOLOGIC FACTORS IN SUBSTANCE USE

There are many factors that play a role in the development of substance use. Accordingly, the use of a holistic framework is important when considering appropriate nursing approaches. Figure 20-1 shows the

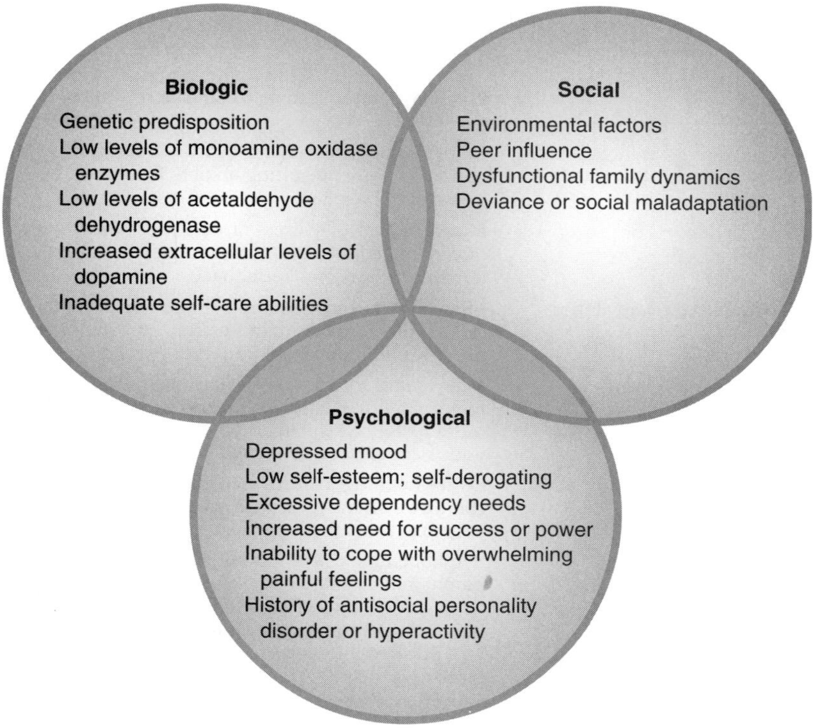

FIGURE 20–1. Biopsychosocial etiologies for patients with substance abuse. (Boyd, M.A., & Nihart, M. A. [1998]. *Psychiatric nursing: Contemporary practice.* Philadelphia: Lippincott Williams & Wilkins.

different biological, psychological, and family/social factors that contribute to the development of substance use disorders.

Table 20-1 further clarifies the psychological issues that research has found to be contributing factors to substance use disorders.

## ◆ SUBSTANCE USE DISORDERS

### SUBSTANCE DEPENDENCE AND SUBSTANCE ABUSE

The diagnostic criteria for each of these disorders fall under two terms: substance dependence and substance abuse.

**Substance dependence** describes a condition in which the individual's symptoms (listed later) have persisted for at least 1 month or occurred at the same time in the same 12-month period. The individual must manifest three of the following symptoms:

## TABLE 20–1. **Psychological issues Leading to Substance Abuse**

| Issue | Psychodynamics Leading to Substance Abuse |
| --- | --- |
| Excessive dependence needs | Excessive dependency needs lead to rejection and a sense of failure. Resulting anxiety is relieved by substance abuse. |
| Need for success or power | Excessive fear of success or failure or appearing weak or challenged. Substance abuse can provide temporary illusion of adequacy and power. |
| Inadequate self-care abilities | Individual has inadequate abilities to self-regulate or self-soothe, or has low self-esteem. Substance abuse provides temporary resolution of psychological pain. |
| Gender identity issues | Males more socialized to externalize stress and feelings by drinking alcohol and using drugs. Women more socialized to "treat" feelings of low self-esteem with alcohol or other drugs. |
| Affect intolerance | Overwhelming, painful feelings from childhood that cannot be tolerated or discussed. Individual may be able to express these feelings when intoxicated. |
| Family systems | Symbolic fusion with parent, failure to separate from parent and develop own self-identity during adolescence can lead to a too rigid or too flexible bonding with substance-abusing peers, leaving individual vulnerable to peer pressure to drink and use drugs. |

From Boyd, M., & Nihart, M. (1998). *Psychiatric nursing: Contemporary practice.* Philadelphia: Lippincott Williams & Wilkins.

1. Tolerance: as defined by either:
   a. Need for markedly increased amounts of the substance to achieve intoxication or desired effect
   b. Markedly diminished effect with continued use of the same amount of the substance
2. Withdrawal, as manifested by either:
   a. Characteristic withdrawal syndrome for the substance
   b. The same (or a closely related) substance is taken to relieve or avoid withdrawal symptoms
3. The substance is often taken in larger amounts or over a longer period than was intended.
4. There is a pattern of persistent desire or unsuccessful efforts to cut down or control substance use.
5. A great deal of time is spent in activities necessary to obtain the substance, use the substance, or recover from its effects.
6. Important social, occupational, or recreational activities are given up or reduced because of substance use.

7. The substance use is continued despite knowledge of having a persistent or recurrent physical or psychological problem that is likely to have been caused or exacerbated by the substance.*

Psychoactive **substance abuse** is a maladaptive pattern of substance use leading to clinically significant impairment or distress, as manifested by one (or more) of the following, occurring within a 12-month period.

1. Recurrent substance use resulting in a failure to fulfill major role obligations at work, school, or home
2. Recurrent substance use in situations in which it is physically hazardous
3. Recurrent substance-related legal problems
4. Continued substance use despite having persistent or recurrent social or interpersonal problems caused or exacerbated by the effects of the substance.†

## ◆ ALCOHOL-RELATED DISORDERS

Alcohol use disorder includes the two categories of substance abuse and substance dependence. The criteria for alcohol substance abuse follow:

1. A pattern of pathologic alcohol use is noted.
   a. Daily use of alcohol is necessary to function.
   b. Person is unable to cut down or stop drinking.
   c. Binges last longer than 2 days.
   d. Person occasionally consumes as much as a fifth of liquor per day.
   e. Amnesia occurs during periods of intoxication (blackouts).
2. Social or occupational functioning is impaired.
3. Disturbance lasts longer than 1 month.

Alcohol dependence includes either a pattern of pathologic alcohol use or impairment in social or occupational functioning. In addition, there is evidence of tolerance or withdrawal symptoms as well as continued use despite knowledge that alcohol consumption causes or worsens a physical or psychological problem.

### TREATMENT APPROACHES TO ALCOHOLISM
The client's body must be detoxified of alcohol before treatment can begin. With the physiologic dependency that results from alcoholism,

---

*Adapted from *Desk reference to the diagnostic criteria from DSM-IV.* (1994). Washington, D.C.: American Psychiatric Association, pp. 108–109.
†Adapted from *Desk reference to the diagnostic criteria from DSM-IV.* (1994). Washington, D.C.: American Psychiatric Association, p. 112.

detoxification usually must be medically supervised to ensure the client's physical and mental well being. This most frequently takes place in a general hospital medical-surgical setting or in an alcohol rehabilitation center, not on a general psychiatric unit. Refer to any standard text on alcoholism treatment for specific information about the treatment and nursing care of this complex physiologic condition. Once detoxification is completed, three major treatment options are most frequently presented to recovering alcoholics—Alcoholics Anonymous, aversive therapy with disulfiram (Antabuse), or an inpatient rehabilitation treatment program.

### Alcoholics Anonymous

Alcoholics Anonymous (AA) is a peer-support, self-help program that has helped millions of recovering alcoholics achieve a life of sobriety. Two recovering alcoholics who banded together to help each other began AA in 1935. They were Bill Wilson, a stockbroker, and Bob Smith, a physician. By supporting each other as peers, they were able to remain sober. Wilson and Smith decided to share this support with others and developed a series of steps to help the alcoholic recover. In this way AA was founded.

Alcoholics Anonymous is an organization that exists worldwide and is readily available in most communities. Its simple, free approach has brought hope to millions of alcoholics and their families. Alcoholics Anonymous has also developed a related organization for the families of alcoholics called Al-Anon. There is also a group available for adolescent children of alcoholics called Alateen.

### Antabuse

Disulfiram or Antabuse therapy is considered a useful adjunct treatment for some types of alcoholics. It is a form of behavior therapy that uses learning principles to cause the client to associate the thought of drinking with an unpleasant stimulus; in this way the client can be motivated to avoid drinking.

Disulfiram (Antabuse) is a drug that causes the metabolism of alcohol to be blocked. The result is a buildup of acetaldehyde, which is a toxic byproduct of alcohol metabolism in the body. Acetaldehyde produces a variety of very unpleasant physical symptoms, such as flushing, sweating, palpitations, dyspnea, hyperventilation, tachycardia, hypotension, nausea, and vomiting.

The body's reaction to even a small amount of alcohol can be violent and, indeed, can be physiologically threatening to the body's homeostasis. Accordingly, this treatment should be used only with a compliant, motivated individual in order to avoid serious complications.

## Inpatient Treatment Programs

Some people with alcoholism and other types of substance-related disorders need more structure in their return to sobriety. A treatment program that has met with increasing success is an inpatient treatment approach in which a therapeutic environment is used (see Chapter 26, Milieu Therapy and Behavior Modification). In many institutions, alcohol and drug abuse clients are treated in the same setting. Following the detoxification period, there is intensive emphasis on individual, group, and family therapy. Counselors in the individual and group therapy sessions frequently are recovered substance abusers. Many of these programs include intensive education and behavior modification to teach new coping skills to these individuals who have previously turned to alcohol because of their inability to cope. The major emphasis of this teaching is on communication skills and stress management.

## Outpatient Treatment Programs

Outpatient treatment programs are increasingly an option for treating alcohol use disorders. After the detoxification period, which usually occurs in the inpatient setting, individuals follow the therapeutic and coping-skills focus outlined in the preceding, but this treatment takes place in an outpatient setting, generally with the client returning to his or her home in the evening.

## NURSING CARE OF CLIENTS WITH ALCOHOLISM

Nursing care planning includes prioritizing the areas of functioning that are most threatening to the client's physical or mental well being. For example, during episodes of acute cognitive disorder, such as intoxication, withdrawal, or withdrawal delirium, it is important to follow the guidelines presented under the nursing care of clients with delirium in Chapter 17, The Client With Delirium, Dementia, Alzheimer's, and Other Cognitive Disorders.

Treatment with the benzodiazepines (minor tranquilizers) or barbiturates is effective in managing the life-threatening and distressing effects of alcohol withdrawal during detoxification. If the drug is administered and its effects are monitored and balanced carefully, the nurse can maintain the client in a calm and wakeful state. The sedative usually needs to be administered over a 24- to 48-hour period and is reduced to smaller doses over 2 to 3 days until it is discontinued.

One of the important nursing functions is maintenance of adequate fluid and nutritional needs. The client, because of nutritional deprivation, usually has inadequate electrolyte and vitamin levels.

Once the acute detoxification stage is over, the client's mid- and long-term needs should be more actively addressed in the nursing care plan. Alcoholic people are at risk for many types of dysfunction. Evaluation of the potential risks in the following list is an essential part of assessing the client and planning nursing intervention. Nursing care planning, including counseling and preventive teaching, increases in importance when there are positive findings in any of the areas described in the following:

Physical state
—Increased susceptibility to infection
—Altered nutritional status
—Interference with sleep activity
—Interference with sexual activity
—Impairment of vital organs
—Diminished energy
—Increased risk of accident and injury
—Substantial reduction in lifespan
—Insufficient exercise
Psychosocial state
—Low self-concept
—Feelings of alienation, guilt, depression, anger
—Increased risk of suicide
—Increased consumption of other drugs that interact with alcohol
—Interferences with interpersonal relationships, including family, friends, coworkers
—Lack of creative diversion such as hobbies, recreational activities
—Thwarted personal growth, learning, and maturity
—Delayed development of potential
—Lack of philosophical or spiritual pursuits
Economic state
—Possible loss of job or demotion
—Indebtedness
Legal entanglements
—Increased incidence of arrest for driving while intoxicated or for assaults, including child abuse, spouse battering, and tavern fights
Factors associated with the diagnosis of alcoholism
—Social stigma with regard to alcoholism
—Lack of acceptance of the diagnosis by all involved

## ◆ AMPHETAMINE-RELATED DISORDER

The drugs included in this category of drug disorder are amphetamines, dextroamphetamine sulfate (Dexedrine), methamphetamine, also known as *speed,* and others that have amphetamine-like action, such as methylphenidate or other substances used as appetite suppressants, also known as diet pills. The abuse and dependence subcategories include the symptoms listed previously in this chapter. In addition, there is a frequent drug use pattern of taking the drug for 10 to 14 days at a time.

Amphetamines are frequently used by dieters to treat obesity, students to stay alert and study, truck drivers to stay awake, and soldiers to decrease fatigue and increase aggression. Evidence today suggests that tolerance *does* develop to their use; they produce both dependency and withdrawal states; they are clearly among the most dangerous drugs presently available. In the most mentally stable person, amphetamines are able to produce a toxic psychosis that is clinically indistinguishable from paranoid schizophrenia. Death from overdose is usually associated with elevated temperature (hyperpyrexia), convulsions, and cardiovascular shock. The intravenous use of these drugs since the 1960s has resulted fairly often in cases of severe serum hepatitis, lung abscess, and endocarditis. In 1970, necrotizing angiitis was first reported as a result of intravenous amphetamine abuse. **Necrotizing angiitis** is the destruction of the lining of blood vessels because of a toxic substance.

In most cases, amphetamine-induced psychotic disorder clears in a matter of days or weeks following withdrawal of the drug, differentiating it from paranoid schizophrenia. Antipsychotic agents (phenothiazine or haloperidol) often help. The withdrawal depression, which may reach suicidal proportions, may be treated with tricyclic antidepressants.

## ◆ CANNABIS-RELATED DISORDER

The substances included in this category are marijuana, hashish, and, occasionally, purified delta-9-tetrahydrocannabinol (THC). Marijuana is the most commonly used substance in this category. It has been a subject of controversy since 500 BC in China. During the 19th century, cannabis was widely prescribed for a variety of ailments and discomforts (coughing, fatigue, migraine, asthma, delirium tremens, etc.). It remained in the U.S. *Pharmacopeia* until 1941.

Its ability to cause euphoria has been of principal interest throughout history. The effects last 2 to 4 hours from smoking marijuana and 5 to 12 hours from ingestion of the drug. Marijuana also has a tendency to produce sedation. There is no substantial evidence in the world literature, however, that cannabis induces either mental or physical deterioration, at least not in well-integrated, stable people.

Adverse reactions to cannabis appear to be dose related and depend on the setting in which the drug is used. Although rare, anxiety states, with or without paranoid thinking, panic states, and toxic psychosis have been reported.

An amotivational syndrome has been discussed in association with cannabis use, but careful studies fail to prove that this syndrome does, in fact, follow the use of the drug. It may be a sociocultural phenomenon that happens to coincide with the regular use of marijuana.

# ◆ COCAINE-RELATED DISORDER

This category includes the general symptoms of substance abuse listed previously in the chapter. In addition, during periods of intoxication, there are delusions and hallucinations with an otherwise clear sensorium.

Cocaine is an alkaloid derived from the leaf of the plant *Erythroxylon coca,* a shrub indigenous to Bolivia and Peru. Natives of these countries have chewed its leaves for many years, producing central nervous system stimulation. The "high" is similar to that achieved by amphetamines (ie, euphoria, exhilaration, and a powerful sense of well-being and confidence).

Cocaine abuse is a problem of almost epidemic proportions in our society today. The pattern of cocaine use has altered from snorting the cocaine intranasally to intravenous injection or smoking. The commonly abused form of cocaine has changed to "freebase." Freebase is available in a product called "crack," an inexpensive, very potent, and readily available substance. Crack has significantly increased the number of cocaine abusers. Excitement, euphoria, restlessness, stereotyped movement, and gnashing, grinding, or clenching the teeth mark cocaine intoxication.

Tolerance develops, as does physical dependency. Acute toxic effects may be treated with a short-acting barbiturate administered intravenously. A toxic psychosis with visual, auditory, and tactile hallucinations and a paranoid delusional system may develop as with amphetamines. When psychosis develops, it is classified as a cocaine-induced psychotic disorder.

# ◆ HALLUCINOGEN-RELATED DISORDER

This subcategory includes abuse of substances structurally related to 5-hydroxytryptamine. These are lysergic acid diethylamine (LSD), dimethyltryptamine (DMT), and substances related to catecholamines (eg, mescaline). The abuse symptoms are those described previously. In addition, episodes of hallucinogen persisting perception disorder (flashbacks) can occur at unpredictable times for years following termination of the drug.

# ◆ NICOTINE-RELATED DISORDER

Tobacco use continues in this country despite widespread knowledge that it is an important factor in the development of cardiovascular disease, cancer, and severe forms of lung disease. In severe cases of tobacco dependence, several signs of nicotine withdrawal symptoms include the following:

Depressed mood
Insomnia
Irritability, frustration, or anger
Anxiety
Difficulty concentrating
Restlessness
Decreased heart rate
Increased appetite or weight gain

## ◆ OPIOID-RELATED DISORDER

The client with an opioid-related disorder experiences the same symptoms as described for barbiturates. Taken in normal, medically supervised doses, the barbiturates and opioids mildly depress the action of the nerves, skeletal muscles, and heart muscle. They slow down heart rate and breathing and lower blood pressure. In higher doses, however, the effects resemble alcoholic drunkenness, with confusion, slurred speech, and staggering. The client finds it difficult to think, concentrate, and work, and emotional control is weakened. Users may become irritable and angry and want to fight someone. Sometimes, they fall into a deep sleep from which it is difficult to arouse them. In addition, episodes of intoxication involve impairments of attention, speech, memory, respiration, and consciousness. The opioid drugs include heroin, morphine, and synthetics with morphine-like action, such as meperidine (Demerol) and methadone.

References to opium smoking can be found so far back in Asian history that we do not know the date of its first use as a producer of pleasant dreams. It is still smoked in some areas in Asiatic countries, but in Western countries, the alkaloids of opium are preferred. Morphine is one of the main alkaloids of opium, and heroin is a derivative of morphine. Heroin is the narcotic most widely used by addicts today. It has been outlawed in the United States because of its strong addictive power and cannot be made, imported, or sold legally.

When a person becomes dependent on heroin, his or her body craves repeated and larger doses of the drug. Once the habit starts, larger and larger doses are required to get the same effects. This happens because the body develops a tolerance for the drug.

One of the signs of heroin addiction is **withdrawal sickness.** When the user stops the drug, he or she sweats, shakes, gets chills and diarrhea, vomits, and suffers sharp stomach pain. In addition to physical dependence on narcotics, there is also a strong psychological dependence.

Typically, the first emotional reaction to heroin is an erasing of fears and a relief from worry. This is usually followed by a state of inactivity bordering on stupor. Heroin, which is a fine white powder, is usually mixed into a liquid solution and injected into a vein. It tends to dull the edges of reality. Addicts report that heroin makes troubles "roll off the mind," and makes them feel more sure of themselves. This drug also reduces feelings of pain.

The drug depresses certain areas of the brain and reduces hunger, thirst, and the sex drive. Because addicts often do not feel hungry, usually they must be treated for malnutrition when hospitalized.

## ◆ PHENCYCLIDINE-RELATED DISORDER

Drugs included in this category are ketamine (Ketalar) and the thiophene analog of phencyclidine (TCP). This subcategory includes the general symptoms of abuse referred to earlier. In addition, with phencyclidine-induced intoxication, the person experiences delirium associated with the drug or a mixed cognitive disorder.

## ◆ SEDATIVE–HYPNOTIC-RELATED DISORDER

The drugs that are most commonly abused in this category are the anxiolytic drugs, including chlordiazepoxide (Librium), diazepam (Valium), and oxazepam (Serax). The sedatives that are regularly abused are pentobarbital sodium (Nembutal), secobarbital (Seconal), phenobarbital (Luminal), and amobarbital (Amytal). Commonly abused hypnotics are ethchlorvynol (Placidyl), flurazepam (Dalmane), glutethimide (Doriden), methyprylon (Noludar), chloral hydrate, paraldehyde, and methaqualone.

The symptoms of the abuse and dependence subcategories are listed earlier in the chapter. The person with this disorder uses the equivalent of 600 mg or more of secobarbital (Seconal) or 60 mg or more of diazepam (Valium) and experiences amnestic periods during intoxication. The person in the dependence category experiences an increasing need or withdrawal symptoms of cognitive disorder occur.

### BARBITURATES

The sedative category includes barbiturates, which belong to a large family of drugs manufactured for the purpose of relaxing (depressing) the central nervous system. They are synthetic drugs made from barbituric acid (a coal-tar product). Doctors prescribe these drugs widely to treat insomnia, high blood pressure, and epilepsy. They are occasionally used in the treatment of mental illness and to sedate clients before and during surgery. They are often used in combination with other drugs to treat many other types of illness and medical conditions. The symptoms of barbiturate abuse are discussed in the section on opioid abuse.

Often barbiturates are obtained illegally. Because doctors prescribe these drugs so frequently, many people consider them safe to use freely. They are not safe drugs. Overdoses can cause death. They are a leading cause of accidental poisoning deaths in the United States. These drugs distort the way that people see things and slow down their reactions and responses. They are an important cause of automobile accidents. When taken with alcohol, they tend to potentiate (enhance) the effects of the alcohol.

Because they are so easily obtained and produce sleep readily, barbiturates are frequently used in suicide attempts. Barbiturates range from the short-acting but fast-starting pentobarbital sodium (Nembutal) and secobarbital (Seconal) to the long-acting but slow-starting phenobarbital (Luminal), amobarbital (Amytal), and butabarbital (Butisol). The short-acting preparations are the ones most commonly abused. In the doses ordinarily taken by the drug abuser, barbiturates produce mood shifts, restlessness, euphoria, excitement, and, in some individuals, hallucinations. The users become confused and may be unable to walk or perform tasks requiring muscular activity.

The barbiturates cause physical dependence. The body needs increasingly higher doses to feel the effects. True dependence, however, requires taking large doses of the drug for more than a few weeks.

Sudden withdrawal of barbiturates from someone dependent on them is extremely dangerous because it may result in death. A physician will hospitalize the person and withdraw the drug slowly in order to alleviate the cramps, nausea, delirium, and convulsions that attend withdrawal. Some experts consider barbiturate dependence more difficult to cure than a narcotic dependency. It takes several months for a barbiturate user's body chemistry to return to normal.

## METHAQUALONE

A nonbarbiturate sedative-hypnotic, methaqualone (Quaalude), was first introduced in the United States in 1966. Marketed as having little potential for abuse and no effect on dream-stage sleep, it rapidly became used as a recreational chemical. It was found, however, to suppress REM sleep (rapid-eye-movement sleep associated with dreaming). Tolerance to the drug may develop. It is capable of producing both considerable psychological and physical dependence.

A withdrawal syndrome has been observed in people using over 600 mg per day for prolonged periods of time. The withdrawal syndrome begins within 24 hours of cessation of use of the drug, persists for 2 to 3 days, and consists of insomnia, headache, abdominal cramps, anorexia, nausea, irritability, and anxiety. Hallucinations and nightmares also have been reported.

The nursing care of this client and clients with the other substance-use disorders in this chapter is essentially the same as for the alcoholic client described earlier. The side effects of drug withdrawal that are most threatening to health and require the greatest vigilance occur during the detoxification period. The cognitive disorders and the nursing care required during withdrawal and detoxification are described in Chapter 21, The Client With a Personality Disorder.

### BENZODIAZEPINES

Chlordiazepoxide (Librium) and diazepam (Valium) are widely used as minor tranquilizers for the control of anxiety. They produce less euphoria than the preceding two hypnotics, but a withdrawal syndrome may occur when large doses (several hundred milligrams per day) are abruptly stopped. Convulsions may be delayed by several weeks and are managed as with meprobamate withdrawal, described below.

### MEPROBAMATE

Introduced as an antianxiety drug in 1954, meprobamate's therapeutic usefulness is in considerable doubt, but it is still widely prescribed and popular. Tolerance develops and withdrawal symptoms can occur. Abrupt withdrawal causes tremors, ataxia, headache, insomnia, and gastrointestinal disturbances lasting for several days. Occasionally, convulsions occur (usually upon withdrawal from 3 g or more daily). A delirium tremens–like state may occur in 36 to 48 hours. Diphenyl-hydantoin sodium (phenytoin) IV is useful in controlling convulsions.

## ◆ NURSING CARE OF CLIENTS WITH SUBSTANCE-RELATED DISORDERS

Because of the wide variety of side effects of substance withdrawal, this chapter will not attempt to recommend nursing actions for each of the nursing care problems that can result from both substance overdose and withdrawal. In addition, the nursing care in each of these types of substance dependence and their acute side effects is different depending on whether the client is in the inpatient or community setting. The reader is referred to textbooks that address the specific care setting and specific nursing problems associated with different types of substances.

### FAMILY AND SOCIAL SYSTEM RESPONSES TO SUBSTANCE-RELATED DISORDERS

A frequent issue for family members and loved ones of people with substance-related disorders is the loss of self-autonomy. Self-autonomy is the capacity of an individual to have a clear sense of his or her identity while also respecting the autonomy of others. **Codependence** is the term that describes relationships in which the role of one individual is highly related to the dysfunction of another. When codependence is occurring within one relationship, it often occurs in all important relationships, such as in the immediate family, social relationships, and at work. A family in which codependence is occurring often has unspoken rules with which family members are expected to comply.

The nurse who observes these behaviors can gently present other options that support the autonomy of each family member. Because of the strength of codependent characteristics, it is possible that the family member may avoid addressing these options; these characteristics have often been present in preceding generations. The continuum of codependence is present in many individuals and can affect well being in many ways. Because of the importance of this issue and its effects on relationships, the reader is encouraged to seek further information on codependence, the subject of many books available to the general public (Box 20-1).

## KEY POINTS

- A person with substance dependence displays at least three of the following symptoms:
  —Tolerance (need for markedly increased amounts or diminished effect with use)
  —Withdrawal (experiencing characteristic symptoms or taking a related substance to avoid withdrawal)
  —Substance often taken in larger amounts or over a longer period than was intended
  —Persistent desire or unsuccessful efforts to cut down or control substance use

---

### BOX 20–1. Web Resources

*http://www.casacolumbia.org/index.htm*
National Center on Addition and Substance Abuse at Columbia University. Provides information on substance abuse and available resources.

*http://www.psyweb.com*
User-friendly resource giving general information on psychiatric disorders, drugs, testing, treatment, and physiology of the brain. Based on DSM-IV criteria.

*http://www.nida.nih.gov*
Sponsored by the National Institutes of Health. Provides general information, publications, and links to other government agencies and programs.

—Great deal of time spent in obtaining, using, or recovering from effects of the substance

—Important social, occupational, or recreational activities given up or reduced owing to substance use

—Continued substance use despite persistent or recurrent physical or psychological problem caused or exacerbated by the substance

■ Substance abuse is more severe than dependence and includes recurrent substance use that results in a failure to fulfill major role obligations at work, school, or home; continues in situations in which it is physically hazardous; and continues despite recurrent substance-related legal, social, or interpersonal problems caused or exacerbated by the effects of the substance.

■ Treatment approaches to alcoholism include Alcoholics Anonymous, Antabuse therapy, and inpatient treatment programs. Nursing care of clients must cover the acute detoxification stage *and* the long-term recovery stage.

■ Substances can produce psychiatric symptoms even in a mentally stable person, for example, toxic psychosis (amphetamines), delusions and hallucinations (cocaine), and flashbacks (hallucinogens).

■ Opioid drugs include heroin, morphine, methadone, and synthetic morphine-like drugs such as Demerol. Withdrawal sickness (sweating, shaking, chills, diarrhea, vomiting) occurs when the regular user stops taking heroin.

■ Barbiturates are physically addictive, requiring larger and larger amounts to create the same effect. Withdrawal, which causes cramps, nausea, delirium, and convulsions, should be medically supervised.

## SELF-AWARENESS ACTIVITY

Many mental health clinicians believe that all people are at risk for one or another type of addictive disorder.

- Do you believe that information?
- Have you known someone among your family members or friends who have had some type of addictive disorder?
- How does or did it affect them personally?
- How does or did it affect others?
- How did it affect you?
- Did you take some action directly with that person?
- Did you take some action indirectly, such as talking with someone about it to gain some support and insight?
- If this problem were to occur in your life with someone you care about, whom can you talk with about your concerns?

- Have you in the past or do you at the current time have concern about having an addictive problem?
- If you do have concerns, whom can you speak with about it?
- If you do have concerns about your own use of an addictive substance, what do you want to do about your use?

## QUESTIONS

1. Stan has been taking Valium, prescribed by his physician for anxiety. He reports that he must take two tablets in order to obtain the same relief he formerly obtained taking one tablet. The nurse recognizes that Stan may be describing
   a. dependence.
   b. tolerance.
   c. addiction.
   d. substance abuse.
2. Gary, a 43-year-old man, is admitted for an appendectomy. When completing an admitting assessment, the nurse should ask about his use of drugs or alcohol, because:
   a. men have an increased risk of substance-related disorders.
   b. there is a relationship between appendicitis and the use of alcohol.
   c. the routine use of drugs or alcohol may place the client at risk for symptoms of withdrawal.
   d. the question is on the form used by the hospital.
3. For the past 18 months, Melanie has been taking a barbiturate nightly to help her sleep. She tells the nurse that she would like to stop using the medication. The nurse's best recommendation would be to suggest that Melanie
   a. discontinue use of the medication immediately.
   b. taper the dose of the medication, gradually, over the next 2 months.
   c. continue using the medication as it has been prescribed by a physician.
   d. discuss it with her physician as she must be withdrawn under medical supervision.
4. Which statement by a client taking Antabuse (disulfiram) indicates the need for additional teaching?
   a. "This medication blocks the metabolism of alcohol."
   b. "I will become ill if I take this medication and drink alcohol."
   c. "Taking this medication will cure my alcoholism."
   d. "I will take this medication, but still need to attend my AA meetings."

BOX 20–2. **Clinical Vignette**

Stan is a 33-year-old stockbroker. He has been addicted to cocaine for 2 years and denies his excessive use of the substance. He has been anorexic with accompanying weight loss for the past 6 months. He is currently sleeping less than 5 hours per night; his customary night's sleep is 7 or 8 hours. Stan's boss is becoming irritated with Stan's aggressiveness with his coworkers. Stan has begun to speak negatively about his boss and is accusing him of spreading rumors about him.

If you were a coworker of Stan and noticed these changes in his behavior and appearance, what would you say to him?

BOX 20–3. **Nursing Diagnoses Associated With Clinical Vignette**

**INEFFECTIVE DENIAL**
**Definition:** The state in which an individual minimizes or disavows symptoms or a situation to the detriment of his health.

Related nursing diagnosis: Ineffective denial related to refusal to acknowledge his abuse of cocaine as evidenced by excessive weight loss, decreasing sleep, and effects of his aggressiveness and suspiciousness on his work responsibilities.

**COPING: INEFFECTIVE INDIVIDUAL**
**Definition:** A state in which an individual experiences, or is at risk to experience, an inability to manage internal or environmental stressors adequately because of inadequate resources (physical, psychological, behavioral, and/or cognitive).

Related nursing diagnosis: Ineffective individual coping related to abuse of cocaine as evidenced by conflicts with fiance, boss, and coworkers.

**SLEEP DEPRIVATION**
**Definition:** The state in which an individual experiences prolonged periods of time without sustained natural periodic states of relative unconsciousness.

Related nursing diagnosis: Sleep deprivation related to cocaine addiction as evidenced by increased wakefulness and decreased number of hours of sleep per day compared to original number of hours of sleep per day.

## BIBLIOGRAPHY

Barry, P.D. (1991). An investigation of cardiovascular, respiratory, and skin temperature changes during relaxation and anger inductions. *Dissertation Abstracts International, 52-09-B,* 5012.

Boyd, M., & Nihart, M. (1998). *Psychiatric nursing: Contemporary practice.* Philadelphia: Lippincott Williams & Wilkins.

> BOX 20–4. **Family Teaching When a Client Has a Substance Use Disorder**
>
> When a family member has a substance use disorder, the following recommendations can provide support for the client and give the family more confidence in knowing how to support their family member. Family members should be encouraged to call the client's mental health caregiver whenever the client appears to be at risk for harm.
> The family responses that will be therapeutic to this client include:
>
> - Support client in seeing mental health care provider, attending groups, and being in contact with sponsor
> - Obtain recommendations from nursing staff at discharge planning meeting about specific types of effective communication with client
> - Encourage client to plan with family around his or her needs and expectations during recovery
> - Support client in seeing mental health care provider and attending groups
> - Avoid statements or behavior that increase agitation in client or provoke potential for violence
> - Assess needs regarding safety, nutrition, hygiene, sleep, and other activities
> - Review medication compliance
> - Review decision making when appropriate
> - Support problem solving about issues that provoke anxiety, helplessness, hopelessness, or other emotional distress
> - Support dignity of client while setting limits and expecting reasonable behavior

Carpenito, L.J. (2000). *Nursing diagnosis: Application to clinical practice* (8th ed.). Philadelphia: Lippincott Williams & Wilkins.

Estes, N., & Heinemann, M. (1986). *Alcoholism: Development, consequences, and interventions.* St. Louis: C.V. Mosby.

Gastfriend, D., Renner, J., & Hackett, T. (1997). Alcoholic patients—acute and chronic. *Massachusetts General Hospital handbook of general hospital psychiatry* (4th ed.). St. Louis: C.V. Mosby.

Mynatt, S. (1999). Effectiveness of intervention into substance abuse disorders in women with comorbid depression. *Journal of Psychosocial Nursing, 37*(5), 16–29.

Renner, J., & Gastfriend, D. (1997). Drug addicted patients. *Massachusetts General Hospital handbook of general hospital psychiatry* (4th ed.). St. Louis: C.V. Mosby.

Sadock, B., & Kaplan, H. (1998). *Synopsis of psychiatry: Behavioral sciences/clinical psychiatry.*Philadelphia: Lippincott Williams & Wilkins.

Timby, B.K. (2000). *Fundamental skills and concepts in patient care* (7th ed.). Philadelphia: Lippincott Williams & Wilkins.

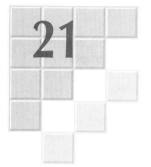

# The Client With a Personality Disorder

## Behavioral Objectives

*After reading this chapter the student will be able to:*

- Explain the differences between people who have a mental illness and those who have a personality disorder.
- List the 11 personality disorders discussed and identify the maladaptive characteristics of each.
- Compare and contrast antisocial and narcissistic personalities.
- Describe the traits and actions of a person who is egocentric.
- Discuss how personality disorders are treated.

## Key Terms

- Egocentricity
- Personality disorder
- Types of personality disorders
  - Antisocial
  - Avoidant
  - Borderline

  - Dependent
  - Histrionic
  - Narcissistic
  - Obsessive–compulsive
  - Paranoid
  - Schizoid
  - Schizotypal

Human needs were discussed in prior units, including psychological needs for tenderness in infancy, participation with others in childhood activities, sharing experiences with peers in the juvenile period, and close friendships and relationships in adolescence. Chapter 13, Stress: Ineffective Coping and Defense Mechanisms, discusses how a person erects defenses against aggressive and sexual tendencies and experiences socially unacceptable feelings and attitudes about important people in his or her life, particularly during childhood. These adaptive defenses allow a person to channel excessive anxiety and balance his or her needs; this person has a healthy personality.

If a person's defenses become pathologically exaggerated or disorganized, he or she can eventually develop a personality disorder. A **personality disorder** is a cluster of personality traits that tend to form in early childhood. These traits form when a child is under increased levels of intolerable stress in the home or social environment. Accordingly, the defenses that form to protect the child from the difficult environment produce personality traits that result in a personality that may become rigid, narrow, and nonspontaneous. A person's basic personality forms during the early years, depending largely on the way he or she learns to adjust to different types of situations, challenges, and threats. The formation of psychological defenses during this time creates the underlying structure of the adult personality. Up to this point, we have discussed mental health and mental illness in considerable detail. We now look at the vast number of people who seem to fit between the classifications of mentally healthy and mentally ill. These are the people whose behavior indicates they have maladapted to life stressors. Because their ego functioning and reality testing remain intact, most of them can adapt socially. Many of these people have personality disorders.

The disorders included in this category are as follows:

Paranoid
Schizoid
Schizotypal
Antisocial
Borderline
Histrionic
Narcissistic
Avoidant
Dependent
Obsessive–compulsive
Not otherwise specified

## ◆ PARANOID PERSONALITY DISORDER

These people tend to be hypersensitive, rigid, suspicious, jealous, and envious. They may have an exaggerated sense of their own importance and generally tend to blame others and ascribe evil motives to them. These characteristics quite often interfere with their ability to maintain satisfactory interpersonal relationships.

## ◆ SCHIZOID PERSONALITY DISORDER

This behavior pattern manifests emotional coldness, sensitivity, fearfulness, inability to socialize well with others, and a tendency to daydream and withdraw from reality. A wide range of behaviors is included in the schizoid group. Most people with a schizoid personality disorder are very sensitive people who feel lonely, imperfectly understood, and isolated. Many of them are timid, shy, self-conscious, and dissatisfied with themselves; others are more secretive, suspicious, and sometimes stubborn. Their feelings are very easily hurt. Playmates who look on him or her as strange or a "sissy" often tease a child of this type. He or she is shy, cries easily, seldom participates in rough play, talks little, and makes no close friendships. Under acute stress he or she may retreat into fantasy and become autistic.

In adolescence, many of these youngsters show patterns of willfulness, disobedience, moodiness, passive stubbornness, and resentfulness. They resent advice, supervision, or correction. Such youngsters are often loners who prefer to get along without strong ties to other people. Although they may be disobedient and moody, they tend to do superior work in school.

In the upper grades and in college, they usually do very well, but tend to be quiet and unsociable. Their love of books may be a substitute for human companionship. They are often imaginative and idealistic and frequently are interested in plans for bettering humanity. They study abstract or philosophical courses in preference to concrete or objective types. Some of these people become artists, poets, or musicians.

Others, although retaining an imaginative attitude toward life and its experiences, lack the fine sensitivity of the preceding group. These people, although kindly and honest, are unsociable, dull, and taciturn; their personalities lack color and sparkle.

Many people have schizoid personalities—the overly sensitive person, the extremely shy person, the recluse, and the dreamer. Often, a sensitive and tender nature hides beneath a cold and unresponsive exterior, or a deeply kind person hides behind a gruff, apparently hostile facade. These types, fearful of hurt and intrusion into their inner world, camouflage their innate tenderness and kindness by erecting barriers that hold people at a distance.

## ◆ SCHIZOTYPAL PERSONALITY DISORDER

A person with this type of personality disorder demonstrates many symptoms related to those of schizophrenia but of a less severe nature. He or she tends to be a loner and has an unusual pattern of talking that is vague and abstract. His or her emotions often do not match the content of a discussion and seem inappropriate for the circumstances. This person may seem preoccupied by his or her thoughts and is superstitious. The person may believe he or she can read the minds of others or that others are reading his or her mind. He or she may be suspicious or paranoid and is unusually sensitive to criticism.

## ◆ ANTISOCIAL PERSONALITY DISORDER

People with this disorder are unable to form any significant attachment or loyalty to other people, groups, or society. They are controlled by their ids and are given to immediate pleasures. They have no sense of responsibility, and in spite of punishment and repeated humiliations, they fail to learn to modify their behavior (i.e., they fail to learn by experience). They are lacking in social judgment and tend to turn their frustrations on society. They are able to rationalize their antisocial actions and consider them warranted, reasonable, and justified. Their character traits seem to be fixed expressions of conflict, and there is certain compulsiveness to their antisocial acts.

The defect in their character structures is their failure to develop a socialized superego and ego ideals; if these do exist, they are directed toward personal acquisition of money and material goods and the control of others for immediate pleasures and satisfactions. The factor, or factors, that produce such an individual are unknown.

As a group, these clients probably cause the most problems in society. They are frequently in trouble with the law, and might first be seen in psychiatric consultation on the recommendation of the court or probation office. They are unable to tolerate frustration, are easily enraged, and can act out violently without feeling remorse. They sometimes describe themselves as cold-blooded and are often described by others as such. They can be ruthless and vindictive and tend to blame others for their behavior.

People with an antisocial personality disorder demand much and give little. They are typically without affection, selfish, ungrateful, and self-centered, and may be exhibitionistic. They are unable to judge their behavior from another's standpoint. Even though such people are inadequate and hostile from a social standpoint, they are quite satisfied with their behavior. To such people, routine is intolerable. They show few feelings of anxiety, guilt, or remorse, and demand immediate and instant gratification of their desires with no concern for the feelings or interests of others. Some use alcohol or drugs. They may react to alcohol poorly and when under its influence become noisy, quarrelsome, and destructive. Their behavior prevents psychosocial adjustment. The personality defect may be limited to a single form of misbehavior, such as stealing, running away, or promiscuity.

# ◈ BORDERLINE PERSONALITY DISORDER

A person with a borderline personality disorder demonstrates unpredictability and instability in many areas of interpersonal and intrapsychic functioning. For instance, he or she may have intense interpersonal relationships that alternate between extremes of love, hate, and dependency. His or her emotional stability is also unpredictable. He or she is impulsive and displays major and inappropriate mood shifts. He or she can experience profound identity disturbances relating to self and body image, sexual identity, life goals, and the nature of relationships and others. In addition, he or she engages in self-harmful activities, such as fighting, self-mutilation, and suicidal gestures. Research on the causes of borderline personality disorder shows an increased incidence of this disorder in individuals who experienced physical, emotional, and/or sexual abuse in childhood.

# ◈ HISTRIONIC PERSONALITY DISORDER

This type of personality disorder is characterized by traits of vanity, self-indulgence, and a flair for dramatization or exhibitionism. These people are immature, self-centered, often vain, and prone to emotional outbursts. Sexual behavior can be provocative and seductive. Actually, most of these people are fearful of sex. Their provocative, attention-getting behavior appears to overlie dependency that is demanding of others. There is reason to suspect that many of these people were spoiled and overprotected in early years. Although they are usually actively engaged in the social world, they respond badly to the frustrations of reality.

Although this disorder is more common in women, the "Don Juan" character represents this personality type in men. His drive for sexual conquest and exhibitionism often hides a feeling of masculine inadequacy. His repeated conquests prove his lack of satisfaction in each successive affair.

# ◈ NARCISSISTIC PERSONALITY DISORDER

These people are egocentric. **Egocentricity** describes a person's attitude and inner feeling that the world exists to meet his or her needs. The egocentric person is grandiose and requires constant attention, although in fact his or her self-esteem is actually poor. When this person's self-esteem is threatened, he or she responds with marked anger or feelings of shame. As could be expected, his or her interpersonal relationships are strongly affected by these personality traits. The egocentric person tends to manipulate and exploit other people in order to meet his or her own needs, and is lacking in empathy to understand the feelings of others.

## ◆ AVOIDANT PERSONALITY DISORDER

People with this type of disorder are basically afraid of rejection. They consciously and unconsciously make choices that help them avoid conflict, humiliation, or shame. They tend to avoid social situations, although they desire affection and close relationships that enhance their sense of worth. They have the capacity to engage in close relationships, but these friendships require constant approval from others.

## ◆ DEPENDENT PERSONALITY DISORDER

A person with dependent personality disorder has a very poor sense of self and demonstrates a low level of self-confidence. He or she cannot make independent decisions or function as a responsible adult. The dependent person consistently defers or represses his or her own needs in order to gain the acceptance and approval of others. Interactions with others are marked by passivity. He or she finds it difficult, if not impossible, to travel alone and be self-reliant, which leads to social limitations.

## ◆ OBSESSIVE–COMPULSIVE PERSONALITY DISORDER

The person with this disorder demonstrates a limited or constricted range of emotions. Warmth, spontaneity, and a feeling of emotional "connectedness" with others seem lacking in his or her personality. He or she ceaselessly strives for perfection and is stubborn. Decision-making is difficult for obsessive–compulsive people, who overly attend to trivial details and are unable to carry through the decision-making process to form a conclusion. Compulsive people are frequently overinvolved with their work to the exclusion of normal pleasure and satisfaction in the workplace. They commonly spend excessive time at work and lose time with family and normal recreational activities.

## ◆ PERSONALITY DISORDER NOT OTHERWISE SPECIFIED

This category is for disorders that do not meet criteria for any of the specific personality disorders listed previously. An example includes mixed personality disorder, in which features of more than one specific disorder are present but do not meet the full criteria for any one disorder. This category also includes disorders not covered by the preceding classifications, such as depressive personality disorder and passive-aggressive personality disorder.

## ◆ TREATMENT OF PERSONALITY DISORDERS

People with personality disorders are rarely hospitalized. Their personality traits may cause difficulty in their relationships with others in the family, at work, or in social settings. Persons with personality disorders are generally resistant to referral to outpatient or private psychotherapy clinical settings. If outpatient psychiatric care is sought, the most appropriate treatment mode is individual or group psychotherapy, depending on the severity of the disorder. There are no specific recommendations for nursing care, because these clients usually are not treated in inpatient settings (Box 21-1).

## K E Y   P O I N T S

- ■ Coping and defense mechanisms allow a person to channel excess anxiety and balance needs. Adaptive mechanisms allow a person to develop a healthy personality.
- ■ If a person builds too many defenses, he or she may not be able to reduce tension and anxiety. Pathologically exaggerated or disorganized defenses can lead to a personality disorder. The kind of disorder a person develops when coping mechanisms fail depends largely on the basic personality structure developed during childhood.

---

### BOX 21–1. Web Resources

*http://www.mentalhelp.net*
Provides information about common psychiatric disorders and treatments, as well as professional resources. Offers links to support groups and other online resources.

*http://www.borderlinedisorders.com/public.htm*
Provides an overview of borderline disorder, diagnosis, treatment, and resources.

*http://www.psyweb.com*
User-friendly resource giving general information on psychiatric disorders, drugs, testing, treatment, and physiology of the brain. Based on DSM-IV criteria.

■ Personality disorders and their characteristics are:
  —Paranoid: suspiciousness, with a tendency to blame others
  —Schizoid: emotional coldness, tendency to withdraw
  —Schizotypal: vague or abstract speech, preoccupation with own thoughts
  —Antisocial: unable to form any significant attachments or tolerate frustration
  —Borderline: instability, inappropriate mood shifts, self-harmful activities
  —Histrionic: exhibitionism, provocative sexual behavior
  —Narcissistic: egocentric, requires constant attention, grandiose
  —Avoidant: fears rejection, humiliation, or shame, and avoids conflict
  —Dependent: consistently represses own needs to gain others' approval
■ Obsessive–compulsive disorder is characterized by a constricted range of emotions with a ceaseless striving for perfection and over-attention to trivial details. This person is often unable to make decisions or form a conclusion.
■ Treatment of personality disorders is rarely conducted on an inpatient basis. The most appropriate treatment mode is individual or group psychotherapy.

## SELF-AWARENESS ACTIVITIES

Many people demonstrate signs of one or another type of personality disorder. It is the intensity of these characteristics, the level of disruption they create in interpersonal relationships, and the additional level of intensification of symptoms that occur when these individuals are under stress that classify them as belonging to a specific type of personality disorder. Indeed, when we ourselves are under stress we may show evidence of tendencies toward one of the personality disorders described above; however, that does not mean we have a personality disorder. Under stress it is normal for all of us to show tendencies of intensification of normal personality traits.

  • If you have a tendency toward one or another of the cluster of characteristics described above, which ones are they?
  • One of the opportunities to observe personality disorders is in the media. Certain individuals in television programs, music videos, and soap operas, for example, may demonstrate characteristics that fit some of the personality disorders described in this chapter. Who are some of the individuals in the media you would identify? And what type of personality disorder might they be representing?

- Which personality characteristics of your own would you like to modify and why?
- How would you begin to modify them?

## QUESTIONS

1. An individual with an antisocial personality disorder
   a. frequently seeks immediate gratification.
   b. is usually quiet and unsocial.
   c. often engages in self-mutilation.
   d. seeks to avoid conflict.
2. Clients with antisocial personality disorders are rarely treated on psychiatric inpatient settings. When they are treated on inpatient units it is frequently as a result of
   a. self-referral for treatment of social isolation.
   b. a recommendation from a court.
   c. a recommendation from a family member.
   d. a referral from a mental health professional.
3. Clients seen in emergency departments for recurrent, self-inflicted burns or cuts may have
   a. Narcissistic Personality Disorder.
   b. Histrionic Personality Disorder.
   c. Antisocial Personality Disorder.
   d. Borderline Personality Disorder.
4. One of the major nursing concerns for clients with histrionic personality disorder may be that the client is at an increased risk for
   a. sexually transmitted disease
   b. self-mutilating behaviors
   c. social isolation
   d. sensitivity to criticism.

### BIBLIOGRAPHY

American Nurses Association. (1995). *Nursing social policy statement.* Kansas City, MO: American Nurses Association.

Barry, P.D. (1996). *Psychosocial nursing: Care of physically ill patients and their families* (3rd ed.). Philadelphia: Lippincott-Raven.

Boyd, M., & Nihart, M. (1998). *Psychiatric nursing: Contemporary practice.* Philadelphia: Lippincott Williams & Wilkins.

Carpenito, L. (1999). *Handbook of nursing diagnosis* (8th ed.). Philadelphia: Lippincott Williams & Wilkins.

Carpenito, L. (2000). *Nursing diagnosis: Application to clinical practice* (8th ed.). Philadelphia: Lippincott Williams & Wilkins.

*Diagnostic and statistical manual of mental disorders* (4th ed.). (1994). Washington, D.C.: American Psychiatric Press.

Paris, J. (1998). Personality disorders in sociocultural perspective. *Journal of Personality Disorders, 12*(4), 289–301.

Sadock, B., & Kaplan, H. (1998). *Synopsis of psychiatry: Behavioral sciences/clinical psychiatry.* Philadelphia: Lippincott Williams & Wilkins.

Trimpey, M., & Davidson, S. (1998). Nursing care of personality disorders in the medical surgical setting. *Nursing Clinics of North America, 33*(1), 173–186.

---

## BOX 21-2. Clinical Vignette

Rhonda is a 45-year-old housewife who has a long-standing borderline personality disorder. She is married to a controlling, emotionally abusive, and unsupportive partner. Recently she has begun to experience dreams and emotional distress related to memories of abuse that had not been known to her. Related to these emerging memories she has experienced a wide range of emotions, including depression and anxiety. She has had difficulty sleeping. Attempts at managing her symptoms with medication have not been effective. She was admitted to the hospital to stabilize her mental symptoms.

What would it be like to sit with Rhonda on the day of her admission? How would you begin to talk with her? What would you say?

Would it be appropriate if Rhonda's clinical treatment plan included family or couple therapy while she is hospitalized? Why?

---

## BOX 21-3. Nursing Diagnoses Associated With Clinical Vignette

**INEFFECTIVE FAMILY COPING: DISABLING**
**Definition:** Domestic abuse is defined as any action that is intended to harm another person (physical, emotional, financial, social, or sexual.

Related nursing diagnosis: Disabling and ineffective family coping related to client's history of emotional abuse and neglect by husband as evidenced by increased emotional instability.

**POWERLESSNESS**
**Definition:** The state in which an individual or group perceives a lack of personal control over certain events or situations that affect outlook, goals, and lifestyle.

Related nursing diagnosis: Powerlessness related to perceived inability of client to address her husband's emotional abuse.

**SLEEP PATTERN DISTURBANCE**
**Definition:** The state in which an individual experiences or is at risk for experiencing a change in the quantity or quality of his rest patterns that causes discomfort or interferes with desired lifestyle.

Related nursing diagnosis: Sleep pattern disturbance related to nightmares associated with emerging memories of childhood emotional abuse.

## BOX 21-4. Family Teaching When a Client Has a Personality Disorder

When a family member has a personality disorder, the following recommendations can provide support for the client and give the family more confidence in knowing how to support their family member. Family members should be encouraged to call the client's mental health caregiver whenever the client appears to be at risk for harm.

The family responses that will be therapeutic to this client include:

- During discharge planning meeting, obtain information about specific issues created by the client's unique type of personality disorder and ask for recommendations about supportive interactions that the family can provide for client
- With client present, plan for reasonable limit setting of targeted undesirable social behavior at home and other settings during discharge planning meeting
- Provide realistic feedback when behavior exceeds predetermined expectations
- Enforce agreed-upon limits when behavior exceeds predetermined expectations
- Renegotiate family roles, relationships, and responsibilities to support the client's rehabilitation
- Support client in seeing mental health care provider and attending groups
- Review medication compliance
- Encourage client to plan with family around his or her needs and expectations during recovery
- Support client's dignity during communication
- Use collaborative problem solving, when appropriate, to reduce anxiety

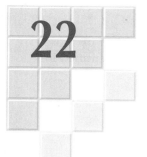

# 22

# The Client With an Eating Disorder

## Behavioral Objectives

*After reading*
*this chapter*
*the student*
*will be able to:*

- Define eating disorder and name the different types currently identified in psychiatric literature.
- Define anorexia nervosa and identify its defining characteristic.
- Name the two types of anorexia nervosa and how they differ.
- Identify the vulnerability factors for anorexia nervosa.
- Define binge eating disorder and identify its vulnerability factors.
- Identify three family dynamics that might contribute to eating disorders.
- Identify treatment options for persons with eating disorders.

## Key Terms

- Anorexia nervosa, restrictive type
- Anorexia nervosa, bulimic type
- Binge eating disorder
- Binging
- Biopsychosocial nursing care
- Bulimia nervosa
- Eating disorder
- Integrated model of treatment
- Purging

Eating disorders have been identified in the medical literature since the 1600s. Although these conditions appear to be on the rise and becoming more prevalent in young persons, research on their prevalence does not support this assumption. An **eating disorder** is a chronic disruption in one's ability to ingest food and derive nutrition from that food because of one or more emotional issues that lasts for 3 or more months. The different types of eating disorders currently identified in the psychiatric literature are the following:

- Anorexia nervosa, restrictive type
- Anorexia nervosa, bulimic type
- Bulimia nervosa
- Binge eating disorder

Currently, it is believed that the incidence of eating disorders is about one to five per 100,000 individuals. The most common type of eating disorders is anorexia nervosa. A second type of eating disorder that develops in 50% of individuals with anorexia nervosa is bulimia nervosa. These conditions are most commonly present in young women in their teens and early twenties; however, young men of the same age range may also develop eating disorders. For example, 40% of persons with binge eating disorder are adolescent men.

**Binging** is the ingestion of large amounts of food followed by purging. **Purging** is the use of self-induced vomiting, laxatives, diuretics, enemas, emetics, or nonpurging methods, such as exercise or fasting, to control weight gain. Persons with bulimia nervosa or binge eating disorder with purging use purging as their method to relieve themselves of excessive food intake.

The Eating Attitudes Test is a self-administered test that provides information about the level of a person's risk of developing or already having an eating disorder. This test is shown in Box 22-1.

## ◆ TYPES OF EATING DISORDERS

### ANOREXIA NERVOSA

Anorexia nervosa is a mental disorder that results in an avoidance of eating because of a cluster of specific emotional issues. Symptoms of anorexia nervosa may begin to manifest as early as 9 years of age. Another defining characteristic of anorexia nervosa is a weight loss of 15% or more of the normal weight of the person, using the height and weight in standardized scales. This mental disorder affects primarily young women between the ages of 12 and 20, but it can continue to be found in women who had the condition as adolescents and carry it beyond their adolescent years. Two types of anorexia nervosa are identified in the literature: restrictive type and bulimic type. In **anorexia nervosa, restrictive type** there is an avoidance of food, resulting in severely diminished nutritional value derived from food accompanied by significant weight loss. The second condition, **anorexia nervosa, bulimic type**, is driven by the same emotional issues as the restrictive type. The difference is that the individual uses purging after eating to

## BOX 22-1. Eating Attitudes Test

Please place an (X) under the column that applies best to each of the numbered statements. All of the results will be strictly confidential. Most of the questions relate to food or eating, although other types of questions have been included. Please answer each question carefully. Thank you.

| | Always | Very Often | Often | Some-times | Rarely | Never |
|---|---|---|---|---|---|---|
| 1. Like eating with other people. | | | | | | X |
| 2. Prepare foods for others but do not eat what I cook. | X | | | | | |
| 3. Become anxious prior to eating. | X | | | | | |
| 4. Am terrified about being overweight. | X | | | | | |
| 5. Avoid eating when I am hungry. | X | | | | | |
| 6. Find myself preoccupied with food. | X | | | | | |
| 7. Have gone on eating binges where I feel that I may not be able to stop. | X | | | | | |
| 8. Cut my food into small pieces. | X | | | | | |
| 9. Aware of the calorie content of foods that I eat. | X | | | | | |
| 10. Particularly avoid foods with a high carbohydrate content (eg, bread, potatoes, rice, etc.) | X | | | | | |
| 11. Feel bloated after meals. | X | | | | | |
| 12. Feel that others would prefer I ate more. | X | | | | | |
| 13. Vomit after I have eaten. | X | | | | | |
| 14. Feel extremely guilty after eating. | X | | | | | |
| 15. Am preoccupied with a desire to be thinner. | X | | | | | |
| 16. Exercise strenuously to burn off calories. | X | | | | | |
| 17. Weigh myself several times a day. | X | | | | | |
| 18. Like my clothes to fit tightly. | | | | | | X |
| 19. Enjoy eating meat. | | | | | | X |
| 20. Wake up early in the morning. | X | | | | | |
| 21. Eat the same foods day after day. | X | | | | | |
| 22. Think about burning up calories when I exercise. | X | | | | | |

*(continued)*

## BOX 22-1. **Eating Attitudes Test** (Continued)

Please place an (X) under the column that applies best to each of the numbered statements. All of the results will be strictly confidential. Most of the questions relate to food or eating, although other types of questions have been included. Please answer each question carefully. Thank you.

| | Always | Very Often | Often | Some-times | Rarely | Never |
|---|---|---|---|---|---|---|
| 23. Have regular menstrual periods. | X | | | | | |
| 24. Other people think I am too thin. | X | | | | | |
| 25. Am preoccupied with the thought of having fat on my body. | X | | | | | |
| 26. Take longer than others to eat. | X | | | | | |
| 27. Enjoy eating at restaurants. | | | | | | X |
| 28. Take laxatives. | X | | | | | |
| 29. Avoid foods with sugar in them. | X | | | | | |
| 30. Eat diet foods. | X | | | | | |
| 31. Feel that food controls my life. | X | | | | | |
| 32. Display self-control around food. | X | | | | | |
| 33. Feel that others pressure me to eat. | X | | | | | |
| 34. Give too much time and thought to food. | X | | | | | |
| 35. Suffer from constipation. | | | | | | X |
| 36. Feel uncomfortable after eating sweets. | X | | | | | |
| 37. Engage in dieting behavior. | X | | | | | |
| 38. Like my stomach to be empty. | X | | | | | |
| 39. Enjoy trying new rich foods. | | | | | | X |
| 40. Have the impulse to vomit after meals. | X | | | | | |

*Scoring:* The patient is given the questionnaire without the X's, just blank. 3 points are assigned to endorsements that coincide with the X's; the adjacent alternatives are weighted as 2 points and 1 point, respectively. A total score of over 30 indicates significant concerns with eating behavior.

From Boyd, M., & Nihart, M. (1998). *Psychiatric nursing: Contemporary practice.* Philadelphia: Lippincott-Raven.

reduce the potential for weight gain. The factors that may contribute to the development of this condition are shown in Box 22-2.

### Vulnerability Factors for Anorexia Nervosa

Research on individuals with anorexia nervosa indicates that numerous biologic, psychological, and sociocultural factors contribute to its development. It is also considered possible that there is a genetic vulnerability that contributes to neurochemical changes. Serotonin and norepinephrine, neurochemicals related to depression, are implicated in eating disorders. Depression affects normal regulation of appetite and satiety.

There may be interrelated biologic factors between depression and eating disorders. For example, a drug developed and used for depression also has been found to be effective in anorexia nervosa. Limited research has shown that fluoxetine hydrochloride (Prozac) reduces the obsessional interest in food and weight, decreases depressive symptoms, and improves the relapse rate of persons with anorexia nervosa.

### BULIMIA NERVOSA

Bulimia nervosa is a condition that was found in 4% of girls and 2% of boys in a study performed by Whitaker and colleagues. The symptoms include recurrent episodes of overeating, also known as binge eating. Generally, binge eating is characterized by eating a volume of food that is significantly greater than another person would eat in the same period of time. The eating is also accompanied by a feeling of being out of control. After the binge, a person with bulimia nervosa engages in

---

**BOX 22-2. Risk Factors for Eating Disorders**

Poor self-image and self-esteem
Inaccurate body image about weight
Rituals and obsessions about food intake
Intense fear of gaining weight or obesity
Emotional issues such as fear of loss of control, rigidly judgmental, high level of dependence on others
Early onset of symptoms: age 9–13
Weighs 85% or less of standard scale for age and body type
Denial and avoidance of discussion of eating issues
Chronic disturbance in family relations
Depression or other mental disorder in self and/or other family members
History of sexual abuse
Amenorrhea

*Note:* Not all factors are present in all persons with eating disorders.

recurrent episodes of purging, as described above. Bulimic episodes occur at least twice a week over a period of 3 months. The bulimic person's self-evaluation is unduly influenced by body shape and weight. He or she does not meet the criteria for anorexia nervosa.

### Vulnerability Factors for Bulimia Nervosa

These individuals usually are within a normal weight range. Between their binging and purging episodes, they may restrict their caloric intake to avoid the types of foods eaten during a binging episode. There may be a higher than average incidence of depression or anxiety when compared with others of the same age. There can also be an increased incidence of substance abuse or dependence involving alcohol or stimulants.

### BINGE EATING DISORDER

**Binge eating disorder** is a type of eating similar to that of bulimia nervosa, without the purging phase. This condition has been recognized in the psychiatric literature for the last decade and is characterized by the use of binge eating with concurrent psychiatric problems, such as depression, wide variations in weight gain and loss cycles, and more severe weight-related distress. The primary difference between the person with a binge eating disorder and one with bulimia nervosa is that there is no purging in the binge eating disorder.

### Vulnerability Factors for Binge Eating Disorder

One of the vulnerability factors for binge eating disorder is a predisposition to obesity. In addition, there is a presence of nonspecific factors for psychiatric disorder, such as parental depression and adverse conditions in childhood, such as a stressful family environment.

## ◆ MEDICAL RISK FACTORS WITH SEVERE EATING DISORDERS

Regardless of the type of eating disorder, when its effects are severe, the eating disorder can become life threatening because of its effects on every body system. Medical intervention is necessary to reduce the physically harmful symptoms. Table 22-1 describes the types of symptoms that occur in different body systems.

## ◆ TREATMENT OPTIONS FOR EATING DISORDERS

Most eating disorders are treated in the outpatient mental health setting by mental health clinicians, such as psychiatrists, psychologists, advanced practice registered nurses, and social workers who have spe-

## TABLE 22–1. **Medical Complications of Eating Disorders**

| Body System | Symptoms |
| --- | --- |
| *Related to Weight Loss* | |
| Musculoskeletal | Loss of muscle mass, loss of fat |
| | Osteoporosis |
| | Pathologic fractures |
| Metabolic | Hypothyroidism (symptoms include lack of energy, weakness, intolerance to cold, and bradycardia) |
| | Hypoglycemia, decreased insulin sensitivity |
| Cardiac | Bradycardia, hypotension, loss of cardiac muscle, small heart, cardiac arrhythmias including atrial and ventricular premature contractions, prolonged QT interval, ventricular tachycardia, sudden death |
| Gastrointestinal | Delayed gastric emptying, bloating, constipation, abdominal pain, gas, diarrhea |
| Reproductive | Amenorrhea, low levels of luteinizing hormone and follicle-stimulating hormone |
| Dermatologic | Dry, cracking skin caused by dehydration, lanugo (fine babylike hair over body), edema, acrocyanosis (bluish hands and feet) |
| Hematologic | Leukopenia, anemia, thrombocytopenia, hypercholesterolemia, hypercarotenemia |
| Neuropsychiatric | Abnormal taste sensation (possible zinc deficiency) |
| | Apathetic depression, mild organic mental symptoms, sleep disturbances |
| *Related to Purging (Vomiting and Laxative Abuse)* | |
| Metabolic | Electrolyte abnormalities, particularly hypokalemia, hypochloremic alkalosis; hypomagnesemia; increased blood urea nitrogen |
| Gastrointestinal | Salivary gland and pancreatic inflammation and enlargement with increase in serum amylase; esophageal and gastric erosion or rupture; dysfunctional bowel with haustral dilatation; superior mesenteric artery syndrome |
| Dental | Erosion of dental enamel (perimyolysis), particularly frontal teeth with decreased decay |
| Neuropsychiatric | Seizures (related to large fluid shifts and electrolyte disturbances), mild neuropathies, fatigue, weakness, mild organic mental symptoms |

Adapted from Yager, J. (1990). Eating disorders. In A. Stoudemire (Ed.), *Clinical psychiatry for medical students.* Philadelphia: Lippincott, p. 324.

From Boyd, M., & Nihart, M. (1998). *Psychiatric nursing: Contemporary practice.* Philadelphia: Lippincott-Raven.

cial expertise in treating eating disorders. The primary reason for partial or inpatient hospitalization of the person with an eating disorder is to stabilize the physical symptoms that are threatening the client's well being and survival. Partial and inpatient hospitalization are important options for persons who are experiencing acute medical symptoms as a result of their eating disorders. The personnel in an eating disorders treatment program, whether outpatient or inpatient, are experts in their field. These clinicians are skilled in assessing the mental, physical, and dental effects of eating disorders that create major health challenges for the person with an eating disorder. A treatment approach that uses both physical and mental assessment and treatment interventions is known as an **integrated model of treatment**.

Studies have shown that cognitive therapy is most effective for persons with eating disorders. Research has also found that general psychotherapy, group therapy, and the use of pharmaceuticals are effective in the treatment of eating disorders. It appears that different eating disorder treatment teams have developed their own unique protocols.

### FAMILY INTERVENTION

Most researchers who have investigated the factors contributing to eating disorders agree that several communication patterns are present in the families of persons who develop these disorders. Box 22-3 shows some of the communication patterns that may lead to eating disorders. Interventions with family members are developed in the treatment setting based on the presenting dynamics contributing to the disorder (see Box 22-4).

## ◆ NURSING CARE OF THE CLIENT WITH AN EATING DISORDER

Clients with eating disorders are rarely treated in the mental health setting. Rather, because of the severe effects of chronic eating disorders on their physical state, they usually are hospitalized in specially designed units. The nursing staff in these units is trained to provide biopsychosocial nursing care. **Biopsychosocial nursing care** is an integrated form that systemically addresses the complex physical, psychological, and family issues involved (see Box 22-5).

### K E Y   P O I N T S

---

- Eating disorders affect approximately 5 out of every 100,000 people.
- Girls are more susceptible to eating disorders than boys.

## BOX 22-3. Family Dynamics That May Contribute to Eating Disorders

**ANOREXIA NERVOSA**
Expectations of perfection by parents
Rigidity of beliefs of parents and family
Enmeshed or unclear boundaries between generations
Other disturbances in family emotional environment
Helplessness and lack of control in children
Sexual abuse
Depression in adult members of family

**BULIMIA NERVOSA**
Families are more overtly conflictual than families of anorexia nervosa clients
Statements of criticism and rejection of family members
Three family types: *the perfect family* (high expectations of female family members); *the overprotective family* (female members are viewed as needing protection from outside the family); and *the chaotic family* (may be extreme violations of boundaries either by sexual or physical abuse)
In this type of family the bulimia can be self-soothing

**BINGE EATING DISORDER**
Parental depression
Adverse conditions for child without adequate parental protection or interpretation

- Young women ages 12 to 20 are most likely to develop anorexia nervosa.
- The age incidence of bulimia nervosa begins at a later age than anorexia nervosa and continues to be more common into one's twenties.
- Teenage boys comprise 40% of individuals with binge eating disorder.
- A variety of emotional issues may contribute to eating disorders:
  —High need for control
  —Obsession with thinness
  —Distorted body image
  —Perfectionist family structure
  —Conflict avoidance
  —Unawareness of own emotional responses
  —Emotional enmeshment with other family members
- All body systems are affected when the effects of eating disorders are severe.

## BOX 22-4. Family Teaching When a Client Has an Eating Disorder

An eating disorder is a potentially fatal condition. Many mental health clinicians who write about the cause of and treatment for eating disorders consider that the original roots of the condition may be found in the family's communication patterns and dynamics.

There are many different approaches recommended for families when they have a member with an eating disorder. Accordingly, the various eating disorder treatment programs and the health care providers who establish these programs or provide clinical mental health treatment for eating disorders are the best source of specific recommendations for the family of the person with an eating disorder. Because of the different theoretical approaches, it is suggested that the family of a person with an eating disorder obtain specific recommendations from the care provider responsible for the client's treatment about appropriate family responses with the client.

## BOX 22-5. Web Resources

*Http://www.mirror-mirror.org*
Dedicated to the memory of a woman who died from an eating disorder. Provides general information, resources, and personal stories about eating disorders.

*http://www.psyweb.com*
User-friendly resource giving general information on psychiatric disorders, drugs, testing, treatment, and physiology of the brain. Based on DSM-IV criteria.

*http://www.mentalhelp.net*
Provides information about common psychiatric disorders and treatments, as well as professional resources. Offers links to support groups and other online resources.

■ Treatment for severe eating disorders uses an integrated model of mental and physical assessment in an eating disorders center.

## SELF-AWARENESS ACTIVITY

• Most people have issues with weight. How do you manifest your own issues about weight? How do you manage these issues?

- Have you known someone who has an eating disorder? What were your concerns for that person?
- Often, a person with an eating disorder has strong psychological defenses that make it difficult to talk about important issues. Sometimes one can feel helpless when trying to address concerns with a friend or family member who has an eating disorder. Were you able to talk with the person about the condition? What communication techniques were effective? What would you do in a similar situation today?

## QUESTIONS

1. Eating disorders may result in a number of physiological changes. The highest nursing priority would be the effects on which system?
   a. Musculoskeletal
   b. Gastrointestinal
   c. Dermatologic
   d. Cardiovascular
2. An 18-year-old female client of normal weight presents to the emergency department with a decreased potassium level. The nurse notices scratches on the back of the client's hand. The client may have
   a. a binge eating disorder.
   b. bulimia nervosa.
   c. anorexia nervosa, restrictive type.
   d. anorexia nervosa, bulimic type.
3. The best treatment for a client with an eating disorder includes
   a. medications such as antianxiety and antipsychotic agents.
   b. intensive group and individual therapy.
   c. restrictive behavioral therapy.
   d. therapy that includes mental and physical interventions.
4. Family dynamics are thought to impact the development of eating disorders. The dynamic seen more often in bulimia nervosa than other eating disorders is
   a. enmeshment.
   b. perfectionism.
   c. overt conflicts.
   d. abusive situations.

## BIBLIOGRAPHY

Becker, A., Grinspoon, S., Klibanski, A., & Herzog, D. (1999). Eating disorders. *New England Journal of Medicine, 340*(14), 1092–1098.

Boyd, M., & Nihart, M. (1998). *Psychiatric nursing: Contemporary practice.* Philadelphia: Lippincott-Raven.

Brusseau Goldenberg, L., & O'Connor, S. (1999). Is your patient starving to death? *Nursing99, 3*(3) (Hospital Nursing), 32hn1–32hn4.

*Diagnostic and statistical manual of mental disorders* (4th ed.). (1994). Washington, D.C.: American Psychiatric Press.

Garner, D., & Garfinkel, P. (1979). The eating attitudes test: An index of the symptoms of anorexia nervosa. *Psychosomatic Medicine, 10,* 647–656.

Sadock, B., & Kaplan, H. (1998). *Synopsis of psychiatry: Behavioral sciences/clinical psychiatry.* Philadelphia: Lippincott-Raven.

Stunkard, A. (1997). Eating disorders: The last 25 years. *Appetite, 29*(2), 181–190.

Walsh, B., & Devlin, M. (1998). Eating disorders: Progress and problems. *Science, 280*(29), 1387–1390.

Whitaker, A., Johnson, J., Shaffer, D., et al. (1990). Uncommon troubles in young people: Prevalence estimates of selected psychiatric disorders in a nonreferred adolescent population. *Archives of General Psychiatry, 47,* 487–495.

Wiseman, C., Harris, W., & Halmi, K. (1998). Eating disorders. *Medical Clinics of North America, 82*(1), 145–159.

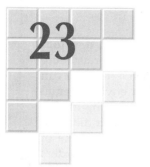

# 23

# The Infant, Child, or Adolescent With a Developmental Disorder

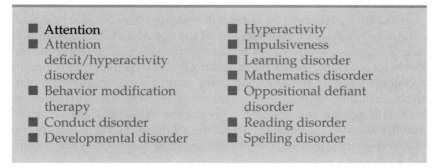

Developmental disorders occur in many children. The term **developmental disorder** describes the origins of the mental disorder as being related to the developmental process of the child. Such a disorder can have its roots in the genetic endowment of the child or environmental influences of the parents and immediate family. This chapter highlights the most frequently occurring developmental disorders, their diagnostic criteria, and the general mental health approaches to the care of these children. The most common types of developmental disorders and their subtypes include:

1. Learning disorders
   a. Reading disorder
   b. Spelling disorder
   c. Mathematics disorder
2. Attention deficit/hyperactivity disorder
   a. Inattention type
   b. Hyperactivity/impulsivity
3. Disruptive behavior disorder
   a. Oppositional defiant disorder
   b. Conduct disorder

## ◆ TYPES OF DEVELOPMENTAL DISORDERS

### LEARNING DISORDERS

Learning disorders are developmental disorders that affect children's abilities to learn subjects that are usually within the intellectual capability of children of their age. It is estimated that approximately 5% of public school children have a learning disorder. Of that number, approximately 40% may drop out of school. Adults with learning disorders often have difficulty with employment and social relations. The different types of learning disorders include:

Reading disorder
Spelling disorder
Mathematics disorder

**Reading disorder** is a condition that affects about 4% of school children. It first becomes noticeable at the age of 6 or 7. The condition affects a child's ability to reach age-appropriate reading achievement levels on standardized tests. Symptoms include an impaired ability to recognize words, slow and inaccurate reading, and poor comprehension. A reading disorder may also contribute to speech difficulties as well as language and spelling achievement. A reading specialist can identify the specific cause of a reading disorder. Remedial education directed at the specific cause of the reading disorder is the recommended course of treatment.

**Spelling disorder** is a condition that affects a child's ability to score at age-appropriate levels on standardized tests. There is no accompanying difficulty with reading or mathematical abilities. A language arts specialist can identify the specific cause of the disorder and recommend a remedial course of education.

**Mathematics disorder** includes difficulties with four different types of mathematical skills. These skills include:

1. Linguistic skills: the ability to understand mathematical terms and convert written mathematical problems into mathematical symbols
2. Perceptual skills: the ability to recognize and understand symbols and order clusters of numbers
3. Mathematical skills: the ability to perform the basic skills of addition, subtraction, multiplication, and division, as well as follow the sequence of basic operations
4. Attentional skills: the ability to copy figures and observe operational symbols correctly

This condition may become known when a child is 6 years of age. Usually, however, the condition is not diagnosed until children reach the age of 8, when mathematical skills become more complex. There is no known cause. Remedial education is the recommended treatment.

## ◆ ATTENTION DEFICIT/HYPERACTIVITY DISORDER

**Attention deficit/hyperactivity disorder (ADHD)** is a condition that can be observed in children as young as 2 years of age. Its formal diagnosis, however, is usually delayed until the child begins school and the cluster of behaviors associated with ADHD can be formally identified. The primary symptoms of this condition are problems with: attention, impulsiveness, and hyperactivity. **Attention** is "a complex mental process that involves concentrating on one activity to the exclusion of others, as well as sustaining that focus over time" (Boyd & Nihart, 1998, p. 882). **Impulsiveness** is "the tendency to act on urges, notions, or desires without adequate consideration of the consequences" (Boyd & Nihart, 1998, p. 883). **Hyperactivity** is "excessive motor activity, as evidenced by restlessness, inability to remain seated, and high levels of physical motion and verbal output" (Boyd & Nihart, 1998, p. 884). Diagnosing this disorder requires careful attention to the specific types of symptoms that a child manifests over a period of 6 months.

The incidence of ADHD in the United States is estimated at 2% to 20% of grade-school children. The condition is more prevalent in boys than girls; the ratio ranges from three to five boys for every girl with the condition. It is most common in firstborn boys. The parents of

ADHD children show an increased incidence of hyperactivity, socially inappropriate behavior, and alcohol use disorders.

## SYMPTOMS OF ATTENTION DEFICIT/HYPERACTIVITY DISORDER

Attention deficit/hyperactivity disorder has been subdivided into two subtypes: inattention and hyperactivity-impulsivity. The determination of which type a child is exhibiting is based on the presence of the symptoms outlined in the *Diagnosis and Statistical Manual of Psychiatric Disorders*, 4th ed. These symptoms are shown in Table 23-1.

## PHARMACOTHERAPY FOR SYMPTOMS OF ATTENTION DEFICIT/HYPERACTIVITY DISORDER

It is theorized that ADHD is related to dysregulation of two different neurochemical groups, norepinephrine and dopamine. These neurochemicals contribute to alertness and the ability to maintain one's attention and concentration. Drugs that stimulate the central nervous system (CNS) are effective in increasing concentration and the ability to maintain attention and decrease impulsivity. The exact mechanism of these drugs is unknown. The most commonly prescribed stimulants used to

---

**TABLE 23–1. Diagnostic Criteria for Attention Deficit/ Hyperactivity Disorder**

Select either type depending on prevalence of symptoms:

Six or more of the following symptoms of inattention have persisted for at least 6 months to a degree that is maladaptive and inconsistent with developmental level:

*Inattention*

Often fails to give close attention to details or makes careless mistakes in schoolwork, work, or other activities

Often has difficulty sustaining attention in tasks or play activities

Often does not seem to listen when spoken to directly

Often does not follow through on instructions and fails to finish schoolwork, chores, or duties in the workplace (and owing to oppositional behavior or failure to understand directions)

Often has difficulty organizing tasks and activities

Often avoids or dislikes or is reluctant to engage in tasks that require sustained mental effort (such as schoolwork or homework)

Often loses things necessary for tasks or activities (eg, toys, school assignments, pencils, books)

Is often easily distracted by extraneous activity

Is often forgetful in daily activities

Six or more of the following symptoms of hyperactivity-impulsivity have persisted for at least 6 months to a degree that is maladaptive and inconsistent with developmental level:

*(continues)*

---

**TABLE 23–1. Diagnostic Criteria for Attention Deficit/ Hyperactivity Disorder** *(Continued)*

*Hyperactivity*

Often fidgets with hands or feet or squirms in seat

Often leaves seat in classroom or in other situations in which remaining seated is expected

Often runs about or climbs excessively in situations in which it is inappropriate (in adolescents or adults, may be linked with subjective feelings of restlessness)

Often has difficulty playing or engaging in leisure activities quietly

Is often "on the go" or often acts as if "driven by a motor"

Often talks excessively

*Impulsivity*

Often blurts out answers before questions have been completed

Often has difficulty awaiting turn

Often interrupts or intrudes on others (eg, butts into conversations or games)

Some hyperactive-impulsive or inattentive symptoms that caused impairment were present before age 7 years

Some impairment from the symptoms is present in two or more settings (eg, at school, home, or work)

There must be clear evidence of clinically significant impairment in social, academic, or occupational functioning

The symptoms do not occur exclusively during the course of a pervasive developmental disorder, schizophrenia, or other psychotic disorder and are not better accounted for by another mental disorder (eg, mood disorder, anxiety disorder, dissociative disorder, or a personality disorder)

---

Adapted from American Psychiatric Association. (1994). *Diagnostic and statistical manual of mental disorders* (4th ed.). Washington, D.C.: American Psychiatric Association.

treat ADHD are dextroamphetamine (Dexedrine) and methylphenidate (Ritalin). The Food and Drug Administration (FDA) has approved dextroamphetamine for children age 3 and over. The FDA has approved methylphenidate for children age 6 and over. The drug of choice for school-age children is methylphenidate; 75% of children who take this medication show significant improvement in their ADHD symptoms.

## THE CLINICAL COURSE OF ATTENTION DEFICIT/HYPERACTIVITY DISORDER

It is not unusual for a child with ADHD to develop depression as an outcome of the condition owing to frustration and poor self-esteem about not being able to perform satisfactorily in school or at home. Symptoms are treated primarily with CNS stimulants. Secondary symptoms of depression and anxiety are treated with medications as indicated. The hyperactivity symptoms of ADHD may begin to decrease at puberty; attention deficit and impulsivity can continue through adolescence, and in 15% to 20% of cases, into adulthood. When ADHD symptoms persist beyond puberty, approximately 50% of the children develop conduct disorders, a subtype of disruptive behavior disorder.

# ◆ DISRUPTIVE BEHAVIOR DISORDER

Two types of disorders are included in this category:

Oppositional defiant disorder
Conduct disorder

## OPPOSITIONAL DEFIANT DISORDER

**Oppositional defiant disorder** is a mental disorder with a cluster of symptoms that form the basis for this diagnosis when these symptoms persist for a period over 6 months. These traits also create significant impairment in social, academic, and occupational settings. These symptoms include a recurrent pattern of negativistic, defiant, disobedient, and hostile behavior toward authority figures. This behavior occurs more frequently than would be expected from someone of the same age or development. The personality traits include the occurrence of at least four of the following characteristics:

- Loss of temper
- Arguments with adults
- Defiance of or refusal to comply with adults' requests or rules
- Deliberately doing things that annoy adults
- Blaming others for personal failings
- General personality traits of touchiness, anger, resentment, and spite

The development of this condition occurs most commonly in children who are strong-willed and whose parents themselves are concerned with maintaining power, control, and autonomy. It is estimated that more girls than boys demonstrate these traits. The primary treatments for this condition are counseling for the child and parents, as well as classes and training in effective parenting skills. **Behavior modification therapy** is an effective therapeutic approach for the child. Ideally this approach is started when the child first shows this behavior pattern. Behavior modification therapy used by the parents socializes the child by reinforcing positive behaviors and ignoring or not reinforcing undesired behavior.

## CONDUCT DISORDER

**Conduct disorder** is a behavioral disorder that evolves over time. Children with this disorder behave in an aggressive manner toward others

BOX 23–1. **Psychosocial Factors That Can Contribute to Conduct Disorder**

Chaotic home environment
Child abuse
Negligence
Lack of supportive environment
Poor social attachments
Presence of attention deficit/hyperactivity disorder
Parental factors:
   Prevalence of hostility, resentment, and bitterness between parents
   Parental psychopathology and substance abuse
   Parents who themselves are the products of abusive homes
   Parental unemployment

Adapted from Sadock, B., & Kaplan, H. (1998). *Synopsis of psychiatry: Behavioral sciences/clinical psychiatry.* Philadelphia: Lippincott Williams & Wilkins.

and violate the rights of others. It is estimated that 6% to 16% of boys and 2% to 9% of girls under the age of 18 show symptoms of this disorder. The ratio of incidence comparing the presence of this condition in boys to its presence in girls is estimated at from 4:1 to as many as 12:1.

### The Cause of Conduct Disorder

No specific factor is associated with the development of conduct disorder. A number of psychosocial factors appear to contribute to the development of this condition. They are shown in Box 23-1.

### Treatment for Conduct Disorder

Because of the multiple causes and symptoms associated with conduct disorder there is no treatment that is curative for all aspects of this condition. Treatment programs that use all available family and community resources and a social environment with consistent rules and expected consequences can help to reduce or control disruptive behaviors. In chaotic families with no potential for change, it may be necessary to remove the child from the home and institute foster care.

### Pharmacotherapy for Conduct Disorder

Conduct disorder is a condition with many symptoms. The presence of symptoms that disrupt the child's ability to respond to treatment are the determining factors that can be responsive to symptom-specific medications. These symptoms include:

- Depression
- Anxiety
- Impulsivity
- Overt explosive aggression
- Lability of mood
- Attention deficit/hyperactivity disorder
- Substance-related disorders

## NURSING CARE OF CHILDREN AND ADOLESCENTS WITH ATTENTION DEFICIT AND CONDUCT DISORDERS

Children and adolescents with attention deficit disorder are rarely institutionalized in the mental health setting. In addition, children and adolescents with mild to moderate conduct disorders usually are not hospitalized. Children and adolescents with severe conduct disorders may be hospitalized, but are rarely seen in traditional mental health settings. This type of disorder requires intervention in child and adolescent treatment facilities where behavioral modification interventions are utilized. Refer to Chapter 26, Milieu Therapy and Behavior Modification, for more information about this form of therapy.

KEY   POINTS

■ Developmental disorders are those disorders whose origin is related to a child's developmental process. The most common types are learning disorders, attention deficit/hyperactivity disorders, and disruptive behavior disorders.

---

BOX 23–2. **Family Teaching When an Infant, Child, or Adolescent Has a Developmental Disorder**

There are a variety of childhood developmental disorders and different family approaches recommended for family members, depending on the child's condition and the theoretical framework of the health care providers responsible for providing the child's care.

Because of the disparity of these views, the nurse who works in an institution that treats children will be trained in the behavioral techniques of the specific clinical model used by the institution. Based on the therapeutic model, nurses will be taught the behavioral interventions that support the child's return to mental health. These nursing approaches are usually similar to the behavioral interventions recommended for family members of a child with a developmental disorder.

■ Learning disorders affect a child's ability to learn subjects that are within the intellectual capacity of other children of the same age. These disorders are classified into three subtypes: reading, spelling, and mathematics.

■ A reading disorder affects a child's ability to reach age-appropriate reading levels on standardized tests and include impaired ability to recognize words, slow and inaccurate reading, and poor comprehension.

■ A spelling disorder affects a child's ability to score at age-appropriate levels on standardized tests.

■ A mathematics disorder is characterized by difficulties with mastering four types of mathematical skills: linguistic (understand symbols and terms); perceptual (understand symbols and terms and order number clusters); mathematical (basic skills such as addition and subtraction); and attentional (copying figures correctly).

■ Attention deficit/hyperactivity disorder is characterized by problems with attention, impulsiveness, and hyperactivity. Generally the disorder is classified as either inattention or hyperactivity-impulsivity. Some children outgrow the symptoms of ADHD by puberty, but some people continue to have symptoms into adulthood.

■ Two medications used to treat the symptoms are dextroamphetamine and methylphenidate. They are believed to regulate brain neurochemicals that contribute to the ability to concentrate and maintain attention.

■ Disruptive behavior disorder is a type of developmental disorder characterized by inappropriate or aggressive behavior. The two subtypes are oppositional defiant disorder and conduct disorder.

■ Oppositional defiant disorder has a cluster of symptoms that occur frequently over a sustained time and significantly impair the child's interactions with family, school, and other settings. Symptoms include loss of temper, argumentativeness, defiance, deliberate refusal to comply with adult requests, and blaming others. These children are also angry, resentful, and spiteful persistently.

■ Behavior modification therapy is the most effective therapeutic mode for a child with oppositional defiant disorder.

■ Conduct disorder is characterized by persistently aggressive behavior and a tendency to violate the rights of others. Treatment usually depends on the child's home environment and community resources.

## SELF-AWARENESS ACTIVITY

Learning disorders and attention deficit/hyperactivity disorders have received a high level of attention during the past two decades.

- Have you or a member of your family been identified as having one or more of these disorders? What was the recommended treatment? Was it effective?
- What is your response to the increased media attention generated by these conditions?
- Take a moment to consider the societal changes that could decrease the incidence of conduct disorders. Name five social changes you recommend that could assist children with this disorder.

## QUESTIONS

1. A client with ADHD is admitted for a tonsillectomy. In providing care for this client the nurse should:
   a. Restrain the client to prevent injury from excessive movement.
   b. Provide detailed information to the client regarding all policies and treatments.
   c. Leave the client alone as much as possible, so as to not embarrass the client.
   d. Provide the client with simple and direct information regarding pertinent policies and treatments.

---

### BOX 23–3. Web Resources

*http://www.psychcentral.com*
A clearinghouse for psychiatric information on the Internet. Provides links and general information on a number of psychiatric disorders.

*http://www.mentalhelp.net*
Provides information about common psychiatric disorders and treatments, as well as professional resources. Offers links to support groups and other online resources.

*http://www.cdc.gov/nceh*
Sponsored by the Centers for Disease Control. Provides information on maintaining a safe environment for children and others.

*http://www.ldonline.org*
Organizational sponsored site for Learning Disabilities. Provides general information, information on current research, and support.

2. A 15-year-old client presents to the emergency department after a fight. The nurse recognizes that the home environment of this client
   a. may be chaotic.
   b. is usually supportive.
   c. provides strong social attachment.
   d. usually includes two working parents.
3. A father talks to the nurse about his child with a learning disorder. The nurse correctly tells the father that:
   a. "All learning disorders can be successfully treated with medication."
   b. "Learning disorders are related to poor home environments and family therapy is the best treatment."
   c. "Children outgrow learning disorders, usually during puberty. It is nothing to worry about until after that time."
   d. "Many remedial specialists are available who may help you develop learning strategies for your child."
4. The primary symptoms for a client with ADHD include
   a. inattention, impulsiveness, and hyperactivity.
   b. activity, impulsiveness, and low intelligence.
   c. inattention, impulsiveness, and high intelligence.
   d. activity, learning difficulties, and behavior problems.

## BIBLIOGRAPHY

Boyd, M., & Nihart, M. (1998). *Psychiatric nursing: Contemporary practice.* Philadelphia: Lippincott Williams & Wilkins.

Buncher, P. (1996). Attention deficit/hyperactivity disorder. *Nurse Practitioner, 21*(6), 43–65.

Carpenito, L.J. (2000). *Nursing diagnosis: Application to clinical practice* (8th ed.). Philadelphia: Lippincott Williams & Wilkins.

*Diagnostic and statistical manual of mental disorders* (4th ed.). (1994). Washington, D.C.: American Psychiatric Press.

Sadock, B., & Kaplan, H. (1998). *Synopsis of psychiatry: Behavioral sciences/clinical psychiatry.* Philadelphia: Lippincott Williams & Wilkins.

Shaywitz, B., Fletcher, J., & Shaywitz, S. (1997). Attention deficit/hyperactivity disorder. *Advances in Practice, 44,* 331–367.

Tannock, R. (1998). Attention deficit hyperactivity disorder: Advances in cognitive, neurobiological, and genetic research. *Journal of Child Psychiatry and Psychiatry and Allied Disciplines, 39*(1), 65–99.

Wissler, K., & Proukou, C. (1999). Navigating the educational system: A practical guide for nurse practitioners. *Journal of Pediatric Oncology Nursing, 16*(3), 145–155.

## DEVELOPING CRITICAL THINKING SKILLS THROUGH CLASS DISCUSSION

### UNIT 4 Case Study
# Nursing the Client With a Mental Disorder

Pat is a 45-year-old single female with a 15-year history of bipolar affective disorder. She recently stopped taking her medication and was brought to the hospital by the police department after a verbal altercation with a bank teller. During the admission process she reports that she no longer needs the medication, as she is now able to control all her symptoms by eating a special diet. Throughout the interview she removes $20 bills from her pockets and undergarment, which she hands to the nurse and states, "Here, you look like you could use this. I have plenty—my stocks have gone through the roof!"

## DISCUSSION QUESTIONS

1. What are the diagnostic criteria for bipolar affective disorder? What evidence do you have that Pat fits these criteria? What other symptoms might you expect Pat to exhibit?
2. What are your nursing priorities for Pat? How were these priorities determined?
3. What nursing assessments do you think ought to be completed on Pat? Why?
4. What nursing interventions would you expect to implement with Pat? Why?
5. What medications might be prescribed for Pat?
6. How would you determine whether Pat was a danger to herself or others?
7. Identify at least one nursing diagnosis that would be appropriate for Pat. What nursing interventions would address this diagnosis?

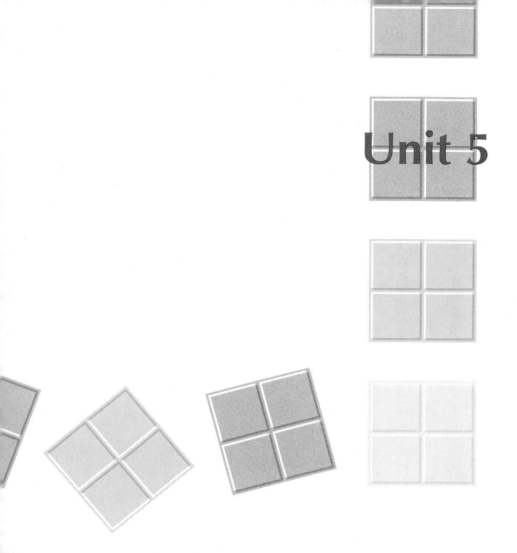

# Unit 5

# INTERVENTION AND TREATMENT OF MENTAL DISORDERS

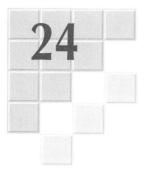

# Crisis Intervention

## Behavioral Objectives

*After reading
this chapter
the student
will be able to:*

- Describe the ways in which events can lead to crisis.
- List the sequence of developments after a critical event that can lead to crisis.
- Explain the symptoms of maladaptation exhibited by a person after crisis.
- Define developmental crisis.
- Identify the six developmental stages and possible results of unresolved issues for each stage.
- Describe the five types of situational events that are most likely to cause crisis.
- Describe the nursing process used with clients in crisis.

## Key Terms

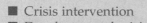

- Crisis intervention
- Developmental crisis
- Situational crisis

- Triage
- Triggering or precipitating event

A crisis of some type usually causes the onset of mental illness. There may be a specific event that triggers a deteriorating capacity for mental functioning—for instance, a new situation with which the person has no previous experience. Accordingly, there are no specific automatic behaviors or coping responses available to respond to or relieve the anxiety associated with such an event.

A number of stressful life experiences, compounded by a new situation, may be "the straw that breaks the camel's back." The person's coping abilities may be already taxed and not responding as well as in earlier difficulties. Finally, the crisis may be one that appears to have no known cause or identifiable **triggering or precipitating event.** In such cases, subtle changes in the client's perception of events often cause distorted or disoriented perceptions that are stressful in and of themselves. These distorted perceptions most often occur in schizophrenia, manic-depressive illness, psychotic depression, and delirium or dementia due to a general medical condition or substance abuse.

## ◆ SEQUENCE OF DEVELOPMENTS FOLLOWING A CRITICAL EVENT

A number of factors determine whether an event has crisis potential:

1. The perception of the event by the person, which is strongly influenced by his or her:
   a. Value system (what is important to the person)
   b. Normal personality style
   c. Normal coping strength
   d. Response to issues of trust, self-esteem, control, loss, guilt, intimacy
   e. Coping skills during normal stresses of living
   f. Level of stress in the past year
   g. Availability of support from family, friends, and caregivers
2. The degree of threat, as perceived by the person, to his or her:
   a. Personal safety
   b. Life goals
   c. Normal role functioning
   d. Family stability
3. The person's coping style: effective versus ineffective coping

When a person is functioning well mentally, his or her ego is able to tolerate the stress of a difficult new event by developing an ever-expanding set of responses to decrease anxiety. Eventually, the new relief behaviors or conscious coping strategies decrease his or her anxiety and crisis is avoided. He or she has adapted to the new event or life change. When effective coping does not occur, a maladaptive response develops. At times maladaptation becomes chronic. Crisis does not occur, but there is a change in the quality of the individual's life and that of his or her family. The quality-of-life changes are caused by diminished capacity to function both psychologically and socially in the way that the person did before the triggering event occurred.

Another possible outcome is that a maladaptive response results in a decreasing ability to deal with anxiety and the emotional, intellectual, and physiologic stresses accompanying it. While this is occurring, the person feels increasingly out of control. His or her awareness of environmental stimuli is decreased. The two possible outcomes of this progressive deterioration are immobility and panic. In either case, the person's capacity to help himself or herself is temporarily lost. Crisis results.

A crisis occurs over a limited period of time. It can last anywhere from a few days to a few weeks. Either it decreases because the client's coping strength gradually returns and he or she has an available support system, or it causes the person's mental functioning to deteriorate to the point at which hospitalization is necessary to protect the client or others.

## ◆ CATEGORIES OF CRISIS

Two main categories of circumstances can challenge a person's ability to cope and adapt. The potential outcomes are developmental crises and life change crises (also known as situational crises).

### DEVELOPMENTAL CRISES

The normal stages of development, as described by Erik Erikson, include many issues that must be worked through and resolved to allow normal progression into the next stage. On occasion, individuals are unable to make the transition, and one or more of these issues are unresolved. When a large number of issues prove too taxing to resolve, **developmental crisis** can occur. Box 24-1 outlines the developmental stages and outcomes that may occur if issues are not resolved.

Although aging from one decade to the next can stress the psyche, it is usually less disruptive than the significant development stages described in the preceding, and the person adjusts to a changed self-image. At times, however, self-esteem temporarily decreases until the person accommodates to the change. Table 24-1 shows examples of different types of approaches and rationales for different types of mental health emergencies.

### SITUATIONAL CRISES

Life change events that can cause crisis include death, divorce, major illness, marriage, childbirth, loss of a job, and retirement. Many times, a life change event occurs at the same time a person is adapting to a new developmental stage. When this happens, the person is at greater risk for inadequate coping and a **situational crisis.** The life change events and their accompanying effects are described in the following sections.

### Death

The death of a loved one or one's own anticipated death is the most severe social stressor that most people encounter in their lives. The

## BOX 24-1. Developmental Stages and Crisis Potential

### INFANCY AND EARLY CHILDHOOD (BIRTH TO 3 YEARS)

**Major Issues (Progressive from Birth)**
Trust, dependence, awareness of separateness from mother, development of autonomy

**When Issues Are Not Resolved**
Distrust, poor self-confidence, fusion of self with caregiver, poor self-control

### CHILDHOOD (3 TO 11 YEARS)

**Major Issues**
Identification with significant elders; development of initiative, security, and acceptance within family and eventually within peer group; mastery of age-appropriate skills and intellectual challenges

**When Issues Are Not Resolved**
Guilt, lack of direction and purpose, self-undermining behavior, feelings of inadequacy

### ADOLESCENCE (12 TO 20 YEARS)

**Major Issues**
Reawakening of oedipal conflicts (see Chapter 8, Stages and Theories of Personality Development), idealization of significant others, resolution of loss of childhood, development of sexual identity, acceptance by peer group, psychological separation from family as adolescent develops his or her own perceptions of the world (physical separation usually occurs a few years later)

**When Issues Are Not Resolved**
Inability to separate from family and assume independence, sexual confusion, self-consciousness, inability to form relationship with person of opposite sex, poor object relations

### EARLY ADULTHOOD (20 TO 30 YEARS)

**Major Issues**
Ability to develop intimacy and commitment within a relationship, commitment to employment, exploration, and clarification of societal norms as they pertain to self

**When Issues Are Not Resolved**
Superficiality in relationships with others, poor goal setting, drifting in and out of relationships and employment, lack of responsibility to self and others

### MIDDLE ADULTHOOD (30 TO 50 YEARS)

**Major Issues**
Maintenance of life goals, creativity, and spontaneity; ability to maintain meaningful relationships, appropriate channeling of emotions

*(continues)*

---

BOX 24-1. **Developmental Stages and Crisis Potential** *(Continued)*

**When Issues Are Not Resolved**
Inability to work or to feel pleasure, poor motivation, egocentrism in relationships and in goal setting

**LATE ADULTHOOD (50 YEARS AND OLDER)**

**Major Issues**
Ability to resolve losses of aging and to integrate ongoing losses, maintenance of hope, acceptance of uncertain future

**When Issues Are Not Resolved**
Continual wishing to relive past experiences, inability to take pleasure in the present, loss of hope, depression

---

losses associated with a death are many. A relationship with a significant other person contains connections to innumerable ongoing experiences and memories, as well as irreplaceable loss of support and caring that the other person provided. In some cases, the relationship with the other person was permeated with conflict. In either a loving or conflicting relationship, the loss results in the eruption of strong feelings of grief, anger, guilt, and fear.

Before a person dies, there is often a period of months or years of physical decline that allows the person and those who know him or her gradually to work through (at least partially) the anticipated death. When this occurs, the coping process commonly follows a pattern similar to that described by Elisabeth Kubler-Ross, including stages of denial, anger, bargaining, depression, and acceptance. The dying person and various family members frequently progress through these stages at different times. One or more family members may deny the illness, express anger, and become depressed, thereby increasing the stress on the family system.

Sudden, unexpected death has even greater crisis potential because family members have had no time to develop their coping ability. Such a death suddenly disrupts their entire world without warning. Even a few days of critical illness allow a family time to adjust, at least minimally, to the imminent death. When sudden death of a loved one occurs, the bereavement process in one or more family members often lasts beyond the normal 1-year period.

## Divorce
Divorce is second in the list of most disruptive events reported by people in the Holmes and Rahe research study on life change stressors.

TABLE 24–1. **Guidelines for Crisis Intervention**

| Approach | Rationale | Example |
|---|---|---|
| Assist the person in confronting reality. | During the crisis experience, the person may use denial as a coping mechanism. Denial is ineffective in resolving the crisis. Emotional support will help the person face reality. | Accompany the husband to view the body of his deceased wife. |
| Encourage the expression of feelings (within limits). | Identification and expression of feelings about the crisis events help the person understand the significance of the crisis. | Encourage a woman who survived a house fire but lost her home to explore the meaning of the lost home. |
| Encourage the person to focus on one implication at a time. | Focusing on all the implications at once can be too overwhelming. | A woman left her husband because of abuse. At first, focus only on living arrangements and safety. At another time, discuss the other implications of the separation. |
| Avoid giving false reassurances, such as, "It will be all right." | Giving false reassurances blocks communication. It may not be all right. | Patient: "My doctor told me that I have a terminal illness." Nurse: "What does that mean to you?" |
| Clarify fantasies with facts. | Accurate information is needed to problem solve. | A young mother believes that her comatose child will regain consciousness, although the medical evidence contradicts it. Gently clarify the meaning of the medical evidence. |
| Link the person and family with community resources, as needed. | Strengthening the person's social network so that social support can be obtained reduces the effect of the crisis. | Provide information about a meeting of a support group such as that of the American Cancer Society. |

Adapted from Lazarus, R. (1991). *Emotion and adaptation.* New York: Oxford University Press, p. 122.

From Boyd, M., & Nihart, M. (1998). *Psychiatric nursing: Contemporary practice.* Philadelphia: Lippincott-Raven.

Divorce, like death, results in multiple changes within the family; however, the dynamic of choice is involved for one or both members of the couple. This element increases the potential for anger, guilt, and loss in both partners. The children, regardless of their ages, can be profoundly affected as well. Increased levels of anxiety and decreased self-esteem and role-functioning ability frequently occur.

## Major Illness
Major illness, mental or physical, presents a moderate-to-severe challenge for individuals and their family members. Usually, they have had no experience with illness in the past, and their ability to cope and adapt is severely challenged. The ongoing effects of psychiatric illnesses, such as schizophrenia and major depressive illness, and chronic physical illnesses, such as cancer and heart disease, involve threats to self-image, body image, and self-esteem; loss of control; issues of dependence and trust; separation from family; and changes in role functioning. Just as the ill person is under increased psychological stress, so are his or her family members, because they must adapt to losses associated with the changed health status and role functioning of their loved one. Communication patterns in the family are often permanently altered as a means of coping with the many changes in the family created by the illness.

## Marriage
Although marriage is usually a happy event for a person and his or her family, it often creates a number of stresses for the couple as well as their families. These include the couple's anticipated role changes and a heightened sense of responsibility. Family members may or may not agree with their loved one's choice of spouse. Often, as the time of marriage approaches, there is a greater awareness of differences in values pertaining to family, tradition, religion, and so on, leading to increased potential for interpersonal and psychological conflict.

Marriage also creates many losses. It may involve the first time a young person has lived apart from his or her family. The anticipated separation is usually accompanied by feelings of sadness and fear in the person about to be married and in his or her parents and siblings. If a man has been excessively emotionally close to his family, he will be unable to reach independent decisions or an agreement with his new wife if her views differ from those of his family. The issue of emotional separation from one's own family is significant in the development of a healthy marital relationship.

## Childbirth
The implications of raising children have become increasingly important to young people during the past two decades. The decision about whether to have children is an important one in the developing relationship between two young people who are contemplating marriage. Values and beliefs about pregnancy, childbirth, and child rearing have strong potential for conflict and are best addressed during the courtship period.

The arrival of a child causes a major shift in the interpersonal dynamics between a husband and wife. Many couples find that the arrival of the first child is a crisis event. Regardless of their psychological preparation, it involves changes in their lives and normal roles that were not anticipated. In most instances, the crisis is short-lived. Adaptation begins to occur within 4 to 6 weeks.

## ◆ TREATMENT SITES FOR CRISIS INTERVENTION

**Crisis intervention** is a series of clinical actions that are effective in reducing the potential for crisis or for stabilizing an individual or social group after a crisis has occurred. There are many sites in which crisis intervention can be effective. These are discussed below.

### THE FAMILY AND SOCIAL NETWORK

Crisis intervention can occur anywhere. Ideally, whatever the precipitating event, the individual in crisis will have a supportive environment that can provide support and problem solving during the crisis period. Social network crisis intervention with the individual can provide needed support. When the individual has adequate inner strength, reserves, and social support, a crisis usually can be averted.

### THE HOME VISITING NURSE CRISIS INTERVENTION TEAM

Visiting nurse and home care organizations in many communities have developed emergency crisis intervention teams that intervene early with individuals and families in crisis. The purpose of early intervention is to decrease the risk of hospitalization by introducing medication, coping support, problem solving, and consultation about community resources to the unique crisis situation. Chapter 5, The Home Care Setting: Client and Family Issues, describes more dimensions of home care crisis intervention.

### COMMUNITY CRISIS INTERVENTION IN OUTPATIENT CLINIC SETTINGS

Community outpatient centers have been created to meet the needs of individuals of all social groups, including the homeless. The purpose of community mental health centers is to provide crisis support by intervening before the crisis requires inpatient hospitalization.

### COMMUNITY CRISIS INTERVENTION IN THE EMERGENCY ROOM

Admission to the emergency room (ER) is an option when the crisis has quickly escalated and immediate stabilization is necessary. Emergency room mental health crisis staff members attempt to gather information about possible family or social network supports available to the individual during the stabilization period. The emergency staff triage the individual to an appropriate inpatient facility when the crisis requires hospitalization.

## GENERAL HOSPITAL EMERGENCY ROOM
## TREATMENT OF PSYCHIATRIC EMERGENCIES
## AMONG THE HOMELESS

The triage of psychiatric clients in general hospital ERs is instituted when community programs are unsuccessful in averting psychiatric hospital admission. **Triage** is the term used to describe how the care of people with mental or physical health problems is prioritized. Those who are most acutely ill with a prognosis of surviving their current illness are prioritized at the highest level. Health care resources are apportioned according to the priority of care assigned to a specific health problem.

In the current health care environment, large numbers of homeless or unemployed people have no health insurance. The use of the general hospital ER as the initial care setting has markedly increased, particularly during the past decade. Many homeless individuals suffer from chronic mental disorders such as schizophrenia, substance abuse, or cognitive mental disorders. Sometimes they are diagnosed with all three disorders concurrently. Adding to their psychiatric distress is their noncompliance in taking the medications that could stabilize their mental conditions.

Changes in the law have allowed law enforcement agencies to involuntarily admit seriously mentally disturbed, antisocial, or dangerous individuals to general hospital ERs for crisis assessment and intervention services. Inner-city hospitals have shown an increase of nearly 100 percent in the number of admissions of mentally ill people to their ERs during the past decade.

Because of deinstitutionalization, transfer of these individuals to mental institutions has been severely restricted by sharp decreases in mental hospital bed capacities. Accordingly, ERs may have to hold these individuals in cramped, inadequate quarters for several days before discharging them to the street or a mental institution. The use of a triage evaluation system prioritizes rapid transfer to the general hospital inpatient unit or mental institution. Those individuals who are not stabilized within 4 hours by psychotropic medication or who pose a high risk of danger to themselves, staff members, or other ER clients will most likely be transferred.

## OTHER RESEARCH FINDINGS ABOUT EMERGENCY
## ROOM PSYCHIATRIC TREATMENT

A study that followed the types of psychiatric admissions to ERs found that there were several groups of clients with specific characteristics.

The findings from this study provide general information about the types of mental health clients who are the frequent users of psychiatric ER services. They include:

Sixty-five percent were self-referrals.

Seventeen percent were unpredictable and violent. Many of these individuals were referred late at night by police departments.

Eight percent were referred by their physicians. The majority of these individuals were referred for depression, anxiety, or other less severe neurotic disturbances.

Seven percent were referred by mental health team referral sources for more serious mental symptoms, such as psychosis, or for additional emotional support.

Another study of psychiatric ER visits found that of 417 persons who were admitted for emergency mental health treatment, 29% were involuntarily returned to the emergency psychiatric service within 12 months. The factors that were most predictive of readmission were the presence of psychotic symptoms and the likelihood of violent behavior toward self or others at the time of the client's first visit to the ER. Another important finding in these individuals was that those who had a brief hospitalization (average stay of 6 days) after their first ER admission showed no difference in their likelihood of returning for another ER admission. The researchers surmised that the short hospital stay was not adequate to resolve the patient's clinical condition.

### PARTIAL HOSPITALIZATION

When crisis is occurring, another option to consider is partial hospitalization. This choice can be useful if the individual requires structure and problem solving as a means of reducing the crisis symptoms. Partial hospitalization is also a helpful choice when the family or social network of the individual is not able to provide 24-hour availability to the person in crisis. Partial day or evening programs can provide the added comfort and safety of being in a supportive environment while the primary support person may be at school or work.

### INPATIENT CRISIS STABILIZATION

When all other options have been considered and the security and acute crisis stabilization resources of the hospital setting are necessary, the hospital is chosen as the treatment setting.

## ◆ THE USE OF NURSING PROCESS WITH CLIENTS IN CRISIS

When a client is admitted in crisis, begin the nursing process immediately. You can provide support while you are admitting the client. Such availability of support from other people is a key factor in the resolution of crisis. The more you understand the frame of reference of a client, the less isolated he or she feels. A major exception to this approach is the client who is suspicious or paranoid.

## ASSESSMENT

In caring for a client who is not coping, remember that each human being perceives the world in a different way from every other person. The unique set of circumstances that each person encounters in his or her development from infancy to adulthood creates different personality dynamics. As a result, the way one person copes with a given situation can be quite different from another.

For example, if you were a passenger in a racecar in the Indianapolis 500, traveling at 120 miles per hour around a curve, you might expect that the perceptions of the driver and passenger regarding the experience are quite different. The passenger might feel a high level of anxiety; the driver, on the other hand, would thrive on the experience. It is the frame of reference of each that determines the overall response. Accordingly, the more you understand about what a particular event means to a person, the more complete will be the data on which you base your care plan.

## PLANNING

Most likely a client in crisis with whom you are working will have been hospitalized by the time you are planning his or her care. One of the most important elements in the client's ability to resolve the crisis is the sense of support he or she feels in the treatment setting. One of the ways you can ensure this is to develop a team plan with members of the various disciplines who are caring for the client. This is also known as systems planning. The caregiving team is usually made up of a psychiatrist, psychologist, family therapist, nurse, occupational therapist, drama therapist, and members of whatever other disciplines your institution uses in the care of clients.

Without such teamwork, each of these caregivers might otherwise work toward opposite goals. The person who suffers is the client. He or she will not feel you are helping if all members of your treatment plan are not working toward similar goals. For this reason, it is important to attend a team conference and understand the treatment plan of the psychiatrist or psychologist in charge of caring for the client. You can ask questions at this conference to clarify your understanding of the client and can also share any information you may have obtained from the client.

In the development of the care plan, be attentive to the client's most active concerns. A short-range care plan can be developed with specific dates to attend to these concerns. A client who is in crisis feels overwhelmed and finds it difficult to think of the mid-term or long-term future. During the planning stage, the short-term and intermediate plan should be reviewed in the team conference with the other caregivers so that all understand the nursing goals.

As the specific goals of the short-term care plan are developed, share them with the client and discuss his or her reaction to each so that he or she will feel less alone and more secure. Share the plan with the client, even if depression makes him or her unresponsive; at the very least, he or she will be listening. If the client is psychotic or violent, wait until medication has increased his or her ability to participate in a discussion about a care plan before you share it.

Never assume that a mentally ill person is helpless; this is countertherapeutic. The more you promote a client's feeling of helplessness and dependency, the longer you are prolonging his or her illness. Accordingly, if the client is able to participate, even in the most minimal way, in the planning of care, his or her sense of control and personal strength will increase.

## IMPLEMENTATION

You begin to undertake what you developed in the nursing care plan during this step of the nursing process. As you implement your plan, watch and listen carefully to the client. His or her verbal and nonverbal responses can indicate whether or not the nursing approach is therapeutic.

## EVALUATION

Use the intermediate goals to review the client's response to nursing intervention during the last step of the nursing process. Usually, however, new information is obtained, the client's condition improves or worsens, new medication is begun, or some other factor intervenes that requires you to use new data to modify or change the original plan. In essence, you must reinstitute the nursing process of assessing, planning, implementing, and evaluating in order to develop a plan that adjusts to the client's changed condition.

K E Y   P O I N T S

---

- A crisis that causes the onset of mental illness may be an event with which the person has no experience and thus has developed no coping responses. It may also be a series of stressful life experiences. In some cases, a crisis may have no identifiable trigger or precipitating event.
- When a person is functioning well mentally, he or she can tolerate the stress of a new event and develop responses to decrease anxiety.

When a person does not cope effectively, a maladaptive response occurs.

■ Maladaptive response results in change to the person's quality of life and capacity to function. It may also result in a person's decreasing ability to deal with anxiety, which may lead to immobility or panic.

■ Crisis results when the person temporarily loses the capacity to help himself or herself.

■ Certain life change events can cause crisis. These situational events are death, divorce, major illness, marriage, and childbirth.

■ Nursing care for a client in crisis includes assessing what events mean to the person, particularly regarding a client's frame of reference about the events that led to the crisis.

■ Nursing care also includes creating a care plan that offers the client consistent support and monitoring the client's responses to the care.

### SELF-AWARENESS ACTIVITY

- It is not unusual to experience a crisis at various times in our lives. Despite our best efforts to avoid them, most of us go through crises at various times in our lives. Have you ever experienced a crisis in your life? As you look at the various types of crises described in this chapter, are you able to identify a specific cause of the crisis?

- Often there are factors operating in our life that cause us to be more vulnerable to crisis. Is it possible to identify one operating factor that caused you to be more vulnerable to the crisis?

- As you look back at how you overcame the crisis, is there one specific factor you can identify that was the most significant cause of your recovery? Often, such a factor is important to use when undergoing a new period of significant life stress.

## QUESTIONS

1. Jane is 24 years old and engaged to be married in 2 weeks. She presents to an emergency department with symptoms of acute stress. She asks the nurse why she would feel this way when she loves her fiance and is "so happy." The best response by the nurse is:
   a. "Perhaps you're too young to be married."
   b. "Even anticipated and happy events in our lives can be stressful; your marriage will bring many changes to your life."
   c. "Your subconscious is trying to tell you not to marry at this time."
   d. "I don't know. What do you think?"

2. The student nurse will be taking her licensure exam in 2 months. The best description of effective coping mechanisms is when she
   a. plans a study schedule that allows time for family, friends, and activities.
   b. tells her friends that she needs to study and asks that they not call her for the next 8 weeks.
   c. realizes that she likely learned all she needs to know while in school and feels confident that additional study is not necessary.
   d. asks her physician to prescribe an antianxiety medication to help her concentrate on her studies.

3. The nurse recognizes that the most severe situational crisis a person will encounter is
   a. joblessness.
   b. death.
   c. marriage.
   d. childbirth.

4. When working with a 27-year-old client, which of the following behaviors indicates that the client has not yet mastered the developmental tasks for his or her age group?
   a. When the client drifts in and out of relationships.
   b. When the client is unable to assume independence.
   c. When the client is egocentric in relationships.
   d. When the client is unable to take pleasure in the present.

## BIBLIOGRAPHY

Aguilera, D.C. (1998). *Crisis intervention: Theory and methodology* (8th ed.). St. Louis: Mosby.

Barry, P.D. (1996). *Psychosocial nursing: Care of physically ill patients and their families* (3rd ed.). Philadelphia: Lippincott-Raven.

Boyd, M., & Nihart, M. (1998). *Psychiatric nursing: Contemporary practice.* Philadelphia: Lippincott-Raven.

Carpenito, L.J. (2000). *Nursing diagnosis: Application to clinical practice* (8th ed.). Philadelphia: Lippincott Williams & Wilkins.

*Diagnostic and statistical manual of mental disorders* (4th ed.). (1994). Washington, D.C.: American Psychiatric Press.

Groves, J.E., & Kurcharski, A. (1997). Brief psychotherapy. In N.H. Cassem (Ed.). *Massachusetts General Hospital handbook of general hospital psychiatry* (4th ed.). St. Louis: Mosby.

Kennedy, G., & Onogu, E. (1999). Psychiatric emergencies: Rapid response and life-saving therapies. *Geriatrics, 54*(9), 40–42, 45–46.

Lazarus, R. (1991). *Emotion and adaptation.* New York: Oxford University Press, p. 122.

Osterman, J., & Chemtob, C. (1999). Emergency psychiatry: Emergency intervention for acute traumatic stress. *Psychiatric Services, 50*(6), 739–740.

Sadock, B., & Kaplan, H. (1998). *Synopsis of psychiatry: Behavioral sciences/clinical psychiatry.* Philadelphia: Lippincott-Raven.

Stefanis, N., Rabe-Hesketh, S., Clark, B., & Bebbington, P. (1999). Evaluation of a psychiatric emergency clinic. *Journal of Mental Health, 8*(1), 29–42.

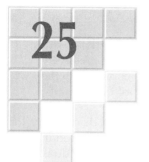

# 25

# Nursing Care of the Older Adult With a Mental Disorder

---

## Behavioral Objectives

*After reading this chapter the student will be able to:*

- Name the percentage of older Americans who are institutionalized.
- Describe why general systems theory is important in assessing the health status of the older adult.
- List the types of losses older adults can experience.
- Name the most common types of mental distress in the elderly and describe each condition and the types of nursing intervention that can reduce the distress.

---

## Key Terms

- Catastrophic reaction
- Cognitive impairment
- Insomnia
- Respite care

---

Advances in health care and government involvement in ensuring adequate care for older adults have resulted in large numbers of people living into their seventies, eighties, and nineties. A majority of elderly persons are self-sufficient and live in their own homes. They are able to maintain an independent lifestyle, often with the involvement of family members who assist them in a variety of supportive ways.

Indeed, although there is a prevalent misconception that the majority of old people are institutionalized, it is not true. It is estimated that 11.7% of the U.S. population—25 million people—are over 65. The number of institutionalized Americans over age 65 is approximately 1,126,000, or only 0.4% of the total population. With few exceptions, the majority of those people were no longer able to live independently or with their families because their mental or physical condition was progressively worsening. The inability of the family system to continue coping with the increasing strain of the infirmity, rather than the severity of the infirmity, determines when institutionalization occurs in most cases.

In considering the nursing care of the elderly with mental disorders, we must remain constantly aware of general systems theory, discussed in Chapter 9, Influences of Family and Social Environment on the Individual.

All systems of human functioning are constantly interacting: physical, psychological, and social. In children and younger adults, the interactions of these three realms of the human being are occurring at all times, although they may not be completely evident. In aged people, it is the effects of these interactions that create the difficulties that they encounter as time progresses.

Most older people remain intellectually aware and capable of independent living until very old age. Despite the losses they encounter, they remain remarkably adaptable and resilient. Their long life experience prepares them to flow with the currents of change that accompany aging rather than be overwhelmed by them.

## ◆ EFFECTS OF LOSS ON THE OLDER ADULT

People of all ages experience losses brought about by physical illness and disabilities. A grieving process in which a variety of mental changes occur accompanies the losses. The grieving process can take up to 1 year when a significant loss occurs. For the elderly, the number of losses they experience can occur in a succession that does not allow them time to adequately resolve one loss before another occurs. Examples of losses frequently encountered in the aging process are shown in Box 25-1.

Losses strain a person's coping abilities. The mastery of the ongoing nature of losses in older age requires well-functioning intellectual and emotional resources; however, age can slowly degenerate these resources.

The body, mind, and social system begin to change at an increased rate as aging occurs. Brain tissue is not immune to the physiologic changes that are occurring throughout the body. The changes in the brain affect our intellectual and emotional capabilities, including abilities to cope.

## ◆ THE MOST COMMON PSYCHOSOCIAL DISORDERS OF THE AGED

It is important to distinguish between the terms *psychiatric* and *psychosocial* when referring to mental disorders in the aged. In order to be termed a psychiatric disorder, a person's mental status must meet the criteria of the

---

BOX 25-1. **Developmental Losses of Older Adults**

- Loss of employment through retirement
- Loss of self-image, if job was a strong source of self-gratification
- Loss of physical health
- Loss of good body image as a result of declining health
- Loss of independence as infirmities increase
- Loss of mobility
- Loss of spouse, friends, or other family members owing to death
- Loss of opportunities for social contact with others
- Loss of home
- Loss of income

---

*Diagnostic and Statistical Manual of Mental Disorders,* fourth edition (DSM-IV) categories of mental disorders (see Chapters 15 to 23). Many people who experience mental distress and emotional pain do not meet these formal criteria. The quality of their lives and that of their families can be severely disrupted, however, because of the impact of decreasing mental abilities on their psychosocial functioning. The following are the most common types of mental distress in the elderly:

Depression
Insomnia
Cognitive impairment
Stress reactions
Decrease in social and daily living skills

## ◆ NURSING CARE OF THE OLDER ADULT WITH DEPRESSION

The incidence of depression in the elderly has never been well documented by research. The number of people of all ages with depression who meet the DSM-IV criteria of major affective illness is approximately 4% to 6%. As described, the elderly experience a number of losses as aging progresses. It is possible that the amount of depression in the elderly is higher than in the general population because unresolved loss is a major factor in many depressive reactions.

Remember that two symptoms of depression are slowing of cognitive functioning and decrease in memory. These are also the symptoms of progressive dementia, a form of cognitive disorder. Unfortunately, primary health caregivers often do not take the time to obtain more information from their clients in order to differentiate between the possible causes of decreased intellectual functioning. Depression is treatable and reversible; dementia generally is not. Too often, the symptoms of depression are assumed to be the signs of dementia; no treatment occurs, and the person's emotional discomfort continues. The symptoms present in older people who meet the criteria of depression are at least 2 weeks of experiencing the following symptoms:

Dysphoric feelings of sadness and hopelessness
Changes in appetite
Changes in sleep patterns
Loss of energy
Lack of interest or pleasure in normal activities
Increased feelings of guilt
Slowed or agitated physical activity
Decreased thinking, concentration, and memory

The most common treatments for depression in the elderly are psychotherapy and antidepressant medication.

The nursing care recommendations given in this chapter should be used as a basis for nursing care planning with depressed older adults. Another nursing care approach that can be considered is nurse-led support groups. This type of group is not the same as a psychotherapy group in which there is more intensive probing and interpretation of a person's statements. Rather, it is a group in which the depressed person has the opportunity to relate with other people who have similar problems.

Often, older people, whether living in their own home, with family members, or in institutions, are isolated from other people. The opportunity to engage in discussion with others in a formal group can provide them with a sense of support and understanding that may have been lacking in their lives. Caring family members, despite their best intentions, cannot provide for all of the psychosocial needs of their aging relative. The sharing of feelings and thoughts with others who are experiencing similar changes can be reassuring and fulfilling.

Nursing care of a depressed older person who is taking antidepressant medication also involves careful observation for the many physical side effects caused by antidepressants (see Chapter 28, Psychopharmacology and Electroconvulsive Treatment of Mental Disorders). These medications can have negative effects on each of the body's major systems. If there is a previously existing physical disorder, these drugs could worsen it. Furthermore, these medications can cause physical symptoms that can be confused with newly emerging illnesses. Elderly individuals often experience a mix of these conditions, which leads to variations in the severity and duration of the distress. Evaluating and determining cognitive abilities may be complicated by age-related changes, such as poor eyesight or hearing, slowed responses, or chronic illness, that make the client's participation in the assessment process more difficult. Remember to document routinely mental and physical status, noting and reporting changes in either.

This will assist the physician in evaluating the therapeutic effects of the medication (see Chapter 14, The Mental Status Exam, and Appendix A, Barry Psychosocial Assessment).

## ◆ NURSING CARE OF THE OLDER ADULT WITH COGNITIVE IMPAIRMENT

**Cognitive impairment** is a decrease in the intellectual aspect of mental functioning; it includes a decrease in problem-solving ability, reasoning, judgment, concentration, and memory. The two most common causes (mentioned in the preceding section) are depression and cognitive disorders.

Remember that some organic brain syndromes are reversible. Ideally, all people suspected of having a dementia type of cognitive disorder should receive a thorough physical examination. Such an examination includes laboratory tests to rule out any other physical condition that could cause a toxic brain syndrome, which might be reversed with treatment. Medication side effects, nutritional deficiencies, different types of physical illness (eg, metabolic disorders, infection, trauma), and so on can cause toxic brain syndromes. Chapter 17, The Client with Delirium, Dementia, Alzheimer's, and Other Cognitive Disorders, describes these conditions.

A psychiatrist should also examine the client when cognitive impairment is suspected. A new subspecialty, geriatric psychiatry, has developed within the field of psychiatry specifically to care for the older adult with mental disorders. Whenever possible, a physician or psychiatric clinical nurse specialist trained in this specialty, who has a systems perspective of the multiple causes of geriatric mental disorders, should perform the psychiatric evaluation.

People with cognitive impairment experience a number of other changes in mental functioning as an outcome of their decreased intellectual ability. Their capacity to cope with stress is decreased, because their ability to solve problems and think through the various events they are encountering is hampered. In addition, they experience a decrease in self-esteem because they can no longer rely on their minds. They may gradually withdraw from relationships and stop attending social functions because they do not want others to notice their decreased mental functioning.

### STRESSFUL EFFECTS ON THE FAMILY OF THE AGED PERSON

Cognitive impairment in an elderly family member places a strain on the entire family system as its members try to adapt. For example, an elderly woman who lives alone may have a physician's appointment, which her son calls to remind her of on the morning of the appointment. When he arrives after a half-hour drive to discover that his mother has forgotten about it and is not ready to leave, he may become frustrated and angry. With the increase in the elderly population also comes an increase in the number of elderly caregivers; in these situations, the person providing the care is experiencing the same kinds of losses and stresses as the identified patient.

As these types of events increase and concern rises about the aging couple's ability to care effectively for each other, or for the safety of the aging person living alone, many families elect to bring the elderly relative into their home. The immediate solution can be positive for all concerned. If the cognitive impairment worsens, however, the level of strain on the family increases.

The children of the aging relative, sometimes called the "sandwich generation," experience increased stress as they attempt to balance the needs of their parents with those of their own children. Communication within the immediate family can become rigid and closed as negative emotions are avoided. Communication in the extended family network of relatives can be equally affected if the person who assumes the caretaking role is resentful. As the mental impairment of the older person increases, it is not unusual for the stress within the family to rise to a critical point, at which point a decision is made to institutionalize the older adult rather than risk what feels like or actually is family disintegration.

Increasingly, support services are being developed in the community to assist families before they reach a crisis point. These services include adult daycare programs or programs designed to relieve the primary caregiver. **Respite care** is the name given to programs designed to temporarily relieve the burden on the primary caregiver. In addition, programs for the primary caregiver are beginning to include group or individual counseling, giving them a chance to relieve themselves of unpleasant feelings such as sadness, anger, or guilt that frequently accompany the care of a cognitively impaired person. Home-based care is another option that is increasingly available. Mental health interventions conducted in the home allow caregivers and family members to participate in these counseling sessions. In-home sessions are particularly useful for clients who find it difficult to get to a doctor's office or mental health clinic. Other helpful programs support coping by increasing knowledge of resources and problem-solving skills for both the older adult and his or her caregivers.

The nursing care of the institutionalized older adult with cognitive impairment is described in Chapter 17, The Client with Delirium, Dementia, Alzheimer's, and Other Cognitive Disorders, under the sections on dementia or delirium, depending on the cause of the mental disorder.

## ◆ NURSING CARE OF THE OLDER ADULT WITH INSOMNIA

Another condition that causes mental distress for many elderly people is **insomnia,** a disturbance in a person's normal sleeping pattern. Insomnia can result from many causes: pain caused by physical conditions, stimulant or diuretic medications, effects of excessive coffee or nicotine, sleeping at other times during the day, poor sleeping environment, or depression or anxiety.

Nearly one-fourth of healthy adults over age 65 report difficulties with their ability to fall asleep, stay asleep, return to sleep if they awaken, or early awakening. In fact, many people overestimate their need for sleep. It should be noted that as a person ages, metabolic rate declines and the need for sleep decreases. In addition, as a person grows older, there are changes in brain wave activity during the various stages of sleep that contribute to increased wakefulness.

Many times, people who experience sleep disturbances of varying levels of difficulty further contribute to the problem by worrying about not sleeping in advance of going to bed. Gradually, they condition themselves so that the thought of not sleeping is accompanied by anxiety.

Generally, it can be helpful to remember that the body maintains regulating mechanisms to ensure its own well being. Sleep occurs when it is necessary to maintain physical and mental equilibrium. An important fact for nurses to know is that hypnotic medications—chronically overused in this country—are effective for no more than 2 weeks, in most cases.

Most people with insomnia are not in institutions and are not recipients of nursing care. Appropriate nursing intervention, regardless of the setting, includes sharing accurate information about sleep hygiene; providing an environment conducive to sleep; reviewing the person's use of caffeinated products, such as coffee, chocolate, tea, sodas, and so on; and recommending modifications where appropriate.

## ◆ NURSING CARE OF THE OLDER ADULT WITH DECREASE IN SOCIAL AND DAILY LIVING SKILLS

An aging person may experience a decrease in his or her normal relationship abilities and living skills. Often, this is the result of cognitive impairment, decreased opportunities for social relationships, and other types of deprivation. Accordingly, as older adults become less able to maintain relationships and to care adequately for nutritional and hygiene needs, it becomes necessary for them to be cared for by relatives, agencies, or institutions.

Some communities offer innovative programs designed to address the needs of two populations: institutionalized clients for whom the goal is discharge, and people who are not institutionalized but whose poor self-care will soon lead to admission if there is no intervention. The programs they designed are aimed at teaching skills—hygiene; self-maintenance skills, such as laundering, meal planning, and money management; normal communication skills; and so on.

Nurses can teach these skills to institutionalized people who lack them and can reinforce their accomplishments with warmth and approval. Also, nurse-led groups that address the topics discussed in the preceding are helpful in teaching social and daily living skills and promoting a supportive group environment in which skill acquisition can take place.

## ◆ NURSING CARE OF THE OLDER ADULT WITH STRESS REACTIONS

As described previously in the chapter, biopsychosocial assessment of older people allows appropriate interventions to be developed that can support adaptation to life's changes. The number of life stressors experienced in old age is usually high. In most cases, adults maintain the same style of coping in old age that they have used throughout their lifetime, but now, a series of life stressors can pile up, undermining coping abilities and overloading coping strength. Examples of these stressors are shown in Table 25-1.

A mild form of cognitive impairment, added to this scenario, can further reduce tolerance for stress. Coping strength is greatly dependent on a person's intellectual capacity. Tolerance for stress may decrease as intellectual capacity diminishes.

The most important external factor in a person's capacity to deal with stress is the availability of support people. Ideally, this support is available from family members or friends. Community support services are hard-pressed to meet the needs of the ever-increasing number of elderly clients.

Some of the primary factors that determine an older person's stress tolerance follow:

Perception of the stressful incident—Does the person view this event as significantly threatening? Why?

History of other stressful incidents during the previous year—Is the current incident the "straw that breaks the camel's back"?

Degree of cognitive impairment due to organic causes

Availability of support people

## TABLE 25–1. Summary of Anxiety Disorders in Later Life

| Characteristic | Changes With Aging |
|---|---|
| Prevalence of anxiety disorders | Lower in later life (5.5%) than in younger years |
| Prevalence of anxiety symptoms | Higher in later life (up to 20%) |
| Differential diagnosis | More difficult in later life because: (1) physical illnesses that often accompany advanced age may mask depression; (2) elders tend to present with physical (somatic) complaints rather than anxiety |
| Treatment | Elders receive disproportionately high numbers of prescriptions for antianxiety drugs (15%). |
| Major causes of anxiety in later life | Medical problems (eg, cardiovascular, pulmonary, thyroid, metabolic, neurologic disorders; vitamin deficiency; sensory deficits); medications (as a side effect or from withdrawal); negative life events (eg, loss of loved ones; physical illness; threat of death; fear of being victimized; diminished self-concept, socioeconomic status, role functioning); psychiatric illness (eg, depression, dementia, hypochondriasis); other (eg, insomnia, chronic pain) |

From Boyd, M., & Nihart, M. (1998). *Psychiatric nursing: Contemporary practice.* Philadelphia: Lippincott-Raven.

## RETIREMENT

The level of stress tolerance for older adults is often related to the issue of retirement. The partner of the retired person can be equally affected. Reichard, Livson, and Peterson proposed the following three basic personality types that adapt well to retirement:

1. The mature type—emotionally well adjusted; life is satisfying for them.
2. The "rocking chair" type—easygoing natures; relieved to be free of responsibilities of work and active family.
3. The "armored" type—actively involved in life to avoid feelings of uselessness; probably have many type A personality characteristics; goal oriented.

They also believe there are two personality types that may not cope well with retirement:

1. The angry type—resentment about unfulfilled goals causes them to resist acceptance of retirement.
2. The self-hating type—feelings of failure cause ongoing guilt and poor self-esteem.

## CATASTROPHIC REACTION

On occasion, if an older person is severely stressed, he or she may be subject to a catastrophic reaction. A **catastrophic reaction** occurs when there is a sudden, unexpected stressor and the person's normal coping mechanisms fail. The result is severe anxiety accompanied by disruption of equilibrium in the physical, intellectual, and emotional realms (see Chapter 12, Stress: Effective Coping and Adaptation). This response is also known as a panic reaction. Frequently it is caused by organic impairment that decreases a person's intellectual capacity to think through and adapt to the stressor.

When an older person is demonstrating decreased tolerance for stress, it often is an indication that his or her problem-solving and decision-making capacities are decreased. Sometimes cognitive impairment is an important contributing factor to catastrophic reactions. Caregivers can help by initiating a discussion of the person's current life situation, with the intention of identifying situations that are problematic. In addition, it is wise to have the person describe potentially stressful circumstances he or she is anticipating. Often, by using the following problem-solving process, solutions can be found that decrease the stress he or she is experiencing.

## PROBLEM-SOLVING PROCESS

1. Identify the problem. Describe why it is a problem and what factors are feeding into it.
2. Describe the possible solutions.
3. Choose the best solution.
4. Implement it.
5. Evaluate the outcome. If not successful, analyze why, choose an alternative from item 2, and implement and evaluate it.

Often, this process relieves the person's distress because it gives him or her the opportunity to describe it. The person then has a stronger sense of mastery of the problem. Recommend the use of this process to the client's family, whether the client is in a hospital or living independently.

It may be necessary to assume a more custodial role if the person is unable to actively participate in this process. Problem solving by the nurse, in consultation with the family, if available, can provide the client with a stronger sense of security.

Generally, it is unwise to routinely administer minor tranquilizers to institutionalized people experiencing chronic stress reactions owing to organic impairment. Instead, whenever possible, it is wise to assess and modify stressors in the environment to minimize the potential for such reactions.

Individual counseling is often helpful for older people living independently and experiencing increasing amounts of stress. This can assist them in identifying both causes and solutions for their stress. In addition, it can help to reduce their anxiety levels. Minor tranquilizers should be avoided, except in the transition period immediately following a severe stressor, such as the unexpected loss of a spouse.

Another stress reliever in the healthy adult is a regular exercise regimen, such as daily walking. The tension-relieving benefits of exercise can have therapeutic effects in chronically stressed individuals.

K E Y   P O I N T S

- Only a small percentage of older adults are institutionalized. Institutionalization often has more to do with lack of family resources for care than with the severity of the elderly person's impairment.
- The losses experienced by an elderly person can occur without time for recovery between losses. This can lead to a strain on the person's coping abilities.
- The most common psychosocial disorders of the elderly are depression, insomnia, cognitive impairment, stress reactions, and decrease in social and daily living skills.

---

BOX 25-2. **Web Resources**

**FOR THE ELDERLY**
*http://www.nih.gov/health/InformationIndex/HealthIndex/Pubincov.htm*
*Sponsored by the National Institutes of Health. Provides general information, publications, and links to other government agencies and programs.*

*http://www.aoa.dhhs.gov*
Administration on Aging website, sponsored by the government. Provides information and links to related resources.

*http://www.aagpgpa.org*
Site sponsored by the American Association of Geriatric Psychiatry. Provides information and resources to support mental health in the elderly.

**FOR FAMILY MEMBERS OF ADULTS WITH MENTAL ILLNESS**
*http://www.nami.org/family/course.html*
Sponsored by the National Alliance for the Mentally Ill, a nonprofit organization. Provides education and information on mental illness and treatment, as well as resources and advocacy support for the client or significant others.

*http://www.nmha.org*
Sponsored by the National Mental Health Association. Provides information and resources for the client and family members.

*http://www.apa.org/psychnet*
Sponsored by the American Psychological Association, provides information on disorders, treatment, and resources for the client and caregivers.

- Slowing of cognitive function and decrease in memory can be caused either by depression or progressive dementia.
- Elderly clients suspected of having a dementia type of cognitive disorder should receive a physical examination to rule out a treatable physical cause.
- Cognitive impairment and other factors of aging place increased strain on the family unit.
- Factors that determine an older person's stress tolerance are perception of the stressful incident, history of other stressful incidents, degree of cognitive impairment, and available support system.
- Three basic personality types that adapt well to retirement are mature (well adjusted), "rocking chair" (relieved to be free of responsibilities), and "armored" (actively involved).
- Two personality types that do not adapt well to retirement are the angry and self-hating types.
- A catastrophic reaction occurs when there is a sudden, unexpected stressor and the person's normal coping mechanisms fail. The response is severe anxiety and disruption of equilibrium, also known as a panic attack.
- Using a problem-solving process (identify the problem, describe possible solutions, choose the best solution, and implement it) can help decrease stress.

### SELF-AWARENESS ACTIVITY

- Are your grandparents still alive?
- Did any of the information in this chapter remind you of concerns that your family has expressed about one or more of your grandparents?
- As you consider getting older, what change or changes in your normal functioning will be the early indicators that you are aging?
- What feelings and thoughts arise as you imagine getting older?
- If you were an elderly person, which of the circumstances common in the lives of elderly people would be of greatest concern to you?

## Q U E S T I O N S

1. When working with an elderly client, the nurse should recognize that
   a. most elderly people are unable to live independently.

    b. loss is a common theme for the elderly.

    c. cognitive deficits are a normal part of the aging process.

    d. the number of life stressors decrease as one ages.

2. When working with an older adult client with insomnia, the nurse should *first*

    a. recommend the use of a sedative-hypnotic medication.

    b. inform the client that most people overestimate their need for sleep.

    c. assess the client's sleep pattern and life factors that may impact sleep quality.

    d. teach the client to avoid the use of caffeine during the late afternoon.

3. Victoria's 88-year-old mother has been having difficulty remembering to take her medication. Victoria is frustrated and vented her feelings with the nurse. Which response would be the best for the nurse to make initially?

    a. "I'm surprised you could say something like that about your mother."

    b. "What do you expect? She's very old."

    c. "Why don't you look at placing her in a nursing care facility?"

    d. "It must be very frustrating for you to see your mother like this."

4. The best nursing approach for elderly clients who are having difficulty making decisions is to

    a. help them identify the problem and possible solutions, and implement the best solution.

    b. assess stressors and make the decisions that would be in their best interest.

    c. consult with family members to make all decisions for the client.

    d. work with health care team members to make the decisions for the client.

## BIBLIOGRAPHY

Adams, T., & Page, S. (2000). New pharmacological treatments for Alzheimer's disease: Implications for dementia care nursing. *Journal of Advances in Nursing, 31*(5), 1183–1188.

Barry, P.D. (1996). *Psychosocial nursing: Care of physically ill patients and their families* (3rd ed.). Philadelphia: Lippincott-Raven.

Boyd, M., & Nihart, M. (1998). *Psychiatric nursing: Contemporary practice.* Philadelphia: Lippincott-Raven.

Carpenito, L. (1999). *Handbook of nursing diagnosis* (8th ed.). Philadelphia: Lippincott Williams & Wilkins.

Carpenito, L. (2000). *Nursing diagnosis: Application to clinical practice* (8th ed.). Philadelphia: Lippincott Williams & Wilkins.

*Diagnostic and statistical manual of mental disorders* (4th ed.). (1994). Washington, D.C.: American Psychiatric Press.

Harrison, A. (1999). Managing acutely disturbed behavior. *Professional Nurse, 15*(3), 183–186.

Krupnick, S., & Wade, A. (1999). *Psychiatric care planning.* Springhouse, PA: Springhouse Corporation.

*Nursing social policy statement.* (1995). Kansas City, MO: American Nurses Association.

Reichard, S., Livson, F., & Peterson, P. (1980). In L. Stein (Ed.). *Aging and personality: A study of 87 older men.* Salem, NJ: Ayer Company Publications.

Sadock, B., & Kaplan, H. (1998). *Synopsis of psychiatry: Behavioral sciences/clinical psychiatry.* Philadelphia: Lippincott-Raven.

Sahr, N. (1999). Assessment and diagnosis of elderly depression. *Clinical Excellence for Nurse Practitioners, 3*(3), 158–164.

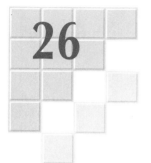

# 26

# Milieu Therapy and Behavior Modification

## Behavioral Objectives

*After reading this chapter the student will be able to:*

- Explain how tranquilizing drugs have helped change the manner of treating mentally ill clients.
- Identify the members of the hospital team who deal with emotionally ill clients.
- Describe the type of atmosphere and attitudes that help establish a therapeutic milieu.
- List the objectives of staff members working with clients who are hospitalized for mental illness.
- Explain why counseling family members is important in the treatment of mentally ill clients.
- Describe the role of halfway houses in the rehabilitation of clients with emotional problems.
- Describe the ways that a client's behavior may be modified or changed by the techniques of relaxation and desensitization, condition avoidance, and operant conditioning (token economy).
- Explain the limitations of behavior modification as a therapeutic modality.

## Key Terms

- Aversive stimulus
- Behavior modification
- Behavioral psychology
- Conditioned avoidance
- Desensitization
- Extinction
- Family therapy
- Major tranquilizers
- Negative reinforcement

- Operant conditioning
- Phenothiazine medications
- Positive reinforcement
- Punishment
- Therapeutic milieu
- Token economy

## ◆ THE THERAPEUTIC MILIEU

The term *milieu* is derived from the French words *ma,* meaning "my," and *lieu,* meaning "place." The phrase "my place" signifies a trusted environment where one can be real and authentic and respected for these qualities. The concept of the **therapeutic milieu** is based on the premise that an individual's current, "here and now" behavior is a reflection of his or her current reality and normal social interactions. This reflection offers insights about why the individual is having difficulty in his or her internal reality or social interactions with others. The treatment team can be most effective by assessing these "here and now" behaviors and designing interventions to modify them so that therapeutic client insights and outcomes can be realized.

Jack has identified several characteristics of a therapeutic milieu. They are as follows:

- Every interaction is an opportunity for therapeutic intervention.
- Clients must assume responsibility for their own behavior.
- Problem solving is achieved by discussion, negotiation, and consensus, rather than a few authority figures.
- Community meetings exist to discuss information and interactions that apply to all staff and clients.
- Peer pressure is a useful and powerful tool.
- Inappropriate behaviors are dealt with as they occur.
- Communication is open and direct between the staff and clients.
- Clients are encouraged to participate actively in their own treatment and decision making on the unit.
- The unit remains in close contact with the community, and there is frequent communication with family and significant members of the client's social network.
- Usually the unit's door is open, and clients have access to areas beyond the unit.

### HISTORY OF DEVELOPMENT OF THE THERAPEUTIC MILIEU CONCEPT

Under the old concept of custodial care for the mentally ill, many clients regressed, relinquished their responsibilities, and were relegated to "back wards." There they were provided with minimal physical care, locked in, and essentially left alone. Most of their decisions were made for them. They were dehumanized, garbed in unattractive clothing, and placed on a rigid institutional routine. When they acted out their hostility, they were subdued with sedative drugs, harsh commands, and, at times, manhandling. If they did not respond to these methods they were put into restraints, such as straitjackets or hand and ankle cuffs. Even those living on the better wards had to submit to regimentation and locked doors and lost their personal belongings and freedom. The staff members who cared for these clients often had little, if any, training in psychology or psychotherapy. The attendants or guards were hired and placed on the wards without in-service training, and they learned to cope with the behavior of their clients to the best of their abilities.

Hermann Simon, a German psychiatrist, introduced the *milieutherapie* approach during the first two decades of the 1900s. Although brief references in historical accounts acknowledge the importance of environment in the treatment of mental disorders, Simon's approach was the first use of the therapeutic milieu on a large scale. The major focus of the *milieutherapie* approach is that a client's social environment can be therapeutic. When all those around the client, staff members and other clients alike, are working to support his or her rehabilitation, restoration to health can be more effectively ensured.

## ACCEPTANCE OF THE THERAPEUTIC MILIEU CONCEPT

The therapeutic milieu concept was not widely adopted in this country until the 1960s. A number of dynamics operating before that time supported its gradual acceptance. The introduction of major tranquilizers during the mid-1900s had the greatest impact on treatment of the mentally ill client, adding another dimension to psychiatric therapy. The **major tranquilizers,** primarily **phenothiazine** pharmaceuticals, were the first medications able to reduce the symptoms of serious mental disorders, such as schizophrenia and bipolar disorder. They lowered the incidence of psychotic symptoms such as delusions, chaotic thinking, severe anxiety, and so on. These medications produced sustained relief of the symptoms of many disturbed mentally ill clients. The amount of disturbed behavior on the nursing units decreased as these drugs became more widely used. The clients became less disorganized and more compliant. Their destructiveness decreased greatly. Accordingly, it became possible to improve the physical surroundings and to gain clients' cooperation in efforts being made for them during their hospitalizations.

As the severity of clients' symptoms yielded to these tranquilizing drugs, great strides were also made in the psychiatric field. Training was begun at all levels to teach hospital personnel the theory of psychiatric care. A client's behavior was regarded as an indication of his or her needs. The different care disciplines began to pool their knowledge and efforts to assess the needs of the client. Thus was born the psychiatric team, which came to include all levels of professionals and paraprofessionals who had actual client contact. Today, in many hospitals, these teams include psychiatrists; psychologists; physicians; nurses; social workers; therapists for drama, art, recreation, and other therapies; teachers; counselors; pastors; and technicians.

When a new client is admitted, he or she is usually apprehensive, upset, and disturbed. He or she is entering a strange new world. Every effort is made to convey that the client will be accepted as he or she is, without criticism, reprimand, or judgment. His or her legal rights are explained. The client is evaluated physically, mentally, and emotionally during the first few days after arrival in order to determine his or her needs. On the basis of these evaluations, the team outlines a treatment program. If the client is able to participate in this planning, he or she is involved and aware of what forms of treatment are being scheduled and why.

## ◆ THE TREATMENT MODEL

Clients are encouraged to set up their own council and form their own rules and regulations. When it is possible for them to do this, they are also expected to enforce these rules. When a resident breaks one of these rules or shows grossly unacceptable conduct, the entire ward then exerts social pressure on this person. This has proved much more effective in reshaping behavior than when the staff has enforced the hospital rules.

Clients are encouraged to be answerable for their behavior as much as possible, but are not required to assume responsibility that they cannot handle. As they improve, more and more responsibilities are offered. Clients should be encouraged to help other clients as much as possible in order to experience responsibility and satisfaction in tasks that hold real meaning.

Clients who tend to withdraw and isolate themselves socially should be placed in a unit that has the interaction of its members as one of its primary goals. The staff should continually reach out toward these withdrawn people and allow them plenty of time to respond. A one-to-one relationship is advisable.

In the past, staff members were cautioned not to become involved in the clients' problems. Their role was that of observing, recording, and controlling the clients' activities. A wide gulf existed between the controlled patient and the controlling staff. Today, emphasis is placed on the necessity of becoming involved with the clients, of participating with them in order to positively influence the course of their illness.

Using the therapeutic milieu approach on clinical units provides a social setting that can socialize clients to the appropriate behaviors expected in the social environments in which they will live following hospitalization. Being socialized to these activities, clients have an opportunity to recognize acceptable and unacceptable behaviors. Box 26-1 shows the outcomes of the therapeutic milieu approach in which behavior modification principles are used as guiding principles for appropriate behavior.

## THERAPEUTIC TEAM TREATMENT

The treatment team is able to develop a comprehensive list of the mental status symptoms, social interactive style, and behaviors that caused the client to be hospitalized by using these "here and now" therapeutic milieu concepts. Therapeutic team treatment includes the following objectives:

1. Develop a team treatment plan to modify specific ineffective coping and social behaviors.
2. Name the objectives or goals of inpatient treatment for each of these ineffective behaviors.
3. Describe the intervention plan for each member of the mental health treatment team with the client.
4. List the mental status and coping criteria necessary for discharge.
5. Describe the outpatient discharge recommendations of the team.

The most therapeutic inpatient hospitalizations are ensured when team planning occurs as described in the preceding. Well-synchronized team planning is the result of good clinical leadership and professional participation by each member of the team. Such planning and therapeutic outcomes can contribute significantly to the ongoing job satisfaction of each team member.

---

### BOX 26-1. Benefits of the Therapeutic Milieu Model

- Clients are accepted.
- Client's rights as individuals are respected.
- Client's treatment needs are explored and addressed.
- Clients are in a more reliable social setting than may be present in their regular social environments.
- Clients are in an environment where they can learn to trust.
- Treatment team efforts are directed toward helping clients.
- The treatment team has a genuine expectation that clients will improve.

## ROLE OF THE NURSE IN THE THERAPEUTIC MILIEU

The nursing staff is one of the most important elements in the hospital environment. Nurses are largely responsible for creating an environment that will produce health for their clients. The interactions that exist among clients and between clients and you are of great importance. The clients must be the focus of interest and concern, so that you may help them to handle stressful situations better. Encourage them to become active participants in all aspects of unit living. Give them the opportunity to discuss fears, problems, observations, successes, and failures openly and frankly with the staff and fellow clients. Group therapy sessions and informal, small, spontaneous interchanges are the best methods.

Each member of a therapeutic staff trained to understand the dynamics of behavior should reinforce each client's strengths and help reduce his or her weaknesses. A client often needs assistance in reestablishing contact with reality. Work and play can be used therapeutically, helping to work off pent-up emotions. A client can be encouraged to satisfy creative needs by making beautiful and useful objects. The social interchange on the unit tends to pull a client back into reality. The nurse's role is directed toward the following:

- Providing the client with a therapeutic milieu that will act as a realistic social setting for his or her therapy
- Encouraging participation in unit activities
- Convincing the client that he or she is a person of worth and dignity
- Reducing the client's anxiety and fear
- Assuring the client that the staff has realistic expectations that he or she can and will improve
- Meeting the client's physical, intellectual, and emotional needs as much as possible
- Emphasizing and providing meaningful tasks and experiences for the client
- Reducing the social distance between the nurse and the client
- Bringing the client slowly but steadily closer to reality and to the community

Although the client is undergoing therapy in the hospital, his or her family should also be involved in family therapy. **Family therapy** provides an environment where family members can explore their own problems and anxieties in relation to their family members with a mental disorder and with each other. Because the client became ill within the family, work, and social settings, these settings should be examined and obvious areas of stress identified. Above all, family, friends, employer, and fellow workers should try to achieve a deeper understanding of the client's feelings and the reasons for his or her behavior if they are going to be able to accept and assist him or her when he or she returns from the hospital. As the client improves, he or she should be allowed short visits home to help re-establish emotional ties there and progress toward eventual complete recovery.

If most of the emotional stress appears to develop within the family setting, complete rehabilitation in a halfway house may be advisable when the client is well enough not to need around-the-clock care. The client can live there for a number of weeks until he or she is able to adjust better to the home setting. Some hospitals have special living units where clients may come and go daily to work. Some clients spend their evenings and nights at a halfway house and return daily to the hospital for therapy.

## ◆ BEHAVIOR MODIFICATION

**Behavior modification** uses systems theory (see Chapter 9, Influences of Family and Social Environment on the Individual) to bring about changes in a client's behavior. What the client *does* is the focus, rather than how he or she feels or why the client is as he or she is.

The field of behavior modification or behavior therapy is strongly based on the psychology of the learning process, as well as conflict resolution theory. Reports of treatment of behavioral disorders by using these methods or related forms of these methods can be found throughout history. It was during the 1960s that behavioral therapy began to be used actively in the treatment of various types of mental disorders. Behavior therapy starts with the assumption that there are one or more types of behavior that create conflict, either within the client or as social system responses to the client's behavior. Accordingly, the client's ability to understand that his or her behavior is causing conflict in the social environment is an essential element in creating a willingness to change his or her behavior. Figure 26-1 shows the different steps in the conflict recognition and resolution process.

For some individuals, insight into the cause of their difficulties in their social environments is not possible. There are a variety of reasons for their inability to develop insight. Generally, these are individuals who have not had reasonable social environments during childhood that interacted with them in a fair and reasonable manner. As a result, they lack the ability to recognize the effects of their actions on individuals in the surrounding environment. When clients are unable to make changes in their behavior as a result of their own insight, behavior modification therapy is one of the options for the treatment team.

Behavior modification therapy differs from the traditional insight-oriented approach to mental illness. It focuses on the behavior of the person rather than on an underlying cause. Behavior modification therapy is an appropriate therapeutic approach for certain types of mental

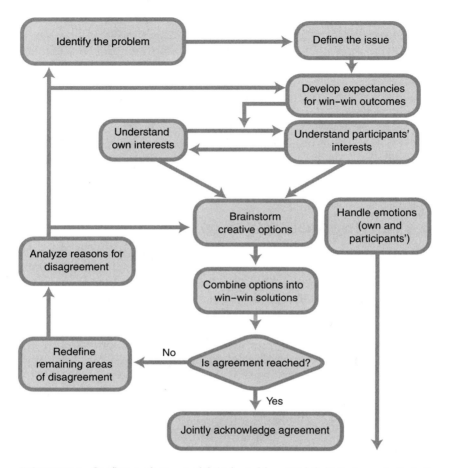

FIGURE 26–1. Conflict resolution model. (Adapted from Littlefield. L., Love, A., Peck, C, C., & Wertheim, E. [1993]. A model for resolving conflict: some theoretical, empirical and practical applicatins. *Australian Psychologist, 28* [3], 80–85.)

disorders. Table 26-1 lists the conditions that have had positive response rates to specific behavioral therapy approaches. The therapy approach appears next to each condition.

The following terms describe the learning principles used in behavior modification or behavior therapy:

**Operant conditioning:** Conditioning or influencing behavior by rewarding a person for positive forms of behavior; also called **behavioral psychology** and behavior modification.

| TABLE 26–1. Behavior Modification Therapy Approaches to Mental Disorders | |
|---|---|
| **Mental Disorder** | **Therapeutic Approach** |
| Phobias or phobic disorders | Desensitization |
| Anxiety or chronic pain | Relaxation |
| | Biofeedback |
| Dependent or passive personality style | Assertiveness training |
| Alcoholism or smoking | Aversive conditioning |
| | Conditioned avoidance |

**Positive reinforcement:** When a person's behavior results in a positive response from others, he or she experiences a feeling of acceptance and internal pleasure and is likely to repeat the same behavior.

**Negative reinforcement:** Rewarding a stoppage of an undesirable event or behavior.

**Aversive stimulus:** Any event that results in an unpleasant feeling.

**Punishment:** A type of reinforcement in which a negative behavior elicits a negative response from the environment. The outcome is a cessation or stopping of negative behavior.

**Extinction:** The complete inhibition of a conditioned reflex as a result of failure of the environment to reinforce it.

Behavioral modification involves modifying the environment of the client in such a way that desirable behaviors are rewarded and undesirable behaviors punished. An example of this is operant conditioning. Using operant conditioning, each client on a psychiatric inpatient unit or partial hospitalization unit has a problem-oriented record on which problem behaviors are listed (such as pacing, excessive smoking, not socializing, talking to voices, and so on). One of the ways that positive behaviors are recognized and rewarded is by using a treatment approach called a **token economy.** Using a token economy therapeutic approach, a schedule is drawn up to provide the client with tokens for desired behavior. For example, a client may be entitled to a token for every half-hour in which he or she does not pace the floor or for every 15-minute conversation he or she holds with another client. These tokens are used to purchase desired things or participation in a desired activity. For example, perhaps the group is planning a picnic or a trip to an amusement park, and each client desiring to go will be charged 30 tokens. If a client does not have enough tokens, he or she is not permitted to go on the excursion. A token economy obviously involves good record keeping, but it does produce desired behaviors.

In a completely developed behavior modification program, the staff, too, may be rewarded for desired behavior (such as coming to work on time and getting the clients to cooperate). In this situation, there is usually a minimal base salary, and the staff can earn more if they produce more.

Another technique of behavior modification is termed **conditioned avoidance.** Here the habit pattern of the client is paired to an unpleasant stimulus so that the client learns to avoid both the stimulus and the habit. The classic example of this technique is the use of disulfiram (Antabuse) in the treatment of the alcoholic.

A classic use of behavior modification techniques is in the treatment of phobias by using relaxation techniques and desensitization. **Desensitization** is a therapeutic approach that involves gradual exposure of an individual to the phobic situation while providing other forms of support and anxiety management. For example, if a client is afraid of flying, the therapist will compile a series of slides or photographs in hierarchical order from the most anxiety-provoking scenes to those that are completely neutral. Such a series may include: (a) a picture looking out of the window of an airplane on take-off (most anxiety-provoking), (b) a picture of the inside of the airplane, (c) the airport waiting room, (d) the airport ticket counter, (e) the airport parking lot, (f) the road to the airport, (g) the client's own car, (h) the client's driveway, and (i) the client's living room (least anxiety-provoking).

In an actual therapy situation there may be 20 or 30 items in the series. Then, the client is taught to relax by a method that is fairly similar to self-hypnosis. While the client is relaxed in the therapist's office, usually on a couch or in a lounge chair, the least anxiety-provoking scene is projected on a screen. The client learns to pair or associate the feeling of relaxation with the picture he or she is viewing. Then the client works his or her way up the series of pictures until he or she comes to one that causes feelings of anxiety. The series is then stopped, the client is assisted to a state of relaxation, and the series is continued (going back a few pictures to a non-upsetting one). After many tries, the client will learn to pair the feeling of relaxation with what was formerly the most anxiety-provoking scene.

Following this desensitization procedure, the client will usually be taken on a field trip to the airport by the therapist. If at any time the client feels anxious, he or she is encouraged to practice relaxation, and the steps are retraced to a non–anxiety-provoking stage. Finally, when the client is ready, he or she may be taken for an actual airplane ride. However, the pattern of relaxation that occurs during the symbolic representation of the feared event usually generalizes to the real-life situation itself, making a field trip unnecessary.

The behavior treated in this example is the fear of flying. Using this therapeutic approach, it is not necessary for the client to ever know *why* he or she became afraid of flying. It is only required that the fear be alleviated.

Although these techniques appear to work on almost anyone, a client with a host of problem behaviors (eg, a chronic paranoid schizophrenic) presents too formidable a task for any behavior therapist. The approach works best with phobias, some sexual disturbances, and some obsessive–compulsive neuroses.

## K E Y    P O I N T S

- Milieu therapy was introduced in the early 1900s. The major focus of this approach is that a client's social environment can be therapeutic for him or her.
- The introduction of major tranquilizers, which lessen anxiety and resulting disturbed behavior by clients, had a tremendous impact on the treatment of the mentally ill client.
- In milieu therapy, the environment acts to help the client function comfortably and encourages improved behavior and self-confidence. It also enables the client to assume responsibility and socialize effectively. This social interchange helps pull clients back into reality.
- In the milieu setting, clients are encouraged to set up and enforce their own rules and regulations. Having residents rather than staff do this is more effective in reshaping behavior. Clients are also encouraged to assume responsibility and to help other clients.
- The nursing staff is largely responsible for creating an environment that is health-producing for the client. Efforts can be directed to emphasizing the client's worth and dignity, meeting the client's needs as much as possible, providing meaningful tasks, and reducing the client's anxiety and fear.
- As the client improves, short visits home help re-establish emotional ties. In some cases, having a client complete rehabilitation in a halfway house may be preferable to discharging the client to an insufficiently supportive family setting.
- Behavior modification focuses on what the client does (behavior) rather than the underlying cause of the behavior. The learning principles used in behavior modification are operant conditioning, positive reinforcement, negative reinforcement, aversive stimulus, punishment, extinction, conditioned avoidance, and desensitization.

## SELF-AWARENESS ACTIVITY

It is natural for all of us to occasionally react to others in our social environments at home, work, school, and different types of group activities, in similar ways to our responses to one or more members of our original families. These reactions can be either positive or negative. Sometimes we are immediately aware of these reactions, and sometimes not. For example, a teacher may remind you of a favorite aunt and you like her before knowing her well. Other times, it is possible to have a negative reaction to a person and wonder why. In the therapeutic milieu of a clinical unit, it is expected that clients respond to the authority figures in the unit, as well as the different group activities in a similar way to his or her current functioning in society as well as within his or her family.

- Have you ever experienced a negative response to a specific person or in a certain group? Where were you and were you able to figure it out at the time or was it later on? How did you resolve it?
- When you are a member of a group, what is your most natural role? Are you an active member who likes to be heard? Do you shy away from being a natural leader of the group or do you dive in to take the leadership? Do you tend to be a peacemaker in a group, or are you one who enjoys "stirring up" people's reactions?
- Are these roles the natural outcome of your group membership in your family and early school experiences?
- Do the principles of behavior modification make sense to you? Is it possible that you have used these concepts in your relationships, without knowing that you were actually attempting to modify someone's behavior? Were you successful? Are there ideas in this chapter that you might consider using the next time that someone's behavior is troubling to you?

## QUESTIONS

1. In a therapeutic milieu, clients would be expected to
   a. follow the treatment plan prescribed by the health care team.
   b. be discharged within 3 months of admission.
   c. participate in only individual therapy.
   d. assume responsibility for his or her own behavior.
2. Nursing staff working in a therapeutic milieu should
   a. encourage the client to participate in activities.
   b. report all client infractions of unit rules to the physician on a weekly basis.
   c. make all decisions for the client regarding his or her nursing care.
   d. All of the above.
3. The social interactions of milieu therapy tend to
   a. let clients feel free to do whatever they wish.

   b. encourage clients to become more dependent on staff.

   c. help clients avoid other clients with more severe mental disorders.

   d. bring the client closer to reality.

4. When working with a structured behavior modification program, the nurse should

   a. encourage the client to explore the origins of his or her mental illness.

   b. reward desired client behaviors.

   c. allow the client to determine the consequences for unacceptable behaviors.

   d. have the client record his or her dreams for evaluation by the psychiatrist.

## BIBLIOGRAPHY

Barker, P. (1998). The behavioral therapies. *Nursing Times, 94*(10), 44–46.

Barry, P.D. (1996). *Psychosocial nursing: Care of physically ill patients and their families* (3rd ed.). Philadelphia: Lippincott-Raven.

Bellus, S., Vergo, J., Kost, P., Stewart, D., & Barkstrom, S. (1999). Behavioral rehabilitation and the reduction of aggressive and self-injurious behaviors with cognitively impaired, chronic psychiatric inpatients. *Psychiatric Quarterly, 70*(1), 27–37.

Boyd, M., & Nihart, M. (1998). *Psychiatric nursing: Contemporary practice.* Philadelphia: Lippincott-Raven.

Carpenito, L. (1999). *Handbook of nursing diagnosis* (8th ed.). Philadelphia: Lippincott Williams & Wilkins.

Carpenito, L. (2000). *Nursing diagnosis: Application to clinical practice* (8th ed.). Philadelphia: Lippincott Williams & Wilkins.

Gerow, J., & Bordens, K. (2000). *Psychology: An introduction.* Carrollton, TX: Alliance Press.

Ogden, J. (2000). *Health psychology: A textbook.* Buckingham, England: Open University Press.

Rathus, S. (2000). *Psychology: The core.* Fort Worth, TX: Harcourt College Publishers.

Sadock, B., & Kaplan, H. (1998). *Synopsis of psychiatry: Behavioral sciences/clinical psychiatry.* Philadelphia: Lippincott-Raven.

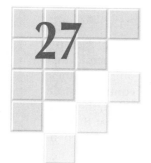

# Group Therapy

---

*After reading*
*this chapter*
*the student*
*will be able to:*

- List the three ways that group therapy can help clients with emotional problems.
- Describe the major patterns of codependent behavior and why people and families use them.
- Describe the differences between group therapy, psychotherapy, and guidance therapy.
- Describe the role of the leader in group therapy.
- Explain why it can be helpful if the members of a therapy group share a degree of similarity in outlook and attitudes.
- Indicate the method by which a qualified member of the health team would set up a therapy group in the hospital.

---

## K e y    T e r m s

- Activity group therapy
- Alcoholics Anonymous
- Art therapy
- Codependence
- Group therapy
- Instructional group
- Occupational therapy
- Play therapy (for children)
- Psychodrama
- Rehabilitation therapy
- Remotivation therapy
- Support group
- Work therapy

There are many definitions and many concepts of group therapy. **Group therapy** is a treatment mode with the guiding principle that individuals function in groups using patterns they acquired in their original families. The purpose of group therapy is to contribute to a change in perception and reality of the group member. In fact, there are many concepts of just what constitutes a group and just what therapy is. Actually, a well-functioning group may consist of as few as four people interacting together; the upper limit is 10 to 12.

## ◆ EARLY SOCIALIZATION IN GROUPS

We become members of many groups throughout our lives. At birth, we become members of the family group. Then come the playgroups, groups in school and church, and the important teenage peer group; then the social groups, business groups, political groups, and parent groups. We remain in some of these groups temporarily, some permanently; some directly, and some indirectly; some voluntarily, and some involuntarily. But always, along life's way, we are involved in group activities.

We are told that our behavior is formed, influenced, and controlled by the dynamic forces existing within groups. If the child's first group—his or her family—fails to provide positive, gratifying interpersonal learning experiences, his or her psychosocial development may well become impaired. For instance, the child who has never learned how to get approval from his or her mother and father tends to develop insecure relationships with authority figures, such as teachers and employers in later life. If he or she fails to relate well with peers in the latency period, and is unable to extract pleasure from association with them, he or she may have trouble in competition and with leadership skills, because it is during this period that leadership and the ability to compete are formed.

## ◆ THE PURPOSE OF GROUPS IN THE THERAPEUTIC SETTING

The concept of structured group interaction, the purpose of which is to promote well-defined therapeutic objectives, is based on the idea that people have a profound effect on one another, both constructive and destructive.

One of the primary treatment modalities in the hospital setting, in addition to medication evaluation and administration, is group therapy. Most hospitalized individuals report that it was the most beneficial aspect of their treatment. Because of the crisis nature of the inpatient experience and the opportunity to meet and talk with others who are also in crisis, the therapeutic group becomes an important vehicle for self-understanding, self-acceptance, short-term planning, and general coping support.

The word *therapy* indicates therapeutic treatment of some sort. Therapeutic refers to any form of treatment or relationship in which the actions, techniques, and practices are purposefully planned and directed toward goals that offer a beneficial effect to the client.

The first clients treated in groups in the United States were tubercular clients. Later, others with various psychosomatic conditions were treated; then the neurotic, the socially maladjusted, and the psychotic. In the early stages of group psychotherapy, it was considered necessary for the therapist to be a psychiatrist. Later, the clinical psychologist was considered sufficiently trained to conduct such sessions. Eventually, nurses assumed this role.

### ◆ THE PURPOSE OF GROUPS IN THE COMMUNITY SETTING

Regardless of the location of a therapeutic group, the purpose is always the same: to provide a safe and supported environment in which individuals can examine their current experiences and options. Many more therapeutic groups occur in the community than the inpatient setting.

The goal of community groups is to support effective coping. A community group may be designed to meet the needs of individuals with specific types of issues, such as recovery from substance dependence, coping with the everyday challenges of chronic depression, or examining the effects of AIDS.

Within the community group setting, individuals have the opportunity to discuss issues that, if left unaddressed, could undermine their decision making and adaptation. Another outcome of group therapy is that it provides additional support to the family or social network of the group member; the availability of group support to an ineffectively coping individual can assist in decreasing the demand on the coping ability of the remaining family members.

### ◆ THE NURSE'S ROLE IN GROUP THERAPY

Three types of groups most commonly have nurse leaders. One type is a support group, in which members explore feelings and thoughts related to a particular subject, such as women's issues or discharge from the hospital. The second is an **instructional group**, in which thoughts and feelings about particular needs related to discharge are discussed within the group. When appropriate, the group leader switches from a leadership to a teaching role. In these first two groups, the major role of the leader is to promote participation from the group members and clarify and paraphrase their statements. This means the leader repeats the statements of others in his or her own words. Such groups have a pre-established structure.

Interpretation and explanation of the causes of clients' conflicts are not undertaken in this setting. A registered nurse functioning as a staff nurse who has had previous group co-leadership and group participation experience is qualified to lead such a group. He or she should discuss the content and process of the group with a supervisor. Ideally, the supervisor should be a certified clinical nurse specialist, a nurse who holds a master's degree in psychiatric/mental health nursing. It is helpful to receive supervision from a person prepared to understand the nursing perspective of client care. Occasionally, people from other disciplines, although skilled as mental health clinicians, lack the ability to integrate the concurrent nursing needs of the client into the group therapy process.

The third type of group, usually called group therapy, has less formal structure than the first two. In it, the members' thoughts and feelings are subject to the analysis and interpretation of the leader. This type of group requires a leader with advanced knowledge of intrapsychic and group dynamics. Customarily, group psychotherapy is led only by people prepared at the master's or doctoral level in one of the mental health disciplines. The nurse-leader, when certified by the Psychiatric/Mental Health Nursing Division of the American Nurses Association, has met the following criteria:

1. Holds a master's degree in psychiatric/mental health nursing
2. Has 2 years' postmaster's experience working in a psychiatric setting
3. Has spent 100 hours in supervision with a board-certified mental health clinician from one of the following disciplines:
   a. Nursing
   b. Social work
   c. Psychology
   d. Psychiatry
4. Has passed a board examination prepared by the American Nurses Association, Division of Psychiatric/Mental Health Nursing

## ◆TYPES OF GROUP THERAPY

Group therapy is a method of treatment in which a number of clients with similar types of problems meet with the therapist in an organized, structured setting for the purpose of arriving at a better understanding of themselves and others, learning how to modify their behavior to a more socially acceptable form, and developing their ability to derive more satisfaction in their relationships with others.

Many varieties of therapy are included today under the general term of group therapy. Among those most commonly used are:

- **Rehabilitation therapy**. The purpose of this form of therapy is to restore a person to his or her pre-illness level of functioning.
- **Remotivation therapy**. The purpose of this form of therapy is to rekindle a person's interest in work, family participation, or type of group or activity to which a person has belonged and lost interest in serving an active role.
- **Occupational therapy**. The purpose of this form of therapy is to prepare an individual to return to his or her prior work role or to prepare to enter a new occupation. In most instances, the individual has experienced some form of physical injury, disability, or mental disorder that renders the person unable to perform his or her prior work responsibilities.
- **Play therapy (for children)**. The purpose of this form of therapy is to provide an environment for children to use traditional children's toys and materials to exhibit, express, and resolve issues and conflicts that are creating increased tension and mental distress.
- **Work therapy**. The purpose of this form of therapy is to provide a working environment where a person can re-enter the work force within a supportive environment to discuss stress-inducing and relationship issues that might otherwise sabotage his or her readiness to return to work.
- **Activity group therapy**. The purpose of this form of therapy is to engage in a specific type of activity as a focal theme, such as attending a play with a group and discussing the activity before and after the experience in a therapeutic group.
- **Psychodrama**. The purpose of this form of therapy is to act out the specific conflicts or life experiences that are important to an individual within a therapeutic group format so that new insights are obtained.
- **Art therapy.** The purpose of this form of therapy is to use artistic materials to express conflicts and discuss those artistic representations within a therapeutic group format led by an art therapist.
- **Alcoholics Anonymous** and other addiction-related groups for persons with the disorder, as well as separate groups for family members. The purpose of these groups is to provide a peer-led program where other individuals experiencing the same types of addictions provide a support group environment to reduce dependence on the substance and its related effects.
- Other **support groups**. The purpose of these groups is to provide a supportive peer-led group in which people who are

experiencing similar types of life adjustments are able to provide encouragement and understanding. There are hundreds of types of peer-led support groups. They include those established by and for parents of children with special needs, such as cerebral palsy, international adoptees, people dealing with life-threatening or altering physical conditions, gay individuals, and so on.

One of the most therapeutic mental health concepts that has developed in the past two decades is **codependence.** In most psychiatric inpatient units there are one or more ongoing therapeutic groups whose purpose is to increase awareness about codependence and how it can affect coping and healthy communication.

Codependence is a cluster of personality traits and patterns that are identified by the chemical dependency field. It is believed that a family coping with an alcoholic member develops codependence as a way to cope with the illness. It is also possible that codependent traits are present in the majority of families as a result of the need to avoid emotional distress or conflict. The characteristics of codependence can create psychological pain in individuals and all of their relationships. Some of the patterns seen in codependence are shown in Box 27-1.

There are a number of groups in clinical settings, as well as self-help groups in the community, that use the codependency concept in their therapeutic approach. These groups include Alcoholics Anonymous; Al-Anon, the group for spouses and loved ones of alcoholics; Adult Children of Alcoholics; similar groups for other types of chemical addiction; and general groups on codependency.

---

### BOX 27–1. **Characteristics of Codependent Relationships**

- Having a strong, compelling desire to solve the problems of others
- Feeling the feelings of others
- Taking responsibility for the choices and actions of others
- Needing to deny one's own feelings
- Needing to please others
- Overcommitting one's time and energy
- Having low self-worth
- Feeling strong guilt and avoiding it by taking care of others
- Worrying frequently
- Feeling emotional turmoil

## ◆ FORMATION OF THE GROUP

The leader should assume the responsibility for making all the arrangements for the group meeting. A treatment goal for the group should be established, as well as plans for its implementation. The nurse should then go to the treatment team and explain the plan for the group, asking for their cooperation in the project. The team members can help choose a balanced group of clients for these sessions, because they are usually quite familiar with the behavioral patterns of the clients under their care.

The next step is to involve the nurse specialist or staff psychiatrists (preferably the team psychiatrist whose clients are to be involved in the therapy) in the project, because supervision is essential to development of therapeutic leadership ability.

The leader should choose a room for the therapy that accommodates the size of the group—one that is well lighted and ventilated and comfortably furnished. The chairs and couches should be arranged in a circle or semicircle. Box 27-2 lists the considerations that promote trust and cohesion within a group.

## ◆ LEADERSHIP STYLE

The way a leader conducts a group can have an important effect on the way the group reaches its objective. The process is what is happening in the group—what dynamics are occurring and why.

---

**BOX 27–2. Factors That Support Group Effectiveness**

- The nurse-leader should interview potential group members to determine their appropriateness for the group.
- The group should consist of 8 to 12 people.
- The group can be homogeneous (people with similar problems, ages, and so on) or heterogeneous (people with a variety of backgrounds, mixed ages, and so on).
- The group meetings in an inpatient setting are usually scheduled from twice weekly to once daily, depending on the purpose of the group.
- The group should be relatively stable in order for the feeling of togetherness to develop. However, it can be "open-ended"; that is, when one or two members leave the group, another one or two can start with the group, so the majority of the group has not changed.
- The length of the therapy is variable. In some instances, it goes on year after year with a few entering and leaving it from time to time. In other instances, if the goal for which it was set up is reached, it may be disbanded.
- The meetings should last from 1 to 1½ hours.

Some group therapists may establish themselves as the authority figure in the group. This might be advisable if the group consists chiefly of withdrawn schizophrenics, where the primary goal is to get them to interact with other members of the group and where a great deal of direct intervention is needed.

However, the method becoming more and more popular is the method by which the group leader, or therapist, sits quietly in the background, controlling the interaction by indirect guidance, sometimes so indirect that it seems as though the clients are running the whole show. The leader invites the clients to share their situations and explain their problems to the entire group. On occasion he or she must quietly redirect the focus to a better solution of the problem, often saying only a word or two.

Unlike psychoanalysis, counseling, or guidance therapy, this form of client interaction does not aim to solve a single, specific situational problem. Rather, its aim is to bring people with similar problems together to help them ventilate their feelings to each other, explore common emotional problems, face their traumatic memories together, and face up to their unacceptable feelings. The leader rarely directs the conversation or suggests remedies for problems but rather acts as a catalyst, helping the ebb and flow of strong emotion, group approval, or group criticism that results from the discussions. The leader encourages clients to express their feelings about people and situations, themselves and their families, their fears and hopes, their hospitalization, and their illness.

## ◆ THE GROUP PROCESS

At times a client expresses deep hostility toward society, a family member, an employer, a fellow worker, and even another member of the group. The other clients can realize, through this anger, that other people can hate and plot revenge and desire to kill, even as they do. They can identify with this destructive form of hate. By assuring the angry client that they, too, entertain similar "bad" emotions, these other clients help restore his or her self-confidence and help channel the destructive impulses without harm to others.

Sometimes a group member receives hostility from fellow members. They may tell the person in no uncertain terms that his or her feeling, behavior, or thinking is wrong. This may result in a behavioral change or a changing concept in the person thus judged by his or her peers.

Slowly, a sense of belonging develops in the group. An increased sense of self-identity is noticeable in most of the participants. Eventually, the clients in the group start behaving like members of a strongly knit family. What threatens one, threatens all. When one member rejoices over a problem worked through there is a sense of elation in the entire group. This is truly a client-administered form of therapy—

clients administer therapy to each other. This form of client-acting-on-client is therapy at its best, and it is a strong deterrent of unacceptable behavior and acting out.

Some people become very anxious as a result of the increased intimacy that such a group formation engenders. Some become overwhelmed and oppressed by shame when they yield to the invitation to disclose the disturbing facts in their past lives. Some cannot tolerate the criticism of their fellow members and may develop antagonism toward those who so criticize them.

On the whole, once a client joins such a therapy group, he or she usually perseveres in it, and very often, members of the group, working out their problems together, become deep friends and carry on these friendships after they leave the hospital.

## KEY POINTS

- The concept of structured group action to promote therapeutic objectives is based on the idea that people have a profound effect on one another, both positive and negative.
- Support groups, instructional groups, and group therapy are often led by nurses.
- In support groups, members explore feelings and thoughts related to a particular subject.
- In instructional groups, members discuss thoughts and feelings about particular needs related to discharge.
- Group therapy is a method of treatment in which clients with similar types of problems meet with a therapist in an organized, structured setting. Their purpose is to better understand themselves and others, learn to modify their behavior, and develop their ability to derive more satisfaction from their relationships with others.
- In group therapy, the members' thoughts and feelings are subject to the analysis and interpretation of the leader. Thus, the leader must have advanced knowledge of intrapsychic and group dynamics.
- When the leader is making arrangements to form a group, he or she should involve the entire treatment team in reviewing the goals for the group and implementation.
- The way the leader conducts the group has an important impact on how the group reaches its objective. Depending on the needs of the group members, the leader may be more or less directive.
- During the group process, members slowly begin to develop a sense of belonging and begin to behave like members of a strongly knit family. The result is "clients-acting-on-clients," which is a strong deterrent to unacceptable behavior.

■ Codependence is a set of personality traits and patterns. It is believed these behaviors are developed as a means to avoid emotional distress or conflict.

### SELF-AWARENESS ACTIVITY

The family is the first group to which we belong. Often, our responses and behavior in a group has similarities to our roles in our original families. For example, a child who is a peacekeeper or an agitator in his or her original family may continue to exhibit similar tendencies in groups during adulthood.

- Stop for a moment and recall your roles and behavior with different people in your family. Is it possible you have similar reactions in different groups to which you now belong? For example, you are now a student nurse and in your nursing program you are in different classes with different groups of people. How would other members of your different groups in nursing school describe your interpersonal style? How would members of your original family describe your interpersonal style?

- Is it possible that you may have different responses to different types of instructors that may relate to your experiences with parents, teachers, and other authority figures when you were a child?

## QUESTIONS

1. A client in an outpatient support group for people with cancer states that she had suicidal thoughts when she was first diagnosed. Another group member interjects that he had similar thoughts. The nurse should:
   a. Separate the clients, so they do not talk about suicide again. One client should be dismissed from the group.
   b. Ignore the comments as the group was established as a support group and the nurse's role is limited.
   c. Realize that these comments allow group members to feel that they are not alone. The risk for suicide should be assessed individually.
   d. Request an emergency psychiatric admission for both clients.

2. The nurse recognizes that a client may be codependent when the client
   a. is addicted to more than one substance.
   b. refuses to be involved in unit activities.

c. has little regard for other clients on the unit.

d. continually tries to please staff and peers.

3. When organizing a group, the nurse should

a. make certain that all group members are the same gender.

b. limit the size of the group to less than six members.

c. schedule the group for a minimum of 2 hours.

d. seek support and cooperation from the treatment team.

4. In support and instructional groups, the nurse leader's role is to

a. promote participation from clients and paraphrase their statements.

b. develop a plan for each client and make sure it is followed.

c. keep the group totally focused on behavior rather than on feelings.

d. write down what everyone says, to discuss it with them later.

## BIBLIOGRAPHY

Barry, P.D. (1996). *Psychosocial nursing: Care of physically ill patients and their families* (3rd ed.). Philadelphia: Lippincott-Raven.

Boyd, M., & Nihart, M. (1998). *Psychiatric nursing: Contemporary practice.* Philadelphia: Lippincott Williams & Wilkins.

Gerow, J., & Bordens, K. ((2000). *Psychology: An introduction.* Carrollton, TX: Alliance Press.

Long, P., & Leach McMahon, A. (1996). Working with groups. In J. Haber, P. Price-Hoskins, A. Leach McMahon, & B. Sideleau (Eds.). *Comprehensive psychiatric nursing* (5th ed.). St. Louis: Mosby–Year Book.

Ogden, J. (2000). *Health psychology: A textbook.* Buckingham, England: Open University Press.

Pollack, L., & Cramer, R. (1999). Patient satisfaction with two models of group therapy for people hospitalized with bipolar disorder. *Applied Nursing Research, 12*(3), 143–152.

Rathus, S. (2000). *Psychology: The core.* Fort Worth, TX: Harcourt College Publishers.

Sadock, B., & Kaplan, H. (1998). *Synopsis of psychiatry: Behavioral sciences/clinical psychiatry.* Philadelphia: Lippincott Williams & Wilkins.

Zupancic, M., & Kreidler, M. (1999). Shame and the fear of feeling. *Perspectives in Psychiatric Care, 35*(2), 29–34.

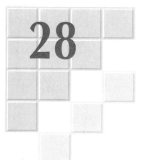

# 28

# Psychopharmacology and Electroconvulsive Treatment of Mental Disorders

---

## Behavioral Objectives

*After reading this chapter the student will be able to:*

- Identify broad classifications of psychotropic medications and their indications for use.
- List at least one medication for each identified classification of psychotropic medication.
- Discuss common side effects and nursing implications for identified psychotropic medications.
- Identify symptoms of significant side effects and nursing implications for identified psychotropic medications.
- Describe electroconvulsive therapy and indications for use.
- Discuss nursing care for the client undergoing electroconvulsive therapy.

---

## Key Terms

- Akathisia
- Antianxiety agents
- Anticholinergic effects
- Anticonvulsants
- Antidepressants
- Antiparkinsonian agents
- Antipsychotics
- Dystonia
- Electroconvulsive therapy
- Extrapyramidal symptoms
- Lithium toxicity
- Mood stabilizers
- Neuroleptic malignant syndrome
- Pharmacokinetics
- Psychotropic drugs
- Pseudoparkinsonism
- Sedative-hypnotics
- Serotonin syndrome
- Tardive dyskinesia
- Therapeutic index

## ◆ GENERAL CONSIDERATIONS ABOUT PSYCHOPHARMACOLOGY

The development of medications that restore brain chemistry to near-normal levels has markedly altered the treatment of mental illness. The availability of these medications has been the single most important contributing factor to the discharge of hundreds of thousands of chronically mentally ill individuals from long-term mental institutions.

The knowledge and clinical use of medications in psychiatry is called psychopharmacology; medications used in the treatment of mental disorders are most commonly called **psychotropic drugs.** Psychotropic medications are those that affect behavior, psychological or cognitive function, or the sensory experience. Development of new, more effective psychotropic agents is ongoing. As the number of new medications or new uses for standard medications increases, nurses must seek appropriate understanding before administering them to clients.

The role of the nurse in the administration of all medications is central and indisputable. Nurses are often the first to perceive the need for medication in a particular client or the need to change the drugs the client is receiving. They may be the first to recognize side effects or adverse reactions and call them to the physician's attention. The nurse instructs the client and significant others about the medication and precautions to observe with certain medications. The psychiatrist, working together with the other members of the mental health team in the area of psychopharmacology, delivers a safer, more comprehensive service to the client as a result of the information received from the nurse about the client's response to medication.

A number of factors may impact the utilization and response of clients to medications. Race and gender have been shown to impact the **pharmacokinetics** (the absorption and action) of psychotropic agents. Compared with whites and African-Americans, Asians are more sensitive to alcohol, **antipsychotics, antidepressants,** and antianxiety medications. African-Americans have impaired metabolism of lithium carbonate, resulting in the need for a lower dose to obtain therapeutic result. Preliminary research indicates that women respond better to serotonin reuptake inhibitors than to tricyclic antidepressants. Medications also may be secreted in breast milk or may pass the placental barrier, so they must be used cautiously in women of childbearing age. Additionally, smoking and the use of caffeine may impact the absorption and distribution of many agents. Psychotropic medications and dosages must be individualized and clients observed frequently for therapeutic response or side effects from these medications.

Another major concern for the client and health care professional is the risk for drug–drug interactions. Many clients take medications for control of both physical and mental illnesses. Many medications are contraindicated when given together. When given together, they may diminish the efficacy of each medication or increase the likelihood of serious side effect. Home or herbal remedies may result in similar problems. Nurses must be certain to review and assess all medications the client is taking in order to identify and address potential problems.

## IMPORTANCE OF CLIENT CONSENT

The drugs used to treat mental disorders have many significant side effects. Because of the nature of these medications and their therapeutic effects and potential side effects, physicians and nurses are required to discuss them with their clients. Through this discussion the health care professional can learn about the client's past experiences with psychotropic medications that may impact current treatment. Clients have the right to know about the risks and benefits associated with a medication before agreeing to take it. Clients have the right to refuse medications or treatment. Refer to Chapter 6, Professional, Legal, and Ethical Issues in Mental Health Nursing, for further discussion of legal-ethical considerations in mental health nursing.

## ◆ MAJOR DRUG CATEGORIES

Seven groups of drugs are used most frequently for clients with mental disorders. These groups and their general functions are shown in Box 28-1.

There are subtle differences in the action of the various medications within a category. For example, some antipsychotic agents are more "alerting," some more sedating. Each drug has particular side effects, and some are more likely than others to cause symptoms mimicking Parkinson's disease. Prescribing health care professionals often base prescriptive decisions on the client's presenting symptoms and the medication profile, in an attempt to "balance" behaviors. However,

---

### BOX 28-1. Drugs Used Most Frequently With Mental Disorders

**Antipsychotics** alleviate psychosis.
**Antidepressants** reduce depression.
**Antianxiety agents** lower anxiety levels.
**Sedative–hypnotics** lower anxiety levels and promote sleep.
**Antiparkinsonian agents** decrease the extrapyramidal symptoms that develop as side effects of major antipsychotics.
**Anticonvulsants** lower the potential for seizures.
**Mood stabilizers** treat the cycles of bipolar disorder.

in terms of drug choice, a client's individual reaction, particular situation, and preference may often cast the deciding vote.

Clients who have taken psychotropic agents can often remember difficulties with drugs. A man who has experienced disturbed sexual functioning on thioridazine (Mellaril) will ask for something else. The person who has a tendency toward pseudoparkinsonism as a medication side effect and has had great difficulty in this regard with haloperidol (Haldol) or fluphenazine (Prolixin) may fear the same reaction will occur with other drugs. If the client's last medication experience was as an inpatient, the doses he or she remembers may be out of line for outpatient care. Too much sedation could make traveling dangerous or might result in the client staying at home in bed.

Nonetheless, wherever possible, the client's wishes are honored and comments about his or her drug experiences are considered. If there is a clear contraindication to the client's drug or dose choice or if the nurse or physician believes that there is great importance in using a different drug, all of the facts are explained to the client and his or her full cooperation is sought.

When a client is started on psychotropic drugs *for the first time*, more caution is required, and a careful history of drug sensitivities in both the client and family must be obtained. A family history of success with a particular psychotropic drug in a blood relative with a similar disease is considered presumptive evidence that the present client may do best with the medication. For example, it is known that amitriptyline (Elavil) is more sedating than imipramine (Tofranil) and usually is a better choice when depression is accompanied by considerable anxiety, agitation, or insomnia. However, if two sisters in a family developed agitated depressions within a few years of each other and the first did well on Tofranil and less well on Elavil, using Tofranil in the second sister should be considered from the beginning. Both constitutional factors and family suggestibility play a role in drug response. Accordingly, information about family drug experience is sought and valued.

## ANTIPSYCHOTICS

Antipsychotic medications are used to treat psychotic symptoms, such as those that exist in a person with schizophrenia. These medications may also be used for clients with psychosis not associated with schizophrenia or those with Tourette's syndrome, severe agitation associated with dementia, mania, and even hiccoughs or nausea and vomiting. They may also be referred to as neuroleptic agents and have been known as major tranquilizers. They are defined as either "typical" or "atypical" agents. Although not fully understood, these agents are thought to exert their effects on dopamine, ultimately reducing the amount of dopamine available or by blocking over-reactive dopamine receptors. They are further categorized by a number of chemical classifications.

Typical, or conventional, antipsychotics are typified by the chemical class phenothiazines. They were introduced in the 1950s and resulted in major changes in the treatment of mental illness. The oldest drug in this category is chlorpromazine (Thorazine). Typical antipsychotics are most effective for clients with positive symptoms of schizophrenia (hallucinations, delusions, bizarre behavior, and inappropriate affect).

Atypical antipsychotics are effective for clients with both positive and negative (lack of motivation, blunted affect, decreased activity, and social isolation) symptoms of schizophrenia. Most atypical antipsychotic medications have been available in the United States since the early 1990s. A comparison of side effects from selected antipsychotic medications is shown in Table 28-1.

TABLE 28-1. **Comparison of Side Effects From Selected Antipsychotic Medications**

| Drug Category (Drug Name) | Sedation | Extrapyramidal | Anticholinergic | Orthostatic Hypotension |
|---|---|---|---|---|
| *Standard (Atypical) Antipsychotics* | | | | |
| Chlorpromazine (Thorazine) | +4 | +2 | +3 | +4 |
| Thioridazine (Mellaril) | +3 | +1 | +4 | +4 |
| Mesoridazine (Serentil) | +3 | +4 | +1 | +3 |
| Fluphenazine (Prolixin) | +1 | +4 | +1 | +1 |
| Perphenazine (Trilafon) | +2 | +3 | +2 | +2 |
| Trifluoperazine (Stelazine) | +1 | +3 | +1 | +1 |
| Thiothixene (Navane) | +1 | +4 | +1 | +1 |
| Loxapine (Loxitane) | +2 | +3 | +2 | +3 |
| Haloperidol (Haldol) | +1 | +4 | +1 | +1 |
| Molindone (Moban) | +2 | +3 | +2 | +1 |
| Pimozide (Orap) | +3 | +4 | +3 | +2 |
| *Atypical Antipsychotics* | | | | |
| Clozapine (Clozaril) | +4 | +/0 | +4 | +4 |
| Risperidone (Risperdal) | +1 | +/0 | +1 | +2 |
| Olanzapine (Zyprexa) | +4 | +/0 | +2 | +1 |

+/0 = lowest likelihood

+4 = highest likelihood

From Boyd, M., & Nihart, M. (1998). *Psychiatric nursing: Contemporary practice.* Philadelphia: Lippincott-Raven.

## Typical Agents

Although therapeutically beneficial, the incidence of side effects in the typical antipsychotic agent is significant. Normal, coordinated, and smooth body movements depend on a critical balance of dopamine and acetylcholine. A disruption of this balance, as a result of medication therapy, may result in the development of movement disorders. Movement disorders are referred to as **extrapyramidal symptoms** (EPS) and have three common reactions: **pseudoparkinsonism, akathisia,** and **dystonia.** Box 28-2 provides descriptions of these reactions. Extrapyramidal side effects require intervention, which generally consists of the administration of **antiparkinsonian agents** on a routine basis or as needed for symptom management.

Other common side effects include photosensitivity and anticholinergic effects. **Anticholinergic effects** are outlined in Box 28-3. These effects are uncomfortable, and many clients stop taking antipsychotic medications because of them. The nurse is responsible for monitoring the client for the presence of EPS as well as teaching the client how to decrease or eliminate other common side effects.

Clients should be taught to avoid prolonged exposure to the sun. They should use sunscreen consistently and wear protective clothing. Clients must also be taught to maintain adequate hydration and stand slowly after sitting or lying down to avoid hypotensive episodes. Activity, diet, and hydration also decrease uncomfortable side effects such as constipation and weight gain.

Another less common, but potentially life-threatening, side effect is **neuroleptic malignant syndrome** (NMS), in which the client experiences dysregulation of cardiovascular function, temperature, and mental status. Neuroleptic malignant syndrome is more frequent in the first 2 weeks of treatment or after an increase in dosage, but it may occur at any time during treatment. Symptoms include fever, severe catatonia, irregular pulse, tachycardia, diaphoresis, change in blood pressure,

---

### BOX 28-2. Overview of Extrapyramidal Symptoms

| SYMPTOM | CHARACTERISTICS |
| --- | --- |
| Pseudoparkinsonism | Symptoms similar to Parkinson's disease. Shuffling gait, masked facies, drooling, tremor, stiff posture, and rigidity. |
| Akathisia | An uncomfortable sense of internal restlessness. Inability to sit still. |
| Dystonia | Muscle spasms of the jaw, tongue, neck or eyes. Potential for laryngospasm. |

## BOX 28-3. Anticholinergic Effects

| | |
|---|---|
| Blurred vision | Urinary retention |
| Photophobia | Decreased sweating (anhidrosis) |
| Dry mouth (xerostomia) | Constipation |

change in mental status, and elevated creatine kinase and myoglobin secondary to muscle breakdown. Not all symptoms may be present, making NMS difficult to diagnose. Treatment includes discontinuation of the antipsychotic medication and supportive therapy to maintain vital function, such as cooling blankets and adequate hydration.

**Tardive dyskinesia** (TD), considered irreversible, is a severe reaction in which the client experiences involuntary movements of the mouth, tongue, and face. It may also progress to involve the client's fingers, arms, trunk, and respiratory muscles. It is usually associated with long-term use of typical antipsychotic agents. Box 28-4 identifies associated risk factors. If tardive dyskinesia develops, the offending medication must be discontinued and the client assisted in maintaining activities of daily living.

An advantage a typical antipsychotic agent may have over an atypical agent is that there are two medications available in decanoate formulations. Decanoate formulations allow the medication to be absorbed slowly, after intramuscular injection, over a period of weeks. Haloperidol (Haldol) and fluphenazine (Prolixin) are available in decanoate. This allows many clients who were not consistent with medication compliance to function on an outpatient basis.

The development of side effects generally depends on the relative potency of the medication.

## BOX 28-4. Risk Factors for Tardive Dyskinesia

Age over 50
Female
Affective disorders, particularly depression
Brain damage or dysfunction
Increased duration of treatment
Standard antipsychotic medication
Possible higher doses of antipsychotic medication

From Boyd, M., & Nihart, M. (1998). *Psychiatric nursing: Contemporary practice.* Philadelphia: Lippincott-Raven.

Typical antipsychotic agents are classified as low-, moderate-, or high-potency agents. Examples of these medications are shown in Box 28-5.

### Atypical Agents

Atypical antipsychotic agents have fewer movement-related side effects than the typical agents. Side effects of these agents may include weight gain, agitation, nervousness, and sexual dysfunction. Although it is generally thought that they have fewer side effects than typical antipsychotic agents, the nurse must be certain to carefully review the medication with the client. Examples of these medications are shown in Box 28-6.

The risk for NMS and TD is thought to be lower with atypical agents, although this has not been fully evaluated with the newer medications. One serious complication seen with clozapine (Clozaril) therapy is agranulocytosis, a deficient number of granulocytic white blood cells, which can result in death if untreated. Clozapine therapy, therefore, is carefully monitored with white blood cell counts before medications are dispensed. Clients should be observed for signs and symptoms of infection and taught to notify their health care provider immediately when they arise.

### ANTIDEPRESSANTS

Antidepressant agents are given primarily to treat the symptoms of depression. These agents are also being used in the treatment of eating disorders, anxiety, pain disorders, and smoking cessation. The effects of these drugs are generally not noticed for 2 to 4 weeks, and the client usually must be encouraged to continue taking his or her medicine, even though at first there is little improvement. Initially, the client's psychomotor retardation, often part of the depressive picture, may seem increased by the drowsiness related to the medication. Once his

---

### BOX 28-5. Examples of Typical Antipsychotic Agents

**LOW-POTENCY AGENTS**
chlorpromazine (Thorazine)
thiodazine (Mellaril)
mesoridazine (Serentil)

**MODERATE-POTENCY AGENTS**
loxapine (Loxitane)
molindone (Moban)
perphenazine (Trilafon)

**HIGH-POTENCY AGENTS**
thiothixene (Navane)
haloperidol (Haldol)
fluphenazine (Prolixin)

---

**BOX 28-6. Examples of Atypical Antipsychotic Agents**

clozapine (Clozaril)                    risperidone (Risperdal)
olanzapine (Zyprexa)                    sertindole (Serlect)
quetiapine (Seroquel)

---

or her depressive symptomatology is relieved, the client tends to discontinue the medication prematurely. However, he or she should ordinarily continue on the antidepressant for 3 to 6 months, and then undergo gradual dosage reduction for up to a total of 1 to 1.5 years.

Another significant nursing consideration is that individuals with suicidal ideations may have an increased risk for suicide as their depressive symptoms lift and they start to have more physical energy. Clients taking antidepressant medications should be routinely evaluated for suicidal ideation or intent. There are four broad categories of antidepressant medication: tricyclics, monoamine oxidase inhibitors, selective serotonin reuptake inhibitors, and novel antidepressants (Box 28-7).

### Tricyclic Antidepressants

Tricyclic antidepressants (TCAs) are related to phenothiazines and frequently have toxic effects on many body systems, most notably the cardiovascular system. A client should have a thorough cardiovascular assessment before these medications are prescribed. They have a significant anticholinergic effect, and the client should also be evaluated for narrow angle glaucoma, prostatic hypertrophy, and urinary retention. The potential for hypotension is also a risk, especially for the eld-

---

**BOX 28-7. Examples of Antidepressant Agents**

**TRICYCLIC AGENTS (TCAs)**
amitriptyline (Elavil)
desipramine (Norpramin)
nortriptyline (Tofranil)
doxepin (Sinequan)

**MONOAMINE OXIDASE INHIBITORS (MAOIs)**
phenelzine (Nardil)
tranylcypromine (Parnate)
selegine (Eldepryl)

**SELECTIVE SEROTONIN REUPTAKE INHIBITORS (SSRIs)**
fluvoxamine (Luvox)
prozac (Prozac)
paroxetine (Paxil)
sertraline (Zoloft)

**NOVEL ANTIDEPRESSANTS**
trazodone (Desyrel)
bupropion (Wellbutrin)
venlafaxine (Effexor)
nefazodone (Serzone)
mirtazapine (Remeron)

erly. These medications also lower the seizure threshold and should be used cautiously in clients with known seizure disorders.

Tricyclic antidepressants work by broadly blocking the reuptake of norepinephrine and serotonin. They tend to produce withdrawal symptoms on abrupt discontinuation of therapeutic dosages taken for 6 to 8 weeks. Withdrawal consists of nausea, vomiting, abdominal cramps, diarrhea, chills, insomnia, and anxiety. Withdrawal begins 4 to 5 days after discontinuation and last 3 to 5 days; it is avoided by gradual withdrawal over 3 to 4 weeks.

Tricyclics cause two types of toxic mental effects. The first consists of a shift from the original depression to a state of manic-like excitement; the second resembles an organic brain syndrome, especially in the elderly, ranging from a transient deficit in recent memory to delirium. Additionally, tricyclics, when taken in overdose, have a high mortality rate.

### Monoamine Oxidase Inhibitors

Monoamine oxidase inhibitors (MAOIs) can be useful in some clients who are not responsive to other medications. However, they cause potentially serious side effects and are considered by some authorities to be unacceptable for general use in a community mental health setting. The nurse should discuss with the physician any cases in which the client's reliability or ability to understand and follow directions is questionable. These medications inhibit enzymes that metabolize serotonin, norepinephrine, and dopamine, resulting in an increase in these neurotransmitters. Common side effects of these medications are daytime sedation, insomnia, weight gain, dry mouth, and orthostatic hypotension.

Hypertensive crisis may result in clients taking MAOIs who eat foods that contain tyramine or dopa. Foods to be avoided when taking MAOIs are outlined in Table 28-2. There also are a number of medications that are contraindicated when a person is taking an MAOI, including asthma tablets or inhalers, weight-reduction aids, selective serotonin reuptake inhibitors (SSRIs), meperidine (Demerol), and products with dextromethorphan or ephedrine.

The symptoms of hypertensive crisis are a sharp elevation in blood pressure, throbbing headache, nausea, vomiting, elevated temperature, sweating, and stiff neck. The client should be positioned with his or her head elevated, have vital signs evaluated, and administered medication to control the hypertension immediately. Additionally, a client scheduled for an elective surgery or being changed to an SSRI should be taken off any MAOIs at least 2 weeks before surgery or before starting an SSRI medication regimen.

### Selective Serotonin Reuptake Inhibitors

Selective serotonin reuptake inhibitors block the reuptake of serotonin, a more selective process than the TCAs, which results in fewer sys-

## TABLE 28–2.  **Example of a Tyramine-Restricted Diet**

| Category of Food | Food to Avoid | Food Allowed |
|---|---|---|
| Cheese | All matured or aged cheese. All casseroles made with these cheeses, pizza, lasagna, etc.<br><br>*Note:* All cheeses are considered matured or aged except those listed under "food allowed." | Fresh cottage cheese, cream cheese, ricotta cheese, and processed cheese slices. All fresh milk products that have been stored properly (eg, sour cream, yogurt, ice cream). |
| Meat, fish, and poultry | Fermented/dry sausage: pepperoni, salami, mortadella, summer sausage, etc. | All fresh packaged or processed meat (eg, chicken loaf, hot dogs), fish, or poultry |
| Fruits and vegetables | Fava or broad bean pods (not beans) | Banana pulp |
|  | Banana peel | All others except those listed in "food to avoid" |
| Alcoholic beverages | All tap beers | Alcohol: No more than two domestic bottled or canned beers or 4-fluid-oz glasses of red or white wine per day; this applies to nonalcoholic beer also; please note that red wine may produce a headache unrelated to a rise in blood pressure. |
| Miscellaneous foods | Marmite concentrated yeast extract | Other yeast extracts (eg, brewer's yeast) |
|  | Sauerkraut | Soy milk |
|  | Soy sauce and other soybean condiments |  |

From Boyd, M., & Nihart, M. (1998). *Psychiatric nursing: Contemporary practice.* Philadelphia: Lippincott-Raven.

temic side effects. Selective serotonin reuptake inhibitors are currently the most frequently prescribed antidepressants. Common side effects include agitation, anxiety, akathisia, insomnia, and sexual dysfunction.

One potentially serious effect is **serotonin syndrome** (SS). Serotonin syndrome is characterized by mental changes, altered muscle tone, fever, and autonomic dysfunction. Serotonin syndrome can present a clinical picture similar to neuroleptic malignant syndrome (NMS). Treatment includes withdrawal of the medication and supportive care. Some over-the-counter remedies such as St. John's Wort, and the co-administration of MAOIs with SSRIs, are thought to increase the risk for SS.

## Novel Antidepressants

These medications do not fit into the other identified classes of antidepressants. Some of them work by blocking serotonin reuptake; others block both serotonin and norepinephrine reuptake. Further information on how these medications exert a therapeutic effect can be found in drug books. In general, giving any of the novel antidepressants during pregnancy and lactation or to individuals with kidney or liver disease is contraindicated. They should also be given cautiously to individuals with known seizure disorders.

## ANTIANXIETY DRUGS

The **antianxiety agents** have limited usefulness in the outpatient setting, unless the anxiety is incapacitating. Anxiety normally accompanies growth and change and is an important ingredient in providing the motivation for most psychotherapeutic work. Most clients can tolerate a moderate level of anxiety without medication. Some antidepressant agents, such as MAOIs and TCAs, are effective when used for individuals with chronic anxiety disorders such as panic disorder or obsessive-compulsive disorder.

Other antianxiety (anxiolytic) agents, such as benzodiazepines and barbiturates, have a high potential for habituation and addiction and carry a danger of withdrawal. These agents reduce activity in the central nervous system (CNS), resulting in a decrease in anxiety. The agents most commonly used for anxiety are the benzodiazepines. Examples of these drugs are found in Box 28-8. These agents are rapidly absorbed and result in sedation, fatigue, reduced motor coordination, impaired memory, and cognitive dysfunction. Maintaining client safety is of prime concern when these medications are prescribed. These agents interact with other CNS depressants, such as alcohol. Severe impairment in cognitive or motor abilities, respiratory depression, or death may result if a client takes benzodiazepines and alcohol together. Conversely, in a controlled medical setting, benzodiazepines may be used to treat alcohol withdrawal.

A non-benzodiazepine anxiolytic is buspirone (BuSpar). It is indicated for generalized anxiety disorder. Buspirone is not effective for

---

| BOX 28-8. **Examples of Benzodiazepine Anxiolytic Agents** | |
| --- | --- |
| alprazolam (Xanax) | diazepam (Valium) |
| chlordiazeproxide (Librium) | lorazepam (Ativan) |
| clonazepam (Klonopin) | |

treating alcohol or benzodiazepine withdrawal and is not used in acute situations for rapid relief of anxiety.

## SEDATIVES AND HYPNOTICS

These drugs have a limited but important place in psychiatry. They are indicated for short-term treatment of insomnia. Barbiturates, benzodiazepines, and non-benzodiazepines are commonly used as **sedative-hypnotics.** An overview of these medications is found in Box 28-9. Barbiturates were the first sedative-hypnotic agents and were introduced in the early 1900s. These drugs are habit-forming and have a narrow **therapeutic index** (the dosage range within which they are effective but above which they are toxic). They have withdrawal effects (eg, convulsions) when discontinued abruptly, especially when they have been taken at high dosages. Withdrawal from severe abuse situations should always be carried out in a monitored hospital setting. Sedative-hypnotic drugs result in depression of the CNS and may impact respiratory function if given in high doses or with other CNS depressants.

## ANTIPARKINSONIAN AGENTS

Parkinsonian symptoms may occur as a side effect of some antipsychotic agents. These symptoms include shuffling gait, masked facies, drooling, tremor, stiff posture, and muscle rigidity. Parkinsonian symptoms are often treated by decreasing the dose of the antipsychotic agent or by switching to an atypical antipsychotic. If these treatment options are not feasible, an antiparkinsonian agent may be added. Some physicians prescribe these medications routinely when an antipsychotic is ordered, whereas others prescribe them only after symptoms arise. Examples of these agents are provided in Box 28-10.

These medications have an anticholinergic effect, resulting in the restoration of an appropriate ratio of dopamine to acetylcholine. Side effects include drowsiness, confusion, constipation, urinary retention,

---

### BOX 28-9. Examples of Sedative-Hypnotic Agents

**BARBITURATES**
pentobarbital (Nembutol)
phenobarbital (Luminal)
secobarbital (Seconal)

**NONBENZODIAZEPINES**
zolpidem (Ambien)
pyrazolopryimidine (Sonata)

**BENZODIAZEPINES**
flurazepam (Dalmane)
temazepam (Restoril)
triazolam (Halcion)

---

> ### BOX 28-10. **Examples of Antiparkinsonian Agents**
>
> benztropine (Cogentin)
> trihexyphenidyl (Artane)
> biperiden (Akineton)

---

blurred vision, dilated pupils, and photophobia. Nursing responsibilities center on management of the associated side effects.

## ANTICONVULSANTS

The use of **anticonvulsants** in psychiatric settings, for control of psychiatric symptoms, is increasing. In addition to being used for clients with underlying seizure disorders, anticonvulsants may be used for treatment of impulse control disorders related to brain injury and to treat seizures related to withdrawal from alcohol or sedative-hypnotic agents. Further, anticonvulsants are frequently used as **mood stabilizers** for clients with bipolar affective disorders. The use of anticonvulsants as mood-stabilizing agents is discussed in the following section. The nurse must know why the medication is being given in order to monitor for therapeutic response.

## MOOD STABILIZERS

### Lithium Carbonate

Lithium carbonate (Eskalith, Lithonate, Lithane) remains the drug of choice for acute manic episodes. It can terminate a manic episode within 10 days in 90% of clients. Lithium is an essential pharmacologic agent in the treatment of bipolar disorders. A bipolar disorder can include acute episodes of psychosis during the manic phase and severe depression during the depressed phase. Often, it is necessary to use antipsychotic and antidepressant medications in conjunction with lithium.

Lithium is also used with varying success in other forms of cyclic illness, whether or not there is a manic phase. Because the effective therapeutic dosage is fairly close to the toxic dosage (narrow therapeutic index), it is important to monitor the lithium blood level regularly. This is done with a laboratory test called a serum lithium level.

A therapeutic serum lithium level is 0.5 to 1.0 mEq/L. A serum lithium level of 1.5mEq/L is considered toxic. Symptoms of **lithium toxicity** are nausea, vomiting, diarrhea, tremor, headache, hypotension, and a change in level of consciousness. The medication should be held and the physician notified if toxicity is suspected. Because lithium is excreted at far different rates in various people, a serum determination must be made frequently at the beginning to be sure the 1.5-mEq/L limit is not exceeded. In the presence of febrile illness or in any situation that causes a loss of fluids (including administration of diuretics), the lithium level must be closely watched.

### Carbamazepine

Carbamazepine (Tegretol) is effective for clients who do not respond to lithium carbonate and those with rapid-cycling or dysphoric mania. Side effects associated with carbamazepine include sedation, drowsiness, and dizziness. A gradual introduction of the drug helps manage these symptoms. A potentially serious side effect is bone marrow suppression, evidenced by agranulocytosis or aplastic anemia. Clients and nurses must watch closely for signs of infection, fever, sore throat, pallor, or easy bruising. Regular monitoring of a complete blood count is also recommended.

### Valproic Acid

Valproic acid (Depakene, Depakote) has also been shown to be effective in the treatment of bipolar affective disorder. Common side effects include gastrointestinal upset, nausea, and heartburn. Taking the medication with food can minimize these effects. A potentially serious side effect is an increase in liver toxicity. Clients should be monitored for signs of liver toxicity, including severe anorexia, weight loss, vomiting, lethargy, jaundice, and edema.

## ◆ ADVERSE EFFECTS OF PSYCHOTROPIC MEDICATIONS

Psychotropic medications have proved effective for many patients. They allow many with mental illness to function in society and enjoy an improved quality of life. With appropriate psychotropic medications, symptoms of psychosis, depression, and mania are diminished or abated and the client is able to pursue life goals and relationships without these distractions. However, these medications are not without risk. Although some of the adverse effects are manageable, others are life threatening. The nurse must be well acquainted with the actions, dosages, forms, characteristics, and complications of the medications he or she administers. Box 28-11 identifies common reasons why many clients do not comply with psychotropic medication regimens.

Many of the potential side effects were discussed under each individual drug heading; however, it is recommended that a current drug reference be consulted prior to the administration of any psychotropic medication. The nurse must be aware that each client will respond differently to medications, and he or she must listen to the client's con-

---

BOX 28-11. **Common Reasons for Medication Noncompliance**

Uncomfortable side effects
Side effects that interfere with quality of life, such as work performance or
   intimate relationships
Lack of awareness of or denial of illness
Stigma
Confusion about dosage or timing
Difficulties in access to treatment
Substance abuse

From Boyd, M., & Nihart, M. (1998). *Psychiatric nursing: Contemporary practice.*
Philadelphia: Lippincott-Raven.

---

cerns and continually assess for therapeutic and nontherapeutic effects
of medications.

The nurse also evaluates appropriate laboratory tests for therapeutic drug levels, complete blood counts, and liver function tests as
indicated. It is also important to remember that potentially life-threatening interactions exist between psychotropic medications and many
over-the-counter medications, medications prescribed for medical illness, illicit drugs, and alcohol. The nurse must be vigilant in assessing
all medications used by the client and teach the client about potential
interactions.

## ◆ THE ROLE OF THE LICENSED PRACTICAL NURSE IN ADMINISTERING PSYCHOTROPIC MEDICATIONS

### MANAGEMENT OF SIDE EFFECTS

Nursing plays an essential role in managing the side effects of psychotropic medications. As previously stated, some side effects are
lethal, whereas others may be uncomfortable. The nurse is responsible
for ongoing assessment of the client. He or she must monitor the client
for behavioral and physical reactions to prescribed medications. Any
sensitivity or toxic reaction to a medication must be immediately
reported and emergency interventions initiated. The client's response
to medications should be carefully documented, because the physician
may rely heavily on the observations of nursing personnel in determining whether changes in medication are needed.

For side effects that are not life threatening, the nurse may implement or facilitate a number of interventions that decrease these side
effects and therefore improve the client's compliance with the pre-

scribed treatment. Nursing interventions for common medication-related complaints are outlined in Table 28-3.

Some side effects may be transient in nature and will resolve within a few weeks, with or without intervention. Other side effects may be long-term, and the physician may consider altering the medication or dosage if comfort measures are inadequate.

### PATIENT TEACHING
Psychotropic medications, no matter how effective, are by no means the final answer for all mental health problems. Drugs cannot in themselves repair all behavioral, physical, and social symptoms of mental illness; however, appropriate medications in addition to other therapy will often allow the client with a mental illness to live a productive and meaningful life.

The nurse is involved in maintaining a therapeutic milieu, implementing therapeutic interactions with clients, and usually is responsible for teaching the client and his or her family members about the client's illness and treatment. When a client understands his or her illness and how medications may provide benefit, he or she may be more likely to comply with the prescribed treatment. The client should be given information specific to his or her situation; however, teaching that is appropriate for any client is outlined in Box 28-12.

## ◆ LEGAL ISSUES IN ADMINISTERING PSYCHOTROPIC MEDICATIONS

Clients with mental illness have the right to refuse treatment (refer to Chapter 6, Professional, Legal, and Ethical Issues in Mental Health Nursing) and must give their consent prior to treatment. The nurse

---

**TABLE 28-3. Nursing Interventions for Common Side Effects to Psychotropic Medications**

| | |
|---|---|
| Dry mouth | Use sugar-free, hard candy. Drink plenty of fluids and rinse mouth frequently. Maintain good oral hygiene (brushing and flossing). Saliva replacements may be prescribed. |
| Weight gain | Increase activity and exercise. Improve diet and avoid high-calorie snacks. |
| Constipation | Increase activity and fluids. Increase fiber (fresh fruits and vegetables) in diet. |
| Sleepiness | Allow for rest periods. Consider taking medication at bedtime (confer with physician). |
| Stomach upset | Take medication with a snack or milk, unless contraindicated. Take medication with a full glass of water. |

---

### BOX 28-12. General Client Teaching on Psychotropic Medications

Notify your physician of any existing medical conditions or if you are breastfeeding.

Take your medication exactly as prescribed.

Keep medication out of the reach of children.

Do not suddenly stop taking your medication.

Report adverse reactions to your physician.

Consult with your physician or pharmacist before taking any over-the-counter medications.

Carry medical information with you at all times (including a list of current medications and your physician's name).

Keep all scheduled appointments with health care providers.

Consult with your physician if you are planning to become pregnant.

Know what medications you are taking and why you are taking them.

Call your health care provider if you have any questions or concerns about your treatment.

Employ medication-specific preventative measures (eg, use of sunscreen or rising slowly when changing positions).

Avoid the use of alcohol.

---

must be careful not to infringe on these rights. Clients are frequently "at the mercy" of health care providers, and nurses should be advocates for them. The nurse should avoid coercive methods in the administration of medication; legal precedents have led to the establishment of policies and procedures related to the forced administration of psychotropic medications in certain situations. The nurse must be aware of the legal statutes and procedures in the state where he or she is employed and comply with these regulations.

### ◆ ELECTROCONVULSIVE THERAPY

One of the alternatives to psychopharmacology when a client does not respond to treatment is **electroconvulsive therapy** (ECT). It is reserved for specific types of mental disorders that do not respond to medications. It is used most effectively in treating moderate to severe depression but may also be used in the treatment of bipolar affective disorder, schizoaffective disorder, catatonic schizophrenia, or severe affective disorder during pregnancy. Electroconvulsive therapy is usually considered when the following conditions exist:

- The client cannot physically tolerate the many toxic physiologic side effects of the psychotropic medications. This client usually has heart disease, allergies, or other types of physical disorders that are aggravated by the medication.

- The client has not responded favorably to treatment with antidepressant medication after a period of several weeks and continues to be moderately to severely depressed.

Electroconvulsive therapy is a relatively safe treatment in which low-level electrical stimulation is used to induce a seizure in the client. It is thought that the seizure alters the levels of neurotransmitters in the brain. Although not fully understood, this results in decreased symptoms of illness. Treatments are generally administered two to three times a week, and the client will have therapeutic effect within six to ten treatments.

The client is anesthetized and his or her vital signs and cardiac function (electrocardiogram) are closely monitored during the procedure. A neuromuscular blocking agent is also given to prevent uncontrolled thrashing from the seizure. An electroencephalogram (EEG) monitors the extent and duration of the induced seizure. Following the treatment, the client's head is held to the side to prevent aspiration of saliva. A short-acting anesthesia is used and the client has a brief recovery period while 100 percent oxygen is given until spontaneous respirations return. Electroconvulsive therapy is an effective treatment for many clients with mental illness; there are no absolute contraindications for the procedure.

## USE OF NURSING PROCESS WITH CLIENTS RECEIVING ELECTROCONVULSIVE THERAPY

Although ECT is an effective treatment, many clients may reject the procedure. Media images of ECT, fear of long-term memory loss, and the stigma associated with the procedure all impact a client's decision about the procedure. The nurse is instrumental in teaching the client and his or her family about ECT, what they should expect, and how the client will be cared for during and after the procedure.

The physical care of the client receiving ECT is similar to that of anyone undergoing general anesthesia. The client must take nothing by mouth for 4 to 8 hours prior to treatment and is given medication to prevent bradycardia or asystole during the procedure. Memory impairment may occur after ECT. Generally, it is self-limiting and involves short-term memories, especially for events immediately surrounding the procedure. Memory loss usually resolves with a few hours or days. Memory loss that persists after a few weeks should be reported to the physician. Informed consent must be obtained prior to the procedure.

### Assessment of Symptoms

A thorough assessment of the client must occur prior to ECT and should include a complete physical examination and blood tests. The nurse should also complete a thorough nursing assessment to provide baseline information regarding the client's symptoms prior to the procedure. Immediately following ECT the nurse is responsible for monitoring the client's vital signs, respiratory status, and orientation. The nurse monitors the client every 5 minutes until the client is fully awake, every 15 minutes until alert, and then every 2 to 4 hours until stable. If the client has had ECT in the past, the nurse should also be aware of how he or she responded to previous treatments.

### NURSING DIAGNOSES ASSOCIATED WITH ELECTROCONVULSIVE THERAPY

In addition to the nursing diagnoses related to the client's mental illness, the nurse needs to consider the psychological and physiological implications of ECT when caring for the client. Although each client must be evaluated on an individual basis, three potential nursing diagnoses related to ECT for clients receiving this therapy follow:

1. Knowledge Deficit
2. Fear
3. Impaired Memory

### NURSING INTERVENTION AND RATIONALE

The nursing diagnoses of Knowledge Deficit and Fear are closely related. The client may have fear as a result of knowledge deficit, and he or she may not seek knowledge out of fear; therefore, the nursing interventions for these diagnoses are similar. Nursing interventions for Knowledge Deficit and Fear may include the following:

1. *Develop a positive rapport with the client.* A positive rapport allows the client to be comfortable with the nurse, allowing more honest communication. The client will also have established a sense of trust and will know that the nurse is honest.
2. *Provide continuity of personnel involved in the care of the client.* Continuity enhances the client's sense of security and contributes to the establishment of a positive rapport. Nursing staffs are also better able to interpret client comments and interactions, based on prior experiences.
3. *Convey acceptance of the client's perceptions.* This validates the client's feelings and facilitates open communication.
4. *Explain all procedures to the client.* An explanation of what will happen, where the client will be, and who will be with the client provides him or her with information necessary for understanding the procedure.

Another nursing concern is that the client may experience memory impairment after ECT that may also contribute to his or her fear about the procedure. It also presents a significant concern for nurses to maintain the client's safety during periods of memory impairment. Nursing interventions for impaired memory may include:

1. *Teach the client and family to expect some temporary, short-term memory loss.* If known in advance, this helps to decrease anxiety related to the memory loss.
2. *Remain with the client.* This provides a sense of security and helps to ensure client safety.
3. *Have familiar items and people around the client.* This reassures the client that he or she has not "forgotten" everything and helps to maintain a calm surrounding.

## EVALUATION

The nurse evaluates the efficacy of his or her interventions through an ongoing process. The nurse knows that the interventions related to Fear and Knowledge Deficit have been effective when the client expresses diminished fear about the procedure and he or she is able to discuss the procedure and explain what happens before, during, and after ECT. The success of nursing interventions related to Impaired Memory is evaluated when the client remains safe and effectively copes with the associated short-term memory loss.

## KEY POINTS

- The development of medications that restore brain chemistry to near-normal levels has markedly changed the treatment of mental illness and allows many individuals with mental illness to function in society.
- The role of the nurse in administering psychoactive medications is central, and nurses should be acquainted with the actions, dosages, forms, characteristics, and complications associated with them.
- Nurses should record and report failure of the drug to produce the desired effect, any sensitivity, or a toxic reaction. Physicians rely on the nurse's observations to decide whether the dosage should be maintained, decreased, or increased.
- Clients have a right to know about the side effects and expected outcomes of prescribed medications. Clients also have the right to refuse to take medications.
- Psychotropic medications have side effects ranging from uncomfortable to life threatening. Nurses are responsible for teaching clients about their medications and monitoring them for side effects.
- Antipsychotic medications are classified as "typical" or "atypical." Typical antipsychotics are more likely to cause extrapyramidal side effects than atypical agents.

- Extrapyramidal effects include pseudoparkinsonism, akathisia, and dystonia. Antiparkinsonian agents may control these symptoms.
- The major classifications of antidepressant medications are tricyclics (TCAs), monoamine oxidase inhibitors (MAOIs), and selective serotonin reuptake inhibitors (SSRIs). Monoamine oxidase inhibitors require the client to adhere to dietary restrictions. Selective serotonin reuptake inhibitors are the most commonly prescribed antidepressants today. It takes 2 to 4 weeks for the client to see results from antidepressant medications.
- Tardive dyskinesia can occur with long-term use of some antipsychotic agents. Rhythmic facial and tongue movements characterize it. It is a permanent, irreversible side effect that is not relieved by antiparkinsonian drugs.
- Electroconvulsive therapy may be used to treat clients who do not respond to medication therapy. The client receives an electrical shock during the procedure. The client is anesthetized and does not remember the treatment.
- Nursing care for clients receiving ECT includes preparing the client for the treatment and closely monitoring his or her vital signs and airway after the treatment. Memory impairment associated with ECT generally is self-limiting.

## SELF-AWARENESS ACTIVITY

Imagine that you have "heard voices" for a number of years. The voices are always there for you. You have become accustomed to them, and you are basically satisfied with your lifestyle. Now imagine that someone tells you that you must take a medication to "control" the voices. Review the side effects of antipsychotic medications and ask yourself:

- How would these medications change my life?
- Would I be willing to take these medications? Why or why not?
- Could anyone convince me that taking these medications would help? If so, how?
- What would I do if someone made me take these medications against my will?

## QUESTIONS

1. The physician has just prescribed haloperidol (Haldol) for a client. The nurse would best describe this medication to the client as

   a. "A medication to help you feel less depressed. It is effective but may lead to extrapyramidal symptoms."
   b. "A medication to help you feel less 'hyper.' It has no known side effects."
   c. "A medication to help you sleep better."
   d. "A medication to help you think more clearly. There are some side effects for which we will monitor you closely."
2. A client complains that the imipramine (Elavil) she is taking makes her mouth "too dry." The nurse should recommend that the client
   a. take the medication with food.
   b. maintain good oral hygiene and use a hard, sugar-free candy.
   c. stop taking the medication and report her symptoms to the physician.
   d. take the medication with a full glass of water.
3. A client reports that he has a "really bad headache." He has been taking phenelzine (Nardil) for 2 weeks. The nurse should
   a. recognize this as a transient side effect and get an order for acetaminophen (Tylenol) to treat the headache.
   b. take the client's blood pressure and get an order for acetaminophen (Tylenol) to treat the headache.
   c. take the client's blood pressure and find out what foods the client has been eating.
   d. have the client lie down in a quiet room and check his or her blood pressure within an hour.

4. A client has just returned from having ECT. He is awake and conversing. The nurse's priority in providing care is to
   a. monitor his vital signs every 5 minutes.
   b. maintain a safe environment.
   c. allow him time to rest and recover from the procedure.
   d. teach him what to expect during this recovery period.

## BIBLIOGRAPHY

Barry, P.D. (1996). *Psychosocial nursing: Care of physically ill patients and their families* (3rd ed.). Philadelphia: Lippincott-Raven.

Boyd, M.A., & Nihart, M.A. (1998). *Psychiatric nursing: Contemporary practice*. Philadelphia: Lippincott-Raven.

Fontaine, K.L., & Fletcher, J.S. (1999). *Mental health nursing* (4th ed.). Menlo Park: Addison Wesley Longman.

Glod, C.A. (1998). *Contemporary psychiatric-mental health nursing: The brain-behavior connection*. Philadelphia: F.A. Davis.

Johnson, B.S. (1997). *Psychiatric-mental health nursing: adaptation and growth* (4th ed.). Philadelphia: Lippincott-Raven.

Keltner, N.L. (1997). Catastrophic consequences secondary to psychotropic drugs, part 1. *Journal of Psychosocial Nursing, 35*(4), 41–45.

Keltner, N.L. (1997). Catastrophic consequences secondary to psychotropic drugs, part 2. *Journal of Psychosocial Nursing, 35*(5), 48–50.

Lilley, L.L., & Aucker, R.S. (1999). *Pharmacology and the nursing process* (2nd ed.). St. Louis: Mosby.

Paradiso, C. (1998). *Lippincott's review series: Pharmacology*. Philadelphia: Lippincott-Raven.

Schultz, J.M., & Videbeck, S.D. (1998). *Lippincott's manual of psychiatric nursing care plans* (5th ed.). Philadelphia: Lippincott-Raven.

Shives, L.R. (1998). *Basic concepts of psychiatric-mental health nursing* (4th ed.). Philadelphia: Lippincott-Raven.

Spratto, G.R., & Woods, A.L. (2000). *PDR nurse's drug handbook*. Oradell, NJ: Medical Economics.

*Taber's cyclopedic medical dictionary* (18th ed.) (1997). Philadelphia: F.A. Davis.

Wilkinson, J.M. (2000). *Nursing diagnosis handbook with NIC interventions and NOC outcomes* (7th ed.). Upper Saddle River, NJ: Prentice-Hall Health.

Wintz, C.J.B. (1998). Nursing management of psychotropic drug reactions. *Nursing Clinics of North America, 33*(1), 217–231.

# 29

# Complementary Health Approaches: Therapies and Philosophy in Mental Health Treatment Settings

---

## Behavioral Objectives

*After reading this chapter the student will be able to:*

- Identify the philosophy that underlies complementary health modalities.
- Name the complementary methods that are effective with mental disorders.
- Name the characteristics of the healer.
- Identify the qualities of a healing relationship.
- Explain how systems theory relates to holistic care.
- Identify the guidelines for holistic relationships

---

## Key Terms

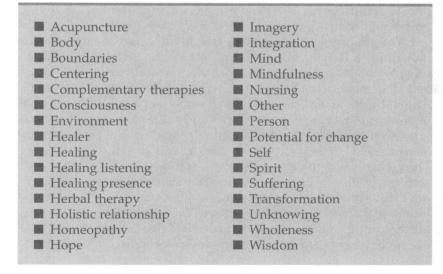

- Acupuncture
- Body
- Boundaries
- Centering
- Complementary therapies
- Consciousness
- Environment
- Healer
- Healing
- Healing listening
- Healing presence
- Herbal therapy
- Holistic relationship
- Homeopathy
- Hope
- Imagery
- Integration
- Mind
- Mindfulness
- Nursing
- Other
- Person
- Potential for change
- Self
- Spirit
- Suffering
- Transformation
- Unknowing
- Wholeness
- Wisdom

# ◆ COMPLEMENTARY THERAPIES

Complementary therapies are healing approaches developed from a variety of sources. The term complementary suggests that these methods be used in conjunction with the allopathic medical approaches used in the Western world—that is, that these methods complement or enhance the use of allopathic medical approaches, such as the use of psychotropic medications for mental disorders. Complementary medical approaches have many sources. Some of these sources include ancient healing practices from China, Tibet, India, and other holistic cultures. Other sources have been developed during the past two or three centuries by individuals who experimented with the use of their own theories of healing mental and physical disorders.

Many individuals with mental disorders have sought relief using complementary therapies during the past decade. Complementary therapies have been used for hundreds or thousands of years, predating the type of allopathic medicine currently practiced in the United States. The National Institutes of Health (NIH), the health care research branch of the federal government, provides funding for research to test the effectiveness of different types of health interventions. The NIH created a new organization in the late 1980s called the National Center for Complementary and Alternative Medicine. One of the purposes of this organization is to research nontraditional medical approaches. Nontraditional medical approaches, also known as **complementary therapies,** are medical interventions whose origins are outside the current allopathic medical treatment approaches that are developed and researched using scientific principles to determine whether they are effective in preventing or treating different types of disease.

The philosophy that underlies the use of complementary health modalities is one of caring and respect for the suffering client. The role of nurses as ministers to those who are suffering faces important challenges in the future of all types of health care, including the mental health arena. These challenges offer opportunities for nurses to enter into partnerships with mental health patients and families who want to understand the meaning of healing and create healing environments. The concepts of holism and healing are complex. These concepts, usually discussed in relationship to physical health settings, offer new hope for healing in the mental health arena. The depth and breadth of their meaning explores some of the most profound questions of human experience. This chapter explores the significant philosophical issues that contribute to the creation of healing environments—in the self, other, and caregiving community.

# ◈ WHAT TYPES OF COMPLEMENTARY METHODS HAVE BEEN FOUND EFFECTIVE WITH MENTAL DISORDERS?

## DEPRESSION AND ANXIETY

Increasing numbers of the U.S. adult population use health approaches that fit into the category of complementary and alternative medicine (CAM). By the mid-1990s approximately 40% of U.S. adults had used at least one type of alternative health care for at least 1 year. Depression is identified as one of the 10 most frequently occurring conditions that results in the use of CAM. The most frequently chosen remedies for depression and anxiety include exercise, relaxation and imagery, acupuncture, herbal remedies, homeopathy, acupuncture, and massage. Descriptions of each of these therapeutic approaches follow.

### Exercise

In research on persons who suffer from depression or anxiety, when compared with other groups with the same conditions who were not exercising, persons with depression or anxiety benefited from regular exercise. Although many hypotheses have been formulated about the beneficial results of exercise, one of them is that exercise alters the physical state of an individual; accordingly, it is believed that neurotransmitters that produce difficult emotional states such as depression and anxiety are brought more into balance by active and reasonable exercise.

### Acupuncture

Acupuncture is an ancient Chinese treatment in which small, very fine needles are inserted into the skin at specific preselected points. These points are believed to be the gatekeepers for healing energy or for the obstruction of that energy. The premise of acupuncture is that two types of energies flow throughout the body in channels called "meridians." It is assumed that illness results when there is an imbalance of these energies. Western acupuncturists believe that the changes brought about by acupuncture are the result of changes in neurophysiology. In order to enhance potential changes in neurophysiology, Western acupuncturists use electrically stimulated acupuncture probes to clear the energy blockages. Many cases of depression and anxiety have shown improvement or full reduction of symptoms using this CAM method. When compared with other groups of individuals who were taking recommended medicine for their mental distress, the groups using acupuncture showed the same rates of improvement as those taking traditional prescribed medicine for depression or anxiety.

### Herbal Therapy

Herbal therapy has been used for thousands of years in many different cultures. Currently St. John's Wort is the only herbal medicine used to treat mild to moderate levels of depression in which research has shown effective outcomes with reduction of symptoms. It should be noted, however, that when an individual has moderate to severe depression and suicide is of concern, herbal therapy should be replaced with supportive psychotherapy and antidepressant medication.

Although there are no reported studies in Western scientific literature on the use of the herbal valerian in persons with anxiety, this herbal has been used since the Middle Ages to reduce the negative effects of anxiety. With the increase in the use of herbals by persons who are also taking traditional allopathic medications, pharmacists have developed an extensive body of knowledge about negative interactions between herbals and prescribed medications. A person who is considering the use of herbal therapies should first check with his or her physician or pharmacist before ingesting an unknown herb.

### Homeopathy

Homeopathy is a type of health approach developed at about the same time that allopathic medicine was becoming popular—around the 1800s. Homeopathic physicians use very small amounts of substances that are known to cause certain conditions to occur to treat the illness. For example, a person who is suffering from food poisoning is given a small amount of a substance known to cause food poisoning. It is believed that the small amount of the causative substance will cause the body to mount a defense as a reaction to the substance. Accordingly, the body is prepared to actively rally to fight off the illness. No scientifically reliable studies have been reported on the effective use of homeopathy in depression or anxiety.

### Imagery and Relaxation Therapy

Imagery is an intervention in which a client is asked to imagine a specific type of situation that then causes changes in the physical state of the client. There are three levels of awareness in imagery: the mental image, a somatic response, and meaning. Generally, imagery techniques involve some aspect of physical and emotional relaxation, and so the two approaches have been combined in this section. There are limited numbers of studies involving the use of imagery or relaxation therapy in persons with depression. A few small studies have been reported in which depressed persons who have used imagery or relaxation have shown improvement when compared to depressed persons with whom there was no formal intervention. The question, when there are limited numbers of studies that report a beneficial effect, is whether it was the actual intervention that caused the change or the attention of the caregiver who provided the intervention that produced the change.

Studies of the effects of imagery or relaxation therapy in individuals with anxiety have shown positive effects of such intervention in a wide number of studies. It should be noted, however, that in persons with high levels of anxiety, such interventions are not as effective as antianxiety medication and psychotherapy or group therapy interventions in reducing debilitating symptoms.

## ◆ CURRENT USE OF COMPLEMENTARY METHODS IN MENTAL HEALTH SETTINGS

The concepts of health, healing, and holism are actively being integrated into the practice of mental health nursing and the therapeutic environment in the mental health setting. The use of complementary methods in the mental health setting is minimal. The primary reason for the minor use of these methods is that the Western world uses a conservative approach in selecting treatment modalities for persons with mental or physical illnesses. Before a new approach is used in the health setting, it usually must demonstrate its efficacy in the research setting.

### WHAT IS HEALING?

In the long continuum of time, many cultures have demonstrated that the body contains the energy and mechanisms to heal many of its ills. In these cultures the unity of mind, body, and spirit within the individual are utilized to draw on these healing powers. **Healing** is the restoration to health, wholeness, or soundness. Others view healing as a cure. Healing potential is enhanced in these cultures with the presence of certain belief systems, spirit, family and community support, the ebb and flow of life and relationships, and in altered states of consciousness.

In primitive cultures and in many current societies, the healing process occurs at times within the self using self-beliefs and practices. At other times when self-practices do not heal or relieve the distress, then the healing presence of the shaman or medicine man may be sought. Healers in these societies serve as a medium between the visible world and the invisible spirit world.

Most societies in the non-Western world believe in the concept of healing, self-healing practices, and empowered healers who can empower the person seeking healing. In many of these societies there is no separation between mental and physical health. Healing refers to restoration of balance in the whole person. Restoration to a prior level of health is the goal of healing practices. These practices occur in the cultures of Native Americans, including Eskimos of North America and Siberia, Indians of the subcontinent, Asian, South American, African, and

Australian aboriginal peoples. Indeed, the number of people worldwide who engage in folk medicine and healing rituals far exceeds those who utilize the principles of Western allopathic medicine.

It is important to note that in these cultures the experience of distress is holistic. The distress of stomach pain, mental illness, or spiritual distress is experienced as whole-person distress. It is not separated anatomically or systemically, as occurs in Western approaches to illness. Although the healing efforts of the shaman may include elixirs that are specific to certain conditions, such as stomach, cardiac, or respiratory ailments, the mission of the healer is to restore the whole person to well being.

## CHARACTERISTICS OF THE HEALER

All persons carry within themselves the capabilities to be healing forces for themselves and others. Although this capacity is present in all people, it may not be self-evident. Early psychic injuries can result in layers of protection over old traumatic hurts that can leave individuals disconnected from their own healing energies. As they work through their own early pain and shed layers of disillusionment and shame, it is possible for one to reconnect with his or her capacity to be a healer. A **healer** is a person who possesses deep intuitive wisdom, compassion and love for others, and the capacity to facilitate the healing process in self and others.

Among the qualities that are most therapeutic for nurses in the mental health setting are those identified as important for all healers. Persons who are viewed as healers possess a range of characteristics that support their healing potential. These include:

1. Gentleness of spirit
2. Compassion for the other
3. Respectfulness of the dignity of the other
4. Respectfulness of choice of the other
5. Mindfulness of the intention of the potential of the healing act to release the healing energies of the other

The healer shares a mutuality of purpose with the other. The healer brings to the encounter a belief that his or her actions can release healing potentials within the other. In order to understand the importance of partnership in the healing process, the words of an aboriginal Australian woman demonstrate the guiding principle of one who wants to be in a healing partnership with a client:

> If you have come to help me
> You are wasting your time
> But if you have come because
> Your liberation is bound-up with mine
> Then let us work together.

The goal of the physician in traditional allopathic medical settings is to treat the diseased part of the human being. Restoration of the whole person to wellness is not the primary goal of the medical caregiver. Attending to the whole person response to illness is and has been the goal of nursing (*American Nurses Association Social Policy Statement*, 1980). The nursing paradigm includes attending to all dimensions of the patient. The core concepts of the nursing paradigm are shown in Box 29-1.

Using the nursing paradigm as a model of health and wellness, healing is the process of restoring a person to health, soundness, or wholeness. The role of being a healing presence and participating with patients and families in this process is a choice that is open to all nurses. The remainder of the chapter explores the physical, mental, and spiritual values that imbue the nurse with a healing presence.

## QUALITIES OF A HEALING RELATIONSHIP

Before a healing relationship can be established, the foundation of the relationship is rooted in several guiding principles. These principles include:

Use of systems theory as a guiding framework
Use of change theory as a guiding framework
Guidelines for therapeutic relationship:
—Characteristics of the caregiver relationship
—Respect for boundaries
—Awareness of potential for over- or under-functioning

---

### BOX 29–1. The Core Concepts of Nursing

**Person:** A human being who contains integrated elements of mind, body, and spirit in dynamic balance.

**Environment:** Those internal or external forces that support or disrupt dynamic balance. These forces include family; community; physical, cultural, political, and economic environments; resources such as health care availability; and the value systems of health care providers.

**Health:** A dynamic state of mind-body-spirit balance that supports the full potential of a human being. It is a subjective state of personal well-being in contrast to a subjective state of distress.

**Nursing:** A process of care whose purpose is to support health.

## ◆ USING SYSTEMS THEORY
   IN HOLISTIC NURSING CARE

Systems theory is more fully explained in Chapter 9: Influence of Family and Social Environment on the Individual. The fundamental concepts of systems theory in a holistic framework follow.

The individual is a complex integrated system composed of interacting subsystem elements of mind, body, spirit, and social relationships. Each element consists of multiple abstract and concrete factors that have mutual feedback loops. Change or stress in any one factor has radiating effects into the subsystem; ultimately the change in the subsystem may create demand or change in the whole body and human system. Changes within the whole body system may then create challenge or threat in the family and/or other social systems, such as work, community, or health care system.

Responses by external systems, such as health care givers, can create changes within one or more of the human subsystem elements. Other types of external system factors that result in challenge or threat include an unlimited range of mental, spiritual, or physical stress factors.

Any type of perceived stressor can set off a cascade of responses in the whole body system. Viewing these responses as mutually interactive in the mind-body-spirit is the focus of a healing intervention.

## ◆ THE IMPORTANCE OF POTENTIAL
   FOR CHANGE IN THE CLIENT

One of the most important challenges that all humans face is their potential for change, particularly during stressful times. **Potential for change** is the inner openness to learning new ways of coping or new ways of perceiving the world. It is a natural human need to resist change. Change stirs up the pot. It creates uncertainty. When an individual and his or her family are facing the presence of mental illness, the resistance to change becomes more active. Recognizing that this is so is an important awareness for the nurse in the mental health setting. The nurse is urged to be clear about the needs of the patient *and* the care plan developed by the mental health team.

Listening empathically to the patient is important—and learning to support the patient within the parameters of the mental health team care plan can be a challenge. Working within these two sometimes-opposite realities can cause a nurse to feel as though he or she is on a tightrope. Supporting the care plan may involve the need for change in the patient's belief system or lifestyle. The following information about the importance of openness to change and the meaning of this change to the client tests the nurse's communication skills.

## ◆ CHANGE THEORY

This section addresses specific concepts associated with change theory that support the mental health healing continuum. The concepts include the following conditions:

1. Shared vision, values, and goals. The caregiver and patient are in agreement about these three important outcome-related criteria.
2. A perceived need for change. The patient recognizes the mind, body, spirit, or social distress that is the focus of the healing work.
3. A perceived ability to change. The patient believes that change in one or more aspects of the mind, body, spirit, or social distress is possible.
4. The availability of concrete options. The patient can be the subject of the healing modality, but actions and attitudes that empower the patient and the potential for healing can be taught and reviewed.

## ◆ GUIDELINES FOR HOLISTIC RELATIONSHIPS

### HOLISTIC RELATIONSHIPS

The ideal foundation of healing in the mental health setting is a holistic relationship. A **holistic relationship** is one in which the caregiver has a posture of respect for the autonomy, dignity, and healing potential that resides in the other. In addition, the following concepts are fundamental to all balanced relationships:

*Boundaries.* **Boundaries** are unwritten, usually unspoken rules about maintaining appropriate roles and relationships with others. Boundaries are learned in the families of origin of the caretaker and patient. It is particularly important that the caregiver be aware of correct, professional boundaries with patients. Because patients may place themselves in a dependent position with caregivers, they are subject to regression to earlier developmental periods. They may, for example, anticipate giving control of their healing process over to the caregiver. One of the principles of therapeutic healing relationships, for example, is that there is respect for the patient's autonomy and decision-making options. Patients may require guidance from the caregiver regarding the roles of each that their work together is mutually supportive of the well being of the patient.

*Overinvolvement/Overfunctioning Versus Underinvolvement/ Underfunctioning.* Persons who enter the healing professions often have been caregivers in their families of origin. They are frequently viewed as "givers." Indeed, one of the sources of self-esteem for most individuals is to be needed. These characteristics, however, can sometimes result in overdoing for the patient or family. There is a general systems effect when this occurs. The patient or family does less. The overdoing on the part of the caregiver results in less control and subsequent socializing of dependent behavior in the patient or family. If the patient or family is not taught self-care principles and supported in their use, there can be erosion of the results of the healing intervention and illness behaviors are again activated. It can be wise to begin a therapeutic relationship by reviewing the guidelines and expectations of each participant or caregiver, patient, or family member. This agreement then becomes an informal contract that sets the stage for a healing and therapeutic relationship.

## WHAT IS HOLISM?

Holism is the theory that living matter or reality is made up of organic or unified wholes that are greater than the sum of their parts (*American Heritage College Dictionary*, 1993, p. 648). Holistic relates to holism. "It . . . emphasizes the importance of the whole and the interdependence of its parts. . . It is concerned with wholes rather than analysis or separation into parts" (Ibid.).

Holism is the belief system that permeates all non-Western cultures and their approaches to life and all living things. Holism is an approach that was prevalent in the Western world until the advent of strong philosophical forces in the world of training to be medical physicians.

## ELEMENTS OF HOLISTIC HEALTH CARE

The dimensions that support the philosophies of holism and healing are the elements at the heart of the self. These are the dimensions that exist in all human beings. They are often of a profound nature that can defy description using traditional terminology. These dimensions include:

Consciousness
Mind
Body
Spirit
Integration or wholeness
Self
Self and other
Suffering
Hope
Healing presence
—Centering
—Listening

—Unknowing
—Wisdom
Complementary healing methods
Transformation

These topics are discussed in the following. Each of these topics is an essential part of the whole human being although presented as specific entities.

*Consciousness.*   **Consciousness** is the sum of the integrated perceptions in the human being. These perceptions include all elements of the mind, body, and spirit. The word consciousness is derived from the Latin words, *con,* memory together, and *scire,* meaning to know. Consciousness encompasses the full range of self-awareness.

*Mind.*   **Mind** is viewed from many perspectives; the basic concept of mind includes all functions within the mental domains. These include cognition, perception, memory, judgment, and regulation and control of emotions and impulses. Each of these functions is based on physiologic processes.

*Body.*   **Body** consists of the whole of all anatomic parts and physiologic processes. The utilization of a holistic model when assessing physiologic responses to stress and their implications for health demonstrates that the vast majority of body responses to "stress" are actually determined by the coping or "mind" response of an individual. In other words, it is the meaning to that individual of the stressor that mediates the type of sympathetic nervous system activation of the full range of body systems, such as cardiovascular, gastrointestinal, muscular, skeletal, and so on. Again, it becomes virtually impossible to discern where the mind response stops and the body response begins.

*Spirit.*   **Spirit** is defined as ". . . the vital principle or animating force within living beings . . . " (*American Heritage College Dictionary,* 1993, p. 1313). It is also viewed by many as a vital center and the essence of the whole being that is at the core of one's spirituality. The North American Nursing Diagnosis Association (NANDA) has described a pattern of distress of the human spirit. The diagnosis is *Spiritual Distress.* It is defined as "the state in which the individual or group experiences or is at risk of experiencing a disturbance in the belief or value system which provides strength, hope, and meaning to life" (Carpenito, 2000, p. 881). The defining characteristic is that the individual is experiencing a disturbance in his or her belief system. Box 29-2 shows other characteristics that may be present in the individual experiencing spiritual distress.

The most recent edition of the *Diagnostic and Statistical Manual of Mental Disorders* (DSM-IV), the manual used to diagnose the different types of mental disorders, has, for the first time, included a spirit-related clinical diagnosis. It is described as a *religious or spiritual problem*. Its definition is:

> . . . the focus of clinical attention is a religious or spiritual problem. Examples include distressing experiences that involve loss of or questioning of faith, problems associated with conversion to a new faith, or questioning of spiritual values that may not necessarily be related to an organized church or religious institution."
>
> (*Diagnostic and Statistical Manual of Mental Disorders* [4th ed.], 1994, p. 300).

The NANDA and DSM-IV diagnostic categories each refer to religion and spirituality. It is important to clarify that spirituality or formal religious beliefs are subjective states that differ from person to person and within families. Some individuals have strong religious beliefs that form the primary structure through which all experience is measured. Others profess no formal religious belief system, but are imbued with the principles of spirit described previously in this section.

The common experiences of persons with spiritual or formal religious orientation include a sense of purpose, future-orientation and hope, and connectedness with others and an internal or external life force. The effects on the spirit can be profound when these experiences of the spirit are threatened. Fortunately, there are many resources within the individual and environment that work to restore spiritual balance. They include conscious coping mechanisms, unconscious defenses (dreaming when the unconscious processes attempt to modify the underlying foundation of the distress), and the critical element of *hope* associated with the spirit. Environmental resources include the natural environment, as well as family, friends, and spiritual advisors.

---

### BOX 29–2. Contributing Factors to Spiritual Distress

Questions credibility of belief system
Demonstrates discouragement or despair
Is unable to practice usual spiritual or religious rituals
Has ambivalent feelings or doubts about beliefs
Expresses that he has no reason for living
Feels a sense of spiritual emptiness
Shows emotional detachment from self and others
Expresses concern, anger, resentment, and/or fear over meaning of life, suffering, or death
Requests spiritual assistance for a disturbance in belief system

Carpenito, L.J. (2000). *Nursing diagnosis: Application to clinical practice* (8th ed.). Philadelphia: Lippincott Williams & Wilkins.

In the field of crisis intervention it is recognized that social support is one of the most important factors in averting crisis.

*Integration or Wholeness.* The next area to be explored is that of **integration**. Full comprehension of the meaning of integration may be beyond the capacities of the finite human mind. The verb integrate is defined as ". . . to make a whole by bringing all parts together . . . to join with something else; unit . . . to make part of a larger unit" (*American Heritage College Dictionary*, 1993, p. 706). Integration is present in human beings when there is an attitude toward **wholeness** and openness within the self. There is an ongoing sense of personal balance or knowledge to assess self-balance and use internal and external resources to correct imbalances.

Integration also may be reflected in a subjective sense of peace, contentment, or internal harmony that may ebb and flow, but is an ongoing experience or goal of the individual. The use of a holistic model in approaching patients and families begins with caregivers who strive for the ideals of holism and integration in their self and worldviews.

*Self.* The concept of **self** in a holistic model can be viewed with two perspectives. The first is the relationship of the self with self, and the second the relationship of self with other. Before one can be fully present with another it is important that the inner life of the self is explored and viewed as an ongoing unfolding of potential. Maslow described the self-actualized person as having fulfilled the primary needs described in his model of self-development and then moving more deeply into self-awareness in order to realize one's fullest potential. Raheem described the experience of self-wholeness as:

> one in which a person operates from a unified consciousness of body, mind, emotions, and soul. As the bonds of conditioning are shed, one begins to gain fuller awareness of a deep self-directed process that moves toward self-actualization and harmony with the cosmos. As in childhood, one becomes vulnerable again—to oneself, to other people, and to the vast mystery of life itself . . . (pp. 16–17).

It can be helpful to realize that the work of unfolding of the self is a life-long journey that consists of many stages: physical, psychological, and spiritual. It is a journey that is *chosen* and that requires hope, spiritual vision and connectedness with a deep life purpose, and courage to delve into painful perceptions to discover the important elements and resources of the self that lie under the layers of human distress.

*Self and Other.* In a holistic framework the **other** is a concept that involves the relationship of self with another living being. The fundamental approach is one of respect for the other's dignity. Another valuable element of the concept of self and other is the intention of mindfulness. **Mindfulness** is a state of self-awareness and openness toward the self in response to the other's state. Another aspect of holistic, therapeutic use of self with other for the nurse in the mental health setting is to approach the other with respect for the intrinsic wisdom and capacities which that individual brings to the encounter.

*Suffering.* One of the primary causes of distress of the human spirit is **suffering**. Suffering can begin as pain in one of the human domains of physical, psychological, spiritual, or social. A sense of helplessness can evolve when the pain is not relieved despite efforts to reduce it. Suffering is distinct from pain. Pain does not always lead to suffering. At the core of suffering is the loss of central life purpose. Some writers on suffering propose that it is suffering that gives guidance to life. Additionally, they view that when a suffering person reaches the point of loss of central purpose, he is unable to help himself and is dependent on caregivers to facilitate the restoration of meaning and purpose in his life.

*Hope.* The contrasting state to suffering and "giving up" is **hope** or optimism. Seligman described optimistic persons as believing that a defeat is only a temporary setback. Its cause is attributed to chance or bad luck rather than to some inherent personal flaw. When confronted with a bad situation, they view it as a challenge rather than one over which they have no control. Indeed, the characteristics of hope and optimism are the operating life principles of optimistic persons.

The nature of hope is more of a fundamental life principle rather than an emotion. It is broader than a cognitive attitude. Hope is experienced at the physical level as a connected energy with the future. It is suggested that hopefulness is a life principle that resides in the spirit. This proposition includes the possibility that the home of hopefulness is in the spirit, but is inherent in the mind and body. Hopefulness within the spirit may be the fuel that supports the central purpose of an individual.

*Healing Presence.* The concept of **healing presence** as a mode of practice in nursing care is a major thread in healing mental health environments. Nursing offers unique opportunities for intimacy and relationship with patients and families. By the nurse's listening and "being with" them in a centered and caring therapeutic relationship, the patient and family may be supported as they restabilize and reintegrate as a response to acute or chronic illness. Four qualities of the caring self that support the experience of healing presence for the other are centering, healing, listening "unknowing," and wisdom.

**Centering** is a conscious act of focusing one's attention to opening one's awareness and finding an internal reference point. The process of centering usually involves the following steps:

- Attentiveness to one's breath by blowing out all of the breath as though blowing out a candle, then deeply breathing in an abdominal breath and focusing inwardly on the self and the depth of the breath within the self
- Awareness of connection with universal energy
- Intentionally choosing to be a healing presence for the other
- Maintaining the experience of centeredness during the time of encounter with the client

A person who employs **healing listening** is one to whom a client is inclined to tell experiences. Out of his or her listening with a "third ear," the nurse develops the basis for therapeutic interventions. This third ear can catch what people do not say, but only feel and think.

**Unknowing** is the perspective of a listener who understands that he or she *does not know* the experience of the other. Accordingly, one adopts an "unknowing" listening posture with the other. Indeed, only the client knows his or her pain. Healing presence or authentic person-to-person connection allows the other to feel understood. Only by asking the other to explain his or her "knowing" about the subjective experience of illness, pain, or suffering is it possible to understand the client's own inner state.

The fourth element of healing presence to be addressed in this section is **wisdom**. Wisdom is defined as "understanding of what is true, right, or lasting; insight . . . common sense; good judgment" (*American Heritage College Dictionary*, 1993, p. 1548). Wisdom, sometimes also referred to as *knowing*, is a deep grounding within the self about which there is a sense of certainty. This certainty is a form of held knowledge about the self; it can also extend to others. Persons who have worked through layers of psychological injuries and defensive patterns often return to their original intuitive wisdom; such a return to the original personal core is usually accompanied by a deep experience of peace and loss of fear of death.

*Transformation.* The human being is in a state of constant change and growth. The emotional blockages from early psychic or physical injuries result in physiologic patterns that underlie a variety of emotional states such as helplessness, helpless and frozen anger, rage, fear, grief, anxiety, depression, hopelessness, and so on. It is hypothesized that the effects of these "caught," conditioned patterns of emotional response can lead to pathophysiologic mechanisms that, over time, may result in physical or mental disorders.

**Transformation** is the process of "working through" or transforming the original body responses to these toxic emotional states. Transformation usually is a challenging, powerful, and sometimes frightening endeavor. It can involve great courage.

The concepts of holism and healing are postures associated with being "with" oneself and with oneself and other. The awareness of general systems effects within the human being utilizes general systems theory to understand the rich connectedness and dynamic interactions between the mind-body-spirit and social and environmental experiences (Box 29-3).

## K E Y   P O I N T S

- Complementary therapies are treatment methods that can be used along with traditional medical practices to treat mental disorders. They embody caring and respect for the client. Complementary methods include exercise, acupuncture, herbal therapy, homeopathy, and imagery.
- The concept of healing, the restoration of the mind, body, and spirit to wholeness or soundness, is at the foundation of complementary therapies.
- A healer is a person who has deep intuitive wisdom, gentleness, and compassion, and is respectful of the dignity and choices of the person who needs healing.
- Healing relationships are rooted in these key principles: use of systems theory and change theory as guiding frameworks.
- The client's potential for change, his or her ability to learning new ways of coping or of perceiving the world, is central for working with persons with mental disorders.
- A holistic relationship is one in which the caregiver respects the autonomy, dignity, and healing potentials that the client possesses. A holistic relationship also recognizes the importance of boundaries and that caregivers can become overinvolved or underinvolved.
- Key concepts of holism include consciousness, mind-body-spirit, integration, self, other, mindfulness, suffering, hope, healing presence, centeredness, healing listening, unknowing, and transformation.

---

BOX 29–3. **Web Resources**

*Http://nccam.nih.gov*
*Http://www.holisticmed.com*
*Http://www.altmedicine.com*
*Http://www.herbmed.org*

This chapter discusses the concept of holism and its related philosophy.

- Explain the meaning of holism in your own words.
- Do you believe that the practice of holistic nursing care in the mental health setting is related to the nurse's own philosophy of holism in his or her life?
- How do you practice holism in your everyday life?
- Choose one idea in this chapter that you would like to incorporate in your own life. How will you implement this idea? How would it look if you were to implement this idea? How would it feel? When will you begin?

## Q U E S T I O N S

1. Brian Jones, who is diagnosed with bipolar affective disorder, wishes to include a complementary therapy in his treatment. The nurse should:
   a. support his decision; all complementary therapies are proven to be effective.
   b. support his decision and carefully review his selected therapies for contraindications.
   c. not support his decision and refer him to his psychiatrist.
   d. not support his decision and remind him that the only effective treatments are drugs approved by the FDA.
2. Celeste, age 24, has asked the nurse for suggestions on how she can improve her symptoms of mild depression without medication. The best recommendation from the nurse would be to
   a. suggest that she not eat any meat or meat byproducts.
   b. tell her that symptoms of mild depression will disappear with time.
   c. suggest that spending time alone will give her time to accept her symptoms.
   d. suggest that she engage in regular exercise.
3. In a holistic nurse–client relationship, boundaries are
   a. based on respect for the autonomy and decision-making options of the client.
   b. based on clearly written rules about maintaining appropriate roles.
   c. not necessary; the client gives total control of the relationship to the nurse.
   d. not an important component of this relationship.

**4.** Characteristics of the nurse as a "healer" includes all of the following *except*
   a. mindful intention.
   b. respect of dignity.
   c. dispassion for the other.
   d. respect of choice.

## BIBLIOGRAPHY

Achterberg, J. (1992). Ritual: The foundation for transpersonal medicine. *Revision 14*(3), 158–164.

American Nurses Association. (1980). *American Nurses Association social policy statement.* Washington, D.C.: American Nurses Association.

Barry, P.D. (1996). *Psychosocial nursing: Care of physically ill patients and their families* (3rd ed.). Philadelphia: Lippincott-Raven.

Carpenito, L. (2000). *Nursing diagnosis: Application to clinical practice* (8th ed.). Philadelphia: Lippincott Williams & Wilkins.

Deltito, J., & Beyer, D. (1998). The scientific, quasi-scientific and popular literature on the use of St. John's Wort in the treatment of depression. *Journal of Affective Disorders, 51*(3), 345–351.

D'Epiro, N. (1997). Mind-body medicine: Expanding the health model. *Patient Care, 31*(14), 133–134.

*Diagnostic and statistical manual of mental disorders.* (4th ed.). (1994). Washington, D.C.: American Psychiatric Association Press.

Ernst, E., Rand, J., & Stevinson, C. (1998). Complementary therapies for depression. *Archives of General Psychiatry, 55*(11), 1026–1032.

Hoffart, M., & Pross Keane, E (1998). The benefits of visualization. *American Journal of Nursing, 98*(12), 44–47.

Jones, J., & Bearley, W. (1987). *Managing change assertively.* Bryn Mawr, PA: Organizational Design and Development.

Nettina, S. (2000). *Lippincott manual of nursing practice* (7th ed.). Philadelphia: Lippincott Williams & Wilkins.

Raheem, R. (1987). *Soul return.* Lower Lake, CA: Aslan.

Reeder, F. (1994). Rituals of healing: Ever ancient, ever new. In D. Gaut & A. Boykin (Eds.). *Caring as healing: Renewal through hope.* New York: National League for Nursing Press.

Seligman, M. (1991). *Learned optimism.* New York: Alfred A. Knopf.

## DEVELOPING CRITICAL THINKING SKILLS
## THROUGH CLASS DISCUSSION

**UNIT 5 Case Study**
# Intervention and Treatment of
# Mental Disorders

David is a 42-year-old male brought to the emergency department by a friend. He had been talking about life "not being worth it any more," and his friend is concerned that he might be suicidal. He had married for the first time approximately 2 years ago, and his wife recently left him. After evaluation by the Crisis Team, it is determined that admission to an inpatient psychiatric unit for further evaluation and treatment is appropriate. His preliminary diagnosis is Major Depressive Episode; this is his first psychiatric admission.

## DISCUSSION QUESTIONS

1. What are your primary concerns when David arrives on the unit? How would you assess David related to your identified concerns?
2. What are some of the developmental issues facing David? How could you assist in addressing these issues?
3. What are the nurse's primary responsibilities in maintaining a therapeutic milieu for David?
4. What type of group therapy would be appropriate for David? What nursing responsibilities are associated with this therapy?
5. What types of medications might be prescribed for David? How do these medications provide therapeutic benefit?
6. What nursing responsibilities are associated with these medications? What risks are associated with them?

# ANSWERS TO CHAPTER QUESTIONS

## Chapter 1
1. d
2. c
3. a
4. d

## Chapter 2
1. a
2. c
3. d
4. c

## Chapter 3
1. c
2. d
3. b
4. d

## Chapter 4
1. c
2. a
3. c
4. c

## Chapter 5
1. b
2. b
3. b
4. a

## Chapter 6
1. d
2. c
3. d
4. d

## Chapter 7
1. b
2. c
3. b
4. a

## Chapter 8
1. c
2. d
3. a
4. c

## Chapter 9
1. b
2. d
3. b
4. a

## Chapter 10
1. d
2. a
3. d
4. d

## Chapter 11
1. a
2. c
3. c
4. a

## Chapter 12
1. b
2. c
3. c
4. a

## Chapter 13
1. c
2. c
3. b
4. c

## Chapter 14
1. c
2. c
3. c
4. d

## Chapter 15
1. a
2. d
3. b
4. b

## Chapter 16

1. c
2. c
3. d
4. a

## Chapter 17

1. d
2. c
3. a
4. b

## Chapter 18

1. b
2. b
3. c
4. c

## Chapter 19

1. a
2. c
3. b
4. b

## Chapter 20

1. b
2. c
3. d
4. c

## Chapter 21

1. a
2. b
3. d
4. a

## Chapter 22

1. d
2. b
3. d
4. c

## Chapter 23

1. d
2. a
3. d
4. a

## Chapter 24

1. b
2. a
3. b
4. a

## Chapter 25

1. b
2. c
3. d
4. a

## Chapter 26

1. d
2. a
3. d
4. b

## Chapter 27

1. c
2. d
3. d
4. a

## Chapter 28

1. d
2. b
3. c
4. b

## Chapter 29

1. b
2. d
3. a
4. c

# Glossary

**abrupt or gradual withdrawal.** Stopping use of a substance, instantly or over time, which induces depression and two or more of the following symptoms: increase in dreaming, disturbed sleep, and fatigue.

**acting out.** The behavioral outcome of conflict between an unconscious need to express anger and a conscious need to deny it; it is classified as an immature defense mechanism.

**"acting out" behavior.** Behavior in which a person projects anger and blame onto others.

**activity group therapy.** A form of therapy whose purpose is to engage in a specific type of activity as a focal theme, for example, attending a play with a group and discussing the activity before and after in a therapeutic group.

**acrophobia.** Fear of high places.

**acupuncture.** The practice of inserting small needles into the skin at preselected points, to correct the obstruction of healing energies in the body.

**acute stress disorder.** A condition that can be precipitated by the same types of catastrophic stressors as posttraumatic stress disorder except that acute stress disorder is accompanied by dissociative symptoms.

**adaptation.** Process of adjusting to one's environment in such a way that growth and development potential of the person and the general balance of the family are enhanced.

**advice giving.** Counseling technique that tells the client what to do instead of encouraging the client to find his or her own solutions. This is generally not a helpful technique, unless a client is experiencing severe anxiety.

**affect.** Another name for feelings.

**affect, blunted.** The normal range of emotions is missing; seen in people with depression, some forms of schizophrenia, and some types of organic brain syndrome.

**aggression.** An emotion compounded of frustration and hate or rage.

**agitation.** Anxiety associated with severe motor restlessness.

**agoraphobia.** Fear of being in an open place, such as outdoors or on a highway.

**agoraphobia without history of panic disorder.** A form of panic disorder in which a person experiences agoraphobic symptoms but has no history of panic symptoms.

**akathisia.** Extrapyramidal symptoms characterized by an uncomfortable sense of internal restlessness and inability to sit still.

**akinesia.** Complete or partial loss of muscle movement.

**Alcoholics Anonymous.** A peer-led group in which other individuals experiencing the same types of addictions provide a support group environment to reduce dependence on the substance and its related effects.

**alcohol intoxication.** A condition in which recent ingestion of alcohol causes negative behavioral effects.

**altruism.** A mature defense mechanism that channels the desire to satisfy one's own needs into the wish to meet the needs of others.

**ambivalence.** Alternating and opposing feelings occurring in the same person about the same object.

**amnesia.** The complete or partial inability to recall past experiences.

**amnestic disorder.** A rare cognitive disorder in which the level of consciousness is not affected as it is in other organic brain disorders. Short-term and long-term memory are impaired, and the client is in an amnestic state.

**anger.** An inborn emotional reaction to loss or to violation. Type of anger include:

justified anger: A physical and mental state in which the individual feels in control and energized to use the angry feeling to correct the "wrong" or to retrieve what was lost.

rage: A state of expressed anger marked by disorganization and loss of control; most commonly expressed outwardly.

hating anger: A type of animosity or intense dislike that can operate at two different levels: resentment/hostility or violence.

helpless anger: An angry state in which the person perceives that he or she is unable to address the cause of his or her anger and feels disempowered.

**anorexia nervosa.** Avoidance of eating because of a cluster of specific emotional issues.

**anorexia nervosa, bulimic type.** Anorexia driven by the same emotional issues as the restrictive type, but which uses purging to achieve weight loss.

**anorexia nervosa, restrictive type.** Anorexia in which there is an avoidance of food resulting in severely diminished nutritional value derived from food accompanied by significant weight loss.

**anticipation.** A mature defense mechanism by which a person intellectually and emotionally acknowledges an upcoming situation that is expected to provoke anxiety. By acknowledging it and working through some of the anxiety in advance, the event will be less stressful when it occurs.

**antianxiety agents.** Medications that lower anxiety levels.

**anticonvulsants.** Medications that lower the potential for seizures.

**antidepressants.** Medications that reduce depression.

**antiparkinsonian agents.** Medications that decrease the extrapyramidal symptoms that develop as side effects of major antipsychotics.

**antipsychotics.** Medications that alleviate psychosis.

**antisocial personality disorder.** A disorder characterized by a person's inability to form any significant attachment or loyalty to other people, groups, or society.

**anxiety.** A vague and unpleasant feeling of apprehension, helplessness, and general distress, without an identifiable cause, which produces many somatic effects or physical sensations in the body such as tenseness, tremors, cardiovascular excitation, gastrointestinal tightening, and restlessness.

**aphasia.** Partial or complete loss of the power of expression or the ability to understand either written or spoken language. The cause may be functional, organic, or both.

**art therapy.** A form of therapy whose purpose is to use art materials to express conflicts and to discuss those artistic representations within a group format led by an art therapist.

**assertive community treatment (ACT).** An intervention model in which mental health care providers assertively and actively reach out to clients who usually avoid coming to a community mental health center.

**assessment.** The first step of the nursing process, which includes gathering all the information needed to diagnose the specific problems that require nursing care and to develop a care plan.

**attention.** Mental process that involves concentrating on one activity and sustaining that focus over time.

**attention deficit/hyperactivity disorder.** A developmental disorder whose primary symptoms are problems with attention, impulsiveness, and hyperactivity.

**auditory hallucinations.** False sensory perceptions characterized by hearing sounds not present in reality.

**authenticity.** Allowing yourself to be known to others (also called genuineness).

**aversive stimulus.** Any event that results in an unpleasant feeling.

**avoidance.** An immature defense mechanism that causes an individual unconsciously to stay away from any person, situation, or place that might cause unwanted sexual or aggressive feelings to occur.

**avoidant personality disorder.** A disorder characterized by fear of rejection. People with this disorder tend to avoid social situations and consciously or unconsciously make choices that help them avoid conflict, humiliation, or shame.

**awareness, level of.** The client's wakefulness or consciousness, ranging on a continuum from coma to mania.

**behavior.** The observable or objective sign of mental functioning.

**behavior modification.** This focuses on what the client does rather than what the client feels, and uses systems theory to bring about a change in the client's behavior.

**behavioral psychology.** Rewarding a person for positive forms of behavior; another term for behavior modification.

**binge eating disorder.** An eating disorder similar to bulimia nervosa, without the purging phase, characterized by the use of binge eating with concurrent psychiatric problems, such as depression, wide variations in weight gain and loss cycles, and more severe weight-related distress.

**binging.** The ingestion of large amounts of food followed by purging.

**biological psychiatry.** The use of biological means to treat mental disorders.

**biopsychosocial.** Drawing on the knowledge of human biology, psychology, and the human social systems.

**biopsychosocial nursing care.** An integrated form of nursing care that systemically addresses the complex physical, psychological, and family issues of a client.

**bipolar disorder.** A condition in which a person exhibits strong, exaggerated, and cyclic mood swings.

**bipolar disorder, Type I.** A condition characterized by the presence of manic episodes, sometimes with a depressed episode.

**bipolar disorder, Type II.** A condition characterized by recurrent major depressive episodes with hypomanic episodes.

**blocking.** Disturbance in thought process characterized by cessation of thought production for no apparent reason.

**blunting.** Coldness of emotional response to others.

**body.** Whole of all anatomical parts and physiological processes.

**body dysmorphic disorder.** A condition in which a normal-appearing person is preoccupied with an imagined physical defect or grossly exaggerates a slight physical defect.

**borderline personality disorder.** A disorder in which a person demonstrates unpredictability and instability in many areas of interpersonal and intrapsychic functioning.

**boundaries.** The unwritten, usually unspoken rules that keep relationships with other people appropriate.

**brief psychotic disorder.** A condition that can occur as the result of an acutely stressful episode before which the person functioned normally and had no other type of physical or mental disorder.

**bulimia nervosa.** An eating disorder that includes recurrent episodes of overeating, also known as binge eating. After the binging, a person with bulimia nervosa engages in recurrent episodes of purging.

**cannabis intoxication.** Symptoms resulting from the use of cannabis (marijuana, hashish, or THC), including tachycardia and at least one of the following psychological symptoms that occur shortly after use: perception of slowed time, intensified subjective perceptions, apathy, and elation. In addition, one or more of the following physical symptoms appear: dry mouth, increase in appetite, and redness of the eyes. Disruption in social and occupational functioning and suspiciousness can result.

**capping.** The practice of allowing a limited dollar amount for psychiatric care.

**case manager/team leader.** Person who supervises or assigns the functions of the health care team in home care and other settings.

**catastrophic reaction.** This occurs when there is a sudden, unexpected stressor, and the person's normal coping mechanisms fail. The result is severe anxiety accompanied by disruption of equilibrium in the physical, intellectual, and emotional realms.

**catatonia.** A type of motor activity observed in some persons with schizophrenia in which there is either violent physical activity or inhibited or paralyzed" physical activity.

**catatonic excitement.** Behavior characterized by impulsive and stereotyped activities, poorly coordinated, and often lacking apparent purpose. Hostility and feelings of resentment are common; unprovoked outbursts of violence and destructiveness may occur.

**catatonic negativism.** Behavior marked by resistance to instructions of others or purposeful action.

**catatonic rigidity.** The holding of a particular posture for long periods of time and resistance to being moved.

**catatonic symptoms.** A person appears to be in a stupor and may be mute.

**catatonic type schizophrenia.** See *catatonia*.

**catchment area.** A geographic area with a population between 75,000 and 200,000.

**centering.** Conscious act of focusing one's attention to opening awareness and finding and internal reference point.

**cerebral arteriosclerosis.** A frequent cognitive disorder caused by hardening of the arteries of the brain.

**cerebrovascular accident (CVA).** The result of when a large blood vessel in the brain becomes occluded by a large clot, or ruptures.

**circumstantiality.** A disturbance in thought process characterized by frequent digressions on the way to eventual conclusion.

**claustrophobia.** Fear of being in an enclosed place.

**clinical director.** The person in charge of an inpatient unit, usually a psychiatrist.

**clinical nurse specialist.** Registered nurses with advanced degree(s) who generally have completed credentialing as specialists in mental health and broad clinical experience in all areas of patient care.

**clinical psychologist.** A person who had attended 4 years of graduate school and usually 1 or 2 years of postdoctoral training; this person can administer psychological tests that can identify specific causes of a person's mental dysfunction.

**closed family.** A family that is rigid and allows little change in the roles and patterns in the family.

**cocaine intoxication.** Occurs within 1 hour of using the drug and includes at least two of the following psychological symptoms: euphoria, grandiosity, excessive wordiness, excessive vigilance, and psychomotor agitation. In addition, at least two of the following physiologic conditions are present: dilated pupils, elevated blood pressure, tachycardia, nausea and vomiting, and chills or perspiration. There also are symptoms of antisocial behavior.

**codependence.** A cluster of personality traits and patterns, including compelling desire to solve others' problems, low sense of self-worth, and needing to deny feelings, that are developed as a result of a family trying to cope with a member who is addicted to alcohol or other substances. Traits may be present in many families as a way to avoid emotional conflict or distress.

**cognitive impairment.** A decrease in the intellectual aspect of mental functioning; includes a decrease in problem-solving ability, reasoning, judgment, concentration, and memory. The two most common causes are depression and cognitive disorders.

**collaborative care plan.** Care plan developed by a multidisciplinary mental health team. A mental health nurse providing psychiatric home care most likely works as part of a collaborative care team.

**collaborative problem.** Nursing diagnoses can be developed within two primary types of clinical problems experienced by mental health clients:

1. A type of problem that registered nurses can identify and treat without medical approval.

2. A type of problem that involves collaborative care planning with a physician or other licensed health care provider.

A collaborative problem is always developed in conjunction with a medical diagnosis and related treatment plan. The nursing diagnosis rounds out and completes the care ordered by a physician. In psychiatric settings the diagnostic codes developed by the American Psychiatric Association are used to describe the condition for which a client is admitted to the inpatient setting. These are the same codes used in outpatient mental health care. In the mental health setting all nursing diagnoses should be developed in conjunction with the identified mental disorder admitting diagnosis. The mental disorder diagnostic codes are published in the *Diagnostic and Statistical Manual of Mental Disorders,* (4th ed.) (DSM-IV). This book can be found in all mental health settings.

The division of nursing care problems into two types: one that the registered nurse can identify and treat independent of other licensed health care providers, and the other, a problem that requires collaboration and care planning with one or more other licensed health care disciplines is called a bifocal clinical practice model.

**community case manager.** A member of the mental health care team who oversees all aspects of support, for example, direct mental health services, housing, physical care, and so forth, for clients using community mental health centers.

**comorbid.** A mental condition that exists in the presence of and may contribute to another mental disorder.

**competency.** In law, the mental status of a person who is capable of sound decision making and management of his or her own life circumstances.

**complementary therapies.** Those healing approaches developed from a variety of sources that can be used in conjunction with traditional medical approaches.

**comprehensive community mental health center.** A community mental health center that provides the five basic services (inpatient, outpatient, partial hospitalization, emergency services, and consultation/education) as well as five additional services (diagnostic, rehabilitation, precare and aftercare, training for professionals and nonprofessionals, and research/evaluation).

**concussion.** A common result of a head injury. Its symptoms are amnesia, loss of consciousness, and nausea.

**conditioned avoidance.** A behavior modification technique that pairs the habit pattern of a client to an unpleasant stimulus so that the client learns to avoid both the stimulus and the habit.

**conduct disorder.** A developmental disorder characterized by aggressive behavior toward others and violation of rights of others.

**confabulation.** Filling in gaps in memory with statements that are untrue.

**conscience.** A person's inner voice that judge whether thoughts and actions are good or bad.

**consciousness.** The sum of the integrated perceptions in the human being, including all elements of body, mind, and spirit.

**consent.** A legal term for the agreement by a person to an act that will affect his or her body, or to disclose about himself or herself.

**consistency.** The experience of a reliable environment in which the client understands what the rules and expectations are.

**constitution.** The basic temperament or disposition inherited by a child.

**context.** Circumstances that contribute to a client's current difficulty.

**continuum of care.** Succession of settings ranging from acute inpatient care to community-based partial hospitalizations to home care.

**contract.** An agreement with another person. It can be direct (formal appointment times and settings) or indirect (flexible and less scheduled, eg, any time during a shift).

**conversion.** A mechanism by which emotional conflicts are channeled into physical symptoms or physical illness.

**conversion disorder.** A disorder in which a person's body part or system is affected by a inner psychological conflict. These disorders frequently mimic neurologic disorders.

**coping.** The way the mind responds to perceptions that are challenging or threatening.

**coping, effective.** The combination of conscious problem-solving strategies and unconscious defense mechanisms that result in the cognitive and behavioral responses to challenging or threatening events.

**coping, ineffective.** A state in which the individual experiences, or is at risk to experience, an inability to manage internal or environmental stressors adequately because of inadequate resources (physical, psychological, behavioral, and/or cognitive).

**correctional nurse.** A nurse who works in a prison or correctional facility.

**cretinism.** Congenital insufficiency of the thyroid gland that results in both mental and physical defects.

**crisis intervention.** A series of clinical actions that are effective in reducing the potential for crisis or for stabilizing an individual or social group after a crisis has occurred.

**critical path.** The use of a specific care protocol for individuals with specific diagnoses.

**cyclothymic disorder.** a disorder in which a person tends to swing between moods of exhilaration and depression, but not to pathological extremes.

**defense mechanisms.** Methods of thinking or acting that resolve conflict or reduce its severity. These protective processes are automatically developed by the unconscious mind when the conscious coping techniques are unable to manage the anxiety or uncertainty of a threatening event and there is a risk of ineffective coping.

**defining characteristics.** The signs or symptoms that the person is manifesting or describing related to the nursing problem.

**deinstitutionalization.** The act of transferring formerly institutionalized individuals to sheltered environments of to homes in the community.

**delirium.** An acute organic brain syndrome that is usually irreversible.

**delusion.** A disturbance in thought content characterized by an inaccurate belief that cannot be corrected by reasoning.

**delusion of grandeur.** Exaggerated belief about one's own abilities or importance.

**delusion of persecution.** A person's false belief that others are seeking or hurt him or her or cause damage either physically or by insinuation.

**delusion of reference.** A person's false belief that he or she is the center of others' attention and discussion.

**delusional projection.** A narcissistic defense mechanism by which the mind forms conclusions and beliefs that are not based on reality. These beliefs, when firmly rooted, form the basis of paranoid delusions, in which a person believes that someone is out to get him or her.

**dementia.** A chronic organic brain syndrome that is usually irreversible.

**dementia of the Alzheimer's type.** The most common degenerative condition that results in significant dementia. It begins with gradual decrease in memory, emotional stability, and general functioning, usually between the ages of 40 and 60. Within a year, profound dementia accompanied by hallucinations and delusions usually occurs. Complete nursing care is required.

**denial.** A narcissistic defense mechanism in which the person sees, hears, or perceives an event but the mind refuses to recognize it consciously.

**dependent personality disorder.** A disorder characterized by inability to make independent decisions or function as a responsible adult.

**depersonalization.** A sense of not feeling personally present in the situation, as though one is watching oneself and not feeling the emotions of the experience.

**depression.** Hopeless feeling of sadness, grief or mourning, or prolonged or excessive sadness associated with a loss.

**derealization.** A sense of unreality about what has happened or is currently happening.

**desensitization.** A therapeutic approach that involves gradual exposure of a client to a phobic situation while providing other forms of support and anxiety management.

**developmental crisis.** This occurs when a large number of issues that arise during normal human growth and the individual is unable to resolve these issues effectively.

**developmental disorder.** A mental disorder whose origin is related to a child's developmental process.

**developmental task.** According to Erikson's theory of personality development, an action that contributes to some vital attribute in the physical body as well as lays the groundwork for the next level of growth.

**diabetes mellitus.** A result of the undersecretion of the islands of Langerhans in the pancreas. Diabetes is characterized by hyperglycemia (excessive amount of sugar in the blood) due to a deficiency of insulin that helps the cells burn up sugars.

**diagnostic related groups (DRGs).** Categories of mental disorders listed with guidelines for normal days expected for inpatient hospitalization.

**direct statements.** Statements that are intentionally focused to elicit a limited or specific response from a client.

**disintegration.** The disruption of the normal influence of the ego on combining thoughts, feelings, memories, and perceptions into a realistic view of self and environment.

**disorganized type schizophrenia.** A subtype of schizophrenia with insidious onset usually in adolescence. The client's emotions become shallow and inappropriate. He or she withdraws from social contacts, appears preoccupied, and smiles and giggles frequently in a silly manner; speech becomes badly fragmented.

**displacement.** A neurotic defense mechanism that occurs when feelings about a person or thing are shifted to another, safer object. Although the feelings are shifted, their original cause remains the same.

**dissociative amnesia.** The inability to recall an important aspect of the trauma.

**dissociative symptoms.** A protective defense mechanism in which the memory of a catastrophic event is separated from the conscious mind.

**distortion.** A narcissistic defense mechanism used to reshape external reality to reduce anxiety and restore a feeling of emotional comfort.

**dress.** The way a person clothes or cares for himself or herself, usually reflecting the appropriateness of his or her social judgment.

**dual diagnosis.** The presence of two major types of mental disorders in one person, for example, schizophrenia and addiction disorders.

**dynamic.** A constantly operating force within a system that results in some type of action or observable result.

**dyskinesia.** Excessive movement of mouth, protruding tongue, and facial grimacing. It is a common side effect of major tranquilizers.

**dysphoria.** A depressed, disquieted, and restless mood.

**dysthymic disorder.** Mood disorder marked by depressed mood for most of the day, more days than not, and that has existed for at least 2 years (adult) or 1 year (children and adolescents). Symptoms are not as severe as a major depressive episode.

**dystonia.** Extrapyramidal symptoms characterized by muscle spasms of the jaw, tongue, neck, or eyes, and potential laryngospasm.


**eating disorder.** A chronic disruption of 3 or more months in one's ability to ingest food and derive nutrition from that food owing to one or more emotional issues.

**echolalia.** The pathologic repetition or imitation of another's speech. Seen in some forms of schizophrenia.

**echopraxia.** The pathologic repetition or imitation of another's movements. Seen in some forms of schizophrenia.

**ego.** The part of the self that is most closely in touch with reality. The ego's role is to balance a person's biological urges with the person's conscience or the expectations of the social environment.

**egocentricity.** A person's attitude and inner feeling that the world exists to meet his or her needs.

**ego ideal.** The high standard within the ego that motivates the person to continued growth and self-actualization.

**electroconvulsive therapy (ECT).** A treatment for mental disorders that do not respond to medication. In ECT a low-level electrical stimulation is used to induce a seizure, which is thought to alter the levels of neurotransmitters in the brain, resulting in decreased symptoms of illness.

**electrolyte imbalance.** An irregular amount of elements or minerals normally contained in the body within a certain measurement range. Examples of electrolytes are calcium, sodium, and so on.

**emotion focused coping.** Creating thoughts or actions to relieve situational emotional stress. These thoughts or actions do not change the external event but alter the internal emotional reaction to the event.

**empathy.** Ability to hear what another person is saying and borrow the person's emotions temporarily, but still maintain one's own.

**environment.** All internal and external forces that affect the well being of the person, including biological, psychological, and social dynamics, as well as external physical surroundings.

**erotomanic delusional disorder.** A disorder in which the individual believes that someone, usually of higher status, is in love with him or her.

**ethics.** The knowledge of the principles of good and evil.

**etiologic risk factors.** Contributing factors to a nursing diagnosis that may potentially place the person under increased stress and require psychosocial nursing interventions.

**euphoria.** Excessive and inappropriate feeling of well being.

**evaluation.** Statement describing the change in behavior that can be used as a measure of whether the nursing intervention is effective.

**exaltation.** Intense elation accompanied by feelings of grandeur.

**exophthalmic goiter (Graves' disease).** The result of an overactive thyroid. Symptoms include nervousness, irritability, anxiety, and apprehension. Acute thyroid intoxication may cause delirium.

**expressive therapist.** Persons trained to use a special medium such as art, music, drama, or other creative modalities, to allow expression of the emotional conflict that has led to the client's need for hospitalization or treatment.

**extended family.** Family members not in the nuclear family, such as grandparents, aunts, uncles, cousins, and so on.

**extinction.** Lack of reinforcement for a particular behavior causes the behavior and the learning process to progressively decrease and then be forgotten.

**extrapyramidal symptoms.** Symptoms caused by disruption of the balance of dopamine and acetylcholine, resulting in development of movement disorders; a possible side effect of psychotropic medications.

**facies.** Facial expression.

**family.** An inclusive term that means a person's immediate and extended relations who are blood relatives and individuals who are not relatives but who reside in the same home and provide significant support.

**family of origin.** The immediate family into which a child is born, usually consisting of mother, father, and siblings.

**family rules.** The unwritten expectations about what types of behavior or roles are acceptable or unacceptable to the family.

**family system.** This term describes the characteristics of a family such as roles, interactions, boundaries, and patterns of communication.

**family therapy.** This provides an environment in which family members can explore their own problems and anxieties in relation to the family member with a mental disorder.

**fear.** A feeling of dread associated with a specific cause that is identifiable.

**feeling states.** Emotions that involve both physiologic and psychological changes.

**fixation.** An arrest of the normal growth pattern of personality, caused by disturbing early experiences or unsatisfied emotional needs, which can result in personality disorders and immature behavior.

**flight of ideas.** A disturbance in the thought process characterized by rapid speaking with changes from one thought to another connected thought; seen in manic clients.

**focusing.** Paying particular attention to a topic that seem important or pertinent to a client.

**fragmentation.** See *word salad*.

**function.** A specific type of activity that belongs within the role expectations of a particular occupation.

**general adaptation syndrome.** A concept developed by Hans Selye, describing the physiologic responses to stress. The general adaptation syndrome includes three stages: the alarm reaction, the stage of resistance, and the stage of exhaustion.

**generalized anxiety disorder.** A condition in which a person experiences excessive and unrealistic worry and anxiety about two or more life circumstances for at least 6 or more months.

**gestures.** Physical movements that indicate what a person is feeling.

**grandiose delusional disorder.** A disorder in which the person has an inflated sense of self-worth, power, identity, knowledge, or special relationship to a famous person or God.

**grandiosity.** Exaggerated sense of one's importance and power.

**group therapy.** A treatment mode with the guiding principle that individuals function in groups using patterns they acquired in their original families, and that other group members are a strong influence on an individual's behavior.

**habeas corpus.** A writ requiring an immediate court hearing to determine a person's sanity.

**hallucination.** A false sensory perception that does not exist in reality. Can be auditory or visual. Usually occurs in psychotic disorders but can occur in both chronic and acute organic brain disorders.

**head nurse/unit manager.** A person, usually a registered nurse, who manages the physical environment and resources of the mental health unit, supervises other registered nurses and nursing personnel.

**healer.** A person who possesses deep intuitive wisdom, compassion, and love for others, and capacity to facilitate the healing process in self and others.

**healing.** The restoration to health, wholeness, or soundness.

**healing presence.** A mode of practice of nursing care in which the nurse listens and is "with" the client in a centered and caring therapeutic relationship.

**health.** State of physical and mental functioning, ranging from wellness to death.

**herbal therapy.** Herbs and other therapeutic plants used to treat mental disorders.

**histrionic personality disorder.** A disorder characterized by traits of vanity, self-indulgence, and a flair for dramatization or exhibitionism.

**holistic.** A model of care that is geared to the whole person.

**holistic health care priorities.** Qualities such as life sustenance, security, family balance, integrity of the person, discovery of inner strengths, and contributions to betterment of self and others, which are goals underlying the providing of home health care.

**holistic relationship.** A relationship in which the caregiver has respect for the autonomy, dignity, and healing potential that resides in the other.

**home health aide.** A person who has received training in the basic skills required to support clients in various care settings.

**homeopathy.** A health approach that treats conditions by applying a small amount of the illness-causing substance, to induce the body's defense reaction to the substance.

**homeostasis.** A dynamic, ever-changing state in which a system constantly works to maintain balance.

**hope.** The opposite of suffering; more of a fundamental life principle than an emotion.

**hopelessness.** A self-perception in which individuals believe that they have no choices or alternatives in their current life situations.

**humor.** A mature defense mechanism used when a person cannot fully tolerate a difficult situation. It is used without expense to the self or another person. Humor differs from **wit,** in which the actual anxiety-provoking subject is avoided.

**Huntington's chorea.** A hereditary, sex-linked form of psychosis. It appears chiefly in men, usually in their early thirties, and progresses rapidly so that the client ages mentally in a very short time and becomes helplessly psychotic in a few years.

**hyperactivity.** Excessive motor activity as shown by restlessness, inability to remain still, and high levels of physical activity and verbal activity.

**hypersomnia.** Excessive sleep.

**hypnagogic hallucination.** False sensory perceptions that occur during the twilight period between being awake and falling asleep.

**hypochondriasis.** A condition in which a person magnifies a mild, vague physical symptom into more severe symptoms of potentially serious illnesses.

**hypomanic episode.** A distinct period of elevated mood that is clearly different from a person's usual nondepressed mood, but the behavior and mental state do not classify as a manic episode.

**identification.** An important process in influencing personality development, in which the child molds himself or herself after the parent of the same sex and adopts that parent's characteristics and attitudes. Also, a neurotic defense mechanism that results in a person taking on the thoughts, feelings, or particular circumstances of another person as if they were his or her own.

**imagery therapy.** Having clients visualize a scene of situation that then causes changes in the client's physical response.

**immature defense mechanisms.** Defenses develop during the toddler stage (age 2 to 4) and used by healthy adults under moderate to severe stress and by people with all types of personality disorders.

**immobilization.** A reactive state of paralysis as a response to a crisis or a significant threatening event. Can result in depression or withdrawal.

**implementation/intervention.** A phase of the nursing process whose goal is to decrease or eliminate the symptoms of the specific problems that have been identified.

**indirect statements.** A statement that is intentionally general and nonspecific, used to encourage a client to respond openly and freely.

**informed consent.** When the client hears about his or her choices for treatment and decides to be admitted to the hospital.

**inhalant intoxication.** This follows the use of an inhalant that results in abnormal changes in behavior such as perceptions, impaired judgment, belligerence, and impaired occupational or social functioning.

**insomnia.** A disturbance in a person's normal sleeping pattern. Insomnia can be caused by pain, medications, caffeine or nicotine, poor sleep habits or environment, and depression or anxiety.

**instructional group.** A group in which thoughts and feelings about particular needs related to discharge are discussed within the group. The leader takes on a teaching role.

**integrated treatment model.** A treatment approach that uses both physical and mental assessment and treatment interventions. Often used in treatment of eating disorders.

**integration.** Making whole by bringing all the parts together.

**intense brief intervention.** A type of mental health intervention used when a community-based individual experiences an acute mental health emergency. A variety of mental health services are activated to treat the individual in the community so as to avoid the need for hospitalization.

**internal frame of reference.** The unique perspective and meaning that a person has about his or her own personal circumstances and life experiences.

**intrapsychic stress.** The experience of stressful thoughts and feelings that are generated by conflict or tension within the person, as opposed to a conflict or tension that is generated by the environment.

**involuntary commitment.** The legal authority to hospitalize a person with a mental illness against his or her will.

**involuntary hospitalization.** When a client resists hospitalization but caregivers believe that the client's safety depends on being admitted to an inpatient unit, the client is hospitalized without his or her consent, by court order.

**isolation.** An immature defense mechanism that separates the emotion associated with a thought. The emotion is repressed, however. Also called intellectualization and rationalization.

**job description.** A formal document that defines the expected work functions of an employee of a particular institution, the limits of his or her role, and the role of the supervisor who will evaluate the employee.

**judgment.** The final outcome of thought processes and content, resulting in a person's ability to form conclusions and behave in a socially appropriate manner.

**la belle indifference.** A lack of worry in a difficult situation that ordinarily warrants it.

**lability.** Alternating periods of elation and depression or anxiety in the same person within a limited period of time.

**learning disorder.** A developmental disorder that affects a child's ability to learn subjects (reading, spelling, math) that are usually within the intellectual capability of other children of their age.

**least restrictive environment.** The health care setting that provides the most therapeutic and safe environment for the client.

**levels of consciousness.** According to Freud, the mind has three levels of awareness: conscious (the here and now); the subconscious (just below immediate awareness); and unconscious (closed to immediate awareness). How these levels function and interact is the key to human behavior.

**liaison psychiatry.** Branch of psychiatry that addresses the emotional outcomes of physical illness.

**libido.** Normal energy level; includes one's interest in sex.

**licensed practical/vocational nurse.** A person who is licensed to practice practical or vocational nursing by a state health agency. The licensed practical/vocational nurse assists in the implementation of the nursing care plan, under the supervision of a registered nurse.

**limit setting.** Communication of information about client's behaviors that are acceptable and those that are not.

**lithium toxicity.** The result of too much lithium in the blood, characterized by nausea, vomiting, diarrhea, tremor, headache, hypotension, and a change in level of consciousness.

**loose associations.** A disturbance in thought process characterized by poorly connected or organized thoughts.

**loosening of associations.** A type of thinking in which the normal connections between ideas or thoughts seems haphazard.

**major depressive disorder.** This includes the presence of a major depressive episode but the person has not exhibited a manic episode; may be a single episode or recurrent.

**major depressive episode.** A period of altered emotional state in which five or more or nine symptoms are present and represent a change from previous functioning.

**major tranquilizers.** A category of drugs used to reduce the symptoms of major mental disorders such as schizophrenia and bipolar disorder.

**maladaptation.** The result of chronic ineffective coping on the part of one or both parents that can result in dysfunctional patterns of responses to stress within one or more family members.

**mania.** A distinct period of abnormally and persistently elevated mood, characterized by extreme excitement, restlessness, talkativeness, inflated self-esteem, and decreased sleep.

**manic episode.** This is characterized by a distinct period of abnormally and persistently elevated, expansive, or irritable mood, lasting at least 1 week. Three of seven characteristic symptoms must be persistent and significantly present.

**mathematics disorder.** A developmental disorder in which a child has difficulties with four types of mathematical skills: linguistic, perceptual, mathematical, and attentional.

**mature defense mechanisms.** Coping mechanisms, usually formed after age 6, that are used by the healthy, mature mind when it is under minimal stress. These defenses have a larger conscious component than earlier or less mature defense mechanisms.

**Medicaid.** A health insurance program offered by the federal government to people over 65 years of age.

**Medicare.** A health insurance program funded by both federal and state governments that covers health care costs for children and adults under age 65 who are eligible for public aid programs.

**medication efficacy.** The ability of a medication to work effectively with the unique biochemistry of the effects of a panic disorder and reduce a person's unique emotional symptoms.

**medication technician.** A person, supervised by hospital pharmacists, who prepares and delivers medication to clients.

**melancholic symptoms.** Those in which there is strong evidence of sadness, crying, and despondence.

**memory.** The mind's ability to recall earlier events.

**MEND A MIND.** Mnemonic aid to assist in recalling the various biologic causes of cognitive disorders.

**mental status.** State of mental functioning that a person is demonstrating at a given time.

**mind.** All functions within the mental domain, including cognition, perception, memory, judgment, and regulation and control of emotions and impulses.

**mindfulness.** State of self-awareness and openness toward the self in response to the other's state.

**modulation and flow of speech.** A way of evaluating a person's speech and communication status; indicates whether the speech is lively or dispirited.

**mood.** Another name for feelings.

**mood episode.** Periods of alteration in an individual's normal range of emotions for a period of time.

**mood stabilizers.** Medications that treat the cycles of bipolar disorder.

**motor activity.** The way a person moves his or her body, and an important indicator of mental status.

**myxedema.** A condition resulting from hypoactivity of the thyroid gland. Physical symptoms include lowered blood pressure, temperature, respiration and pulse rate; cold hands and feet; slowed physical activity; and dullness of facial expression. Mental symptoms include slowness in thinking and ability to grasp ideas.

**narcissistic defense mechanisms.** The earliest-formed defense mechanisms (birth to age 3) characterized by self-centeredness. They are employed by the healthy adult mind only during periods of extreme stress.

**narcissistic personality disorder.** A disorder characterized by extreme egocentricity. See egocentricity.

**necrotizing angiitis.** The destruction of the lining of blood vessels owing to a toxic substance.

**need.** A fundamental requirement for something or someone.

**negative reinforcement.** Rewarding a stoppage of an undesirable event or behavior.

**neologism.** A word that is invented or made up by condensing other words into a new one. This is typical in schizophrenia.

**neuroleptic malignant syndrome.** A potentially life-threatening side effect of some psychotropic medications, characterized by dysregulation of cardiovascular function, temperature and mental status.

**neuropsychiatric changes.** Changes caused by physical deterioration in the anatomy and physiology of the brain, for example, in persons with AIDS and older adults, resulting in changes in mental status that result in one or more types of mental disorder.

**neurotic defense mechanisms.** Defense mechanisms developed after age 4; they can cause a significant level of psychological distress such as depression or anxiety, but usually do not result in the need for psychiatric hospitalization.

**neurotransmitters.** Biochemical substances that send messages from the central nervous system to the body tissues.

**neurovegetative signs of depression.** Specific changes in physical functions, the basis of which are neurotransmitter alterations driven by depression.

**North American Nursing Diagnosis Association (NANDA).** An organization formed by a group of nurses in 1973 in order to identify the types of health problems that nurses are clinically prepared to diagnose and treat.

**no-suicide contract.** A written or verbal agreement between a mental health professional and a client in which the client agrees that he or she will not engage in suicidal behavior for a specified period of time. Also called a no-harm contract.

**nuclear family.** The immediate family into which a child is born.

**nursing.** A role that includes the dimensions of person centered care, including comfort, emotional care, and monitoring of safety and hygiene.

**nursing diagnosis.** A statement of a specific type of patient care problem that a nurse is clinically prepared to diagnose and treat.

**nursing goal or priority.** Statement about the expected measurable client behavior that demonstrates that the original clinical problem has been resolved or is decreased so that discharge is possible.

**nursing intervention.** Statement about the nursing behavior/action that can alter the client's clinical problem and achieve the nursing goal or priority.

**Nurse Practice Acts.** Laws enacted by each state that describe the roles and responsibilities of nurses.

**Nursing Practice Standards of the Licensed Practical/Vocational Nurse.** The rules that govern the role and scope of practice of the LPN/LVN.

**nursing process.** The steps involved in organizing and implementing nursing care of clients.

**nursing rationale.** A statement developed in conjunction with each nursing intervention that provides the reasoning to support the nursing plan for each diagnosis.

**obsessive-compulsive disorder.** A disorder in which a person experiences thoughts and actions that are repugnant, but his or her attempts to stop the pattern result in extreme anxiety.

**obsessive-compulsive personality disorder.** A disorder characterized by limited or constricted range of emotions; a lack of warmth, spontaneity, or feeling of emotional connectedness" with others; and a ceaseless striving for perfection.

**obsessive thought.** A disturbance of thought content characterized by an unwelcome idea, emotion, or urge that repeatedly enters the consciousness.

**occupational therapy.** A form of therapy whose function is to prepare an individual to return to his or her prior work environment, or to prepare him or her to enter a new occupation.

**occupational therapist.** A person who designs activities to provide structured outlets for a client's emotional or physical tensions; they can also use these activities to test a client's abilities to solve problems, set goals, maintain concentration, and perform purposeful tasks.

**open family.** One in which the members, especially the parents, have had the opportunity to develop as healthy, active members of society with positive self-esteem.

**operant conditioning.** Influencing behavior by rewarding positive forms of behavior; also called behavior modification.

**opioid intoxication.** Result of recent use of opioid drug such as heroin, morphine, and the morphine-like drugs, such as meperidine (Demerol) and methadone. Symptoms include constriction of pupils, or dilation if there is a major overdose; and the presence of one or more emotional or neurologic signs: euphoria, dysphoria, apathy, or psychomotor retardation.

**opioid withdrawal.** Result of stopping regular use of opioids. Symptoms include at least four of the following signs: tachycardia, mild hypertension, fever, lacrimation, dilated pupils, rhinorrhea (running nose), piloerection (hairs of skin standing on end), sweating, diarrhea, and yawning.

**oppositional defiant disorder.** A mental disorder with symptoms that include a recurrent pattern of negative, defiant, disobedient, and hostile behavior that significantly impairs a person's social, academic, and occupational settings.

**orderly.** Member of the psychiatric team who helps deter loss of control of a client or clients on a unit.

**orientation.** A person's ability to identify who he or she is, where he or she is and the date and approximate time.

**other.** The concept of a relationship between the self and another living being.

**pain disorder.** Condition in which a person is consistently preoccupied with pain for over 6 months but examination reveals no physiologic basis for pain or that if pathology exists, the pain exceeds what is normally expected for that condition.

**panic disorder with agoraphobia.** Condition in which a person experiences intense fear or discomfort along with a fear of public places.

**panic disorder without agoraphobia.** A condition in which a person meets the criteria for panic disorder but does not experience agoraphobia.

**paranoia.** Beliefs—with no basis in reality—that someone is going to purposely injure another.

**paranoid personality disorder.** A mental disorder in which a person tends to be hypersensitive, rigid, suspicious, jealous, and envious. They may have an exaggerated sense of their own importance and generally tend to blame others and ascribe evil motives to them.

**paranoid type schizophrenia.** A subtype of schizophrenia which adds suspiciousness, projection, and delusions of persecution to other basic schizophrenic traits. Delusions occupy a prominent place in mental concepts, and hallucinations are tied in with these delusions.

**parkinsonian movements.** A fine tremor accompanied by muscular rigidity.

**patterns of human response.** The specific patterns of human functioning, such as exchanging, communicating, relating, valuing, choosing, moving, perceiving, knowing, and feeling, that are evaluated whenever nursing assessment occurs.

**pellagra.** A condition resulting from a lack of vitamin B, owing to alcoholism, inadequate nutritional intake, or absorption disorders. Clients with advanced pellagra exhibit symptoms of mental confusion and delirious states. Irritability, distrust, anxiety, and depression are also common.

**perception.** The way that a person experiences his or her environment through the senses, and his or her frame of reference within that environment. This is equivalent to a person's sense of reality.

**pernicious anemia.** A type of anemia that can result in symptoms of mental fatigue, memory loss, irritability, depression, and apprehension.

**persecutory delusional disorder.** A disorder in which the person becomes increasingly suspicious of people and situations, and feels that people are spying on him or her with harmful intentions. The client with a persecutory disorder assumes anything other people are talking about concerns him or her.

**perseveration.** A disturbance in thought process characterized by repetition of the same word in reply to different questions.

**person.** A human being composed of biological, psychological, and social functions or domains, blended in a complex system that results in a unique individual.

**personality.** The total of all individual tendencies, including strengths, weaknesses, attributes, aspirations and drives, that determines the person's adjustment to his or her material and social environment.

**personality disorder.** A mental disorder in which the ego overuses certain types of defense mechanisms that result in a variety of exaggerated personality or character traits. The category includes paranoid, schizoid, schizotypal, histrionic, narcissistic, antisocial, borderline, avoidant, dependent, and obsessive-compulsive personality disorders.

**pharmacokinetics.** The absorption and action of psychotropic agents.

**phencyclidine (PCP) intoxication.** The result of ingestion of this substance. Following ingestion at least two of the following physiologic symptoms occur: decreased pain response, tachycardia and elevated blood pressure, dysarthria, decrease in voluntary muscle coordination, and horizontal or vertical nystagmus. In addition, there should be at least two of the following psychological symptoms: severe anxiety, mood swings, elation, grandiosity, psychomotor agitation, and sensation experienced in a different part of the body than where pressure is applied.

**phenothiazine medications.** Major tranquilizers used to reduce the symptoms of serious mental disorders, such as schizophrenia and bipolar disorder.

**phobia.** A strong fear of a particular situation.

**planning.** The second stage of the nursing process, involving problem-solving to create a plan for patient care.

**play therapy.** A form of therapy whose function is to provide an environment for children to use traditional toys and materials to exhibit, express, and resolve issues and conflicts that are creating tension and mental distress.

**positive reinforcement.** A feeling of acceptance or pleasure that a person feels when his or her behavior results in a positive response from others, which makes the person more likely to repeat the behavior.

**postpartum onset.** Symptoms of depression that develop after childbirth.

**posttraumatic stress disorder.** A condition in which a person has experienced a catastrophic event that anyone would perceive as very stressful. The person is unable to work through and release dysphoric feelings that follow the event and instead suppresses them into his or her unconscious.

**posture.** The way a person holds his or her body, often indicating how he or she is feeling.

**potential for change.** Inner openness to learning new ways of coping or new ways of perceiving the world.

**powerlessness.** A self-perception that one's own actions cannot change the outcome of a current negative life situation.

**preoccupation of thought.** A disturbance in thought content characterized with connecting all occurrences or experiences to a central thought, usually one with strong emotional overtones.

**primary appraisal.** The mind's constant monitoring of the environment in order to provide safety.

**proactive reaction.** Energy generated by anxiety is used to seek other growth-producing solutions.

**problem focused coping.** Taking action to change the external event that is causing emotional stress. These thoughts or actions attempt to change the environmental stressor.

**production of speech.** A way of evaluating a person's speech and communication status; indicates the ability to produce words.

**projection.** An immature defense mechanism, which is a less pathologic form of delusional projection. It occurs when a person is unable to acknowledge his or her own thoughts or feelings and attributes them to others.

**pseudoparkinsonism.** Extrapyramidal symptoms characterized by effects similar to those of Parkinson's disease: shuffling gait, masked face, drooling, tremor, stiff posture, and rigidity.

**psychodrama.** A form of therapy whose purpose is to allow individuals to act out specific conflicts or life experiences that are important to the individual within a therapeutic group format, so that insights are obtained.

**psychomotor agitation or retardation.** Level of activity in a person's normal actions.

**psychosis.** The mental state caused by a loss of contact with reality. Usually psychosis occurs when the actual external reality is too threatening or anxiety provoking to be acknowledged.

**psychiatric aide.** Member of the therapeutic team who receives his or her training through a program developed by the institution.

**psychiatric social worker.** Member of the mental health treatment team who is knowledgeable about the effect of the family on development and treatment of mental disorders and community resources available to the client.

**psychiatrist.** A physician who has attended medical school and also completed 4 years of residency training as a psychiatrist.

**psychogenic.** A cause of a physical disorder whose etiology is related to painful or conflicting emotions held at the unconscious level.

**psychopathology.** A disease of the mind.

**psychotic behavior.** The most severe manifestation of ineffective coping, caused by psychosis.

**psychotropic medications.** Pharmaceuticals used to treat psychiatric disorders.

**punishment.** A type of reinforcement in which a negative behavior elicits a negative response from the environment, resulting in a cessation or stopping of negative behavior.

**purging.** The use of self-induced vomiting, laxatives, diuretics, enemas, emetics, or nonpurging methods, such as exercise or fasting to control weight gain.

**quality assurance programs.** Review of health care provided, using guidelines about assessment, diagnosis, effectiveness of care planning, and evaluation of outcomes, to monitor the quality of health care delivered in hospitals and communities.

**question, close-ended.** A question that elicits a one-word or limited response because of the way that the question is phrased. For example, "Did you go to school?"

**question, open-ended.** A question that invites the client to give as much information as he or she wants. For example, "Where did you go to school and how was that experience for you?"

**rate of speech.** One way of evaluating a person's speech and communication; how fast or slow a person speaks, which should be consistent with overall motor status.

**reaction formation.** A defense mechanism, also known as compensation, used when a thought, feeling, or impulse is unacceptable to the conscious mind. As a result, the defense causes the person to behave in the exact opposite manner.

**reading disorder.** A developmental order that affects a child's ability to reach age-appropriate reading achievement levels on standardized tests.

**reality.** A person's accurate perception of what is really happening within his or her own experience or environment.

**reappraisal.** The process of the mind continuously evaluating the outcome of its coping efforts and being ready to develop new strategies if those currently in use are not working.

**recent memory.** Ability to recall events that occurred during the previous few days.

**registered nurse.** Person who has an associate or baccalaureate degree in nursing or a nursing diploma who is licensed as a registered nurse by a state health agency. The registered nurse is a member of the mental health team; the registered nurse collaboratively assesses client's present problem and resources and develops a nursing care plan for that client's needs.

**regression.** An immature defense mechanism that occurs when the mind is unable to tolerate severe intrapsychic or environmental stress. A person's psychosocial functioning returns to an earlier developmental stage as a way of reducing anxiety.

**rehabilitation therapy.** A form of therapy whose purpose is to restore a person to his or her pre-illness level of functioning.

**reinforcement.** The reward that follows acting on a stimulus and thus the process by which behavior is learned.

**remote memory.** The ability to recall events that occurred from early childhood through adolescence and adulthood, up until the current week.

**remotivation therapy.** A form of therapy whose purpose is to rekindle a person's interest in work, family participation, or group or activity to which a person once belonged.

**repression.** A defense mechanism created by the unconscious mind to minimize the negative effects of emotion on both mental and physical functioning; an important mechanism in the process of adaptation.

**resentment.** A feeling of hostility and dislike expressed toward another person as the result of an actual or perceived violation.

**residual type schizophrenia.** Classification used when the client has had at least one episode of schizophrenia but does not display acute psychotic symptoms. Other symptoms of schizophrenia are present, however.

**respite care.** Extended family or community resources that can be called on to provide care for the ill individual in the home, to allow rest and recovery for the primary caregiver.

**response.** The action that follows a stimulus.

**role.** The expected behaviors of a person engaged in a particular activity.

**schizoaffective disorder.** A condition that manifests a mixture of symptoms of a major depressive episode or a manic episode of bipolar disorder, as well as some of the symptoms that meet the criteria of schizophrenia.

**schizoid personality disorder.** A disorder that manifests emotional coldness, sensitivity, fearfulness, inability to socialize well with others, and a tendency to daydream and withdraw from reality.

**schizophreniform disorder.** A disorder that meets some of the criteria of schizophrenia; however, the condition lasts less than 6 months, disallowing the schizophrenia diagnosis.

**schizotypal personality disorder.** A disorder in which a person demonstrates many symptoms related to those of schizophrenia but of a less severe nature.

**scope of practice.** A set of functions performed by a person working in a particular occupational role.

**secondary appraisal.** The stage of monitoring during which the mind decides whether it is safe or in trouble.

**sedative–hypnotics.** Medications that lower anxiety levels and promote sleep.

**self.** The concept of the inner core of the individual.

**self-actualization.** The inborn need of all people to fully develop their potential.

**self-esteem.** The feeling of self-acceptance and positive self-image.

**serotonin syndrome.** Potentially serious side effect caused by use of selective serotonin reuptake inhibitors (SSRIs), characterized by mental changes, altered muscle tone, fever and autonomic dysfunction.

**shared psychotic disorder** (formerly induced psychotic disorder). A condition in which a second person takes on a delusion similar to that of another who has a delusional (paranoid) disorder.

**sheltered environment.** A setting that is away from the mentally disordered person's normal family, social, and community (eg, a custodial- or community-based setting).

**sibling position.** Birth order in a family; strongly influences the way a person behaves and communicates in that family.

**situational crisis.** The result of a life change event; occurs when a person is not able to effectively cope; situational crises include death, divorce, major illness, marriage, and childbirth.

**social breakdown syndrome.** A syndrome developed by chronically mentally ill people who were institutionalized for long periods of time, characterized by lack of initiative, submission to authority, withdrawal, and excessive dependence on the institution.

**social network.** All the people whom an individual views as an important source of support.

**social phobia.** A condition in which a person experiences excessive anxiety when exposed to the scrutiny of others, such as the classroom, public speaking, or a social setting.

**social system.** Includes an individual's family and social network, as well as the general social environment in which he or she lives.

**socialization.** The shaping of an individual to the communication style, beliefs, and emotional patterns of a social group; a developmental process during which the young child gains acceptance from his or her parents and other authority figures by conforming to their rules.

**somatic delusional disorder.** A disorder in which the individual believes he or she has some physical disease, disorder, or defect.

**somatization.** A defense mechanism of converting mental awareness of stress into actual physical symptoms or illness.

**somatization disorder.** A condition that usually strikes persons before age 30, in which the person has a history of vague symptoms related to a particular body system, frequently accompanied by depression and anxiety.

**somatoform disorders.** A mental conditions that cause physiologic symptoms.

**specific phobia.** A condition in which a specific object or situation stimulates overwhelming anxiety.

**spelling disorder.** A developmental disorder that affects a child's ability to score at age-appropriate levels on standardized tests.

**spirit.** The vital principle and life force of one's being; the core of a person's spirituality.

**spiritual distress.** A fundamental distress within the self that leads one to question the meaning of one's life.

**standards.** Criteria established by professional nursing organizations for the measurement and evaluation of the quality of nursing care.

**statutes.** Laws enacted by legislative branches of government.

**stimulus.** Something that satisfies a need; leads to a response.

**stress.** The subjective feeling of tension experienced in the physiologic, intellectual, and emotional realms as a response to environmental events that are perceived as threatening.

**stressor.** Those environmental events that result in internal feelings of stress.

**sublimation.** A defense mechanism that operates in association with the defense of repression. In sublimation, a repressed urge or desire is expressed in a socially acceptable or useful way.

**substance abuse.** A maladaptive pattern of substance use leading to clinically significant impairment or distress, as manifested by failing to fulfill major role obligations, hazardous substance use, substance-related legal problems, or substance use despite recurrent social or interpersonal problems caused by the substance use.

**substance dependence.** Describes a condition in which the individual's symptoms have persisted for at least 1 month or occurred at the same time in the same 12-month period. Symptoms include tolerance, withdrawal, increased amount of substance taken, unsuccessful attempts to decrease use, significant time spent in activities to obtain substance, reduced social of work activities because of use, and continued use of drug despite problems caused or made worse by use.

**substance intoxication delirium.** A syndrome caused by recent intake of one or more psychoactive substances. The result is abnormal behavior, such as impairment of judgment, occupational functioning, or social functioning.

**substance-related disorder.** Term used in place of psychoactive substance-use disorder and the term *drug addiction.* It is used for clients whose mental states are altered by alcohol, drugs, tobacco, caffeine-containing beverages, and the side effects of medically prescribed drugs taken as medically indicated.

**substance withdrawal delirium.** A syndrome caused by the reduction or cessation of ingestion of a psychoactive substance following its regular use.

**subsystem.** A concrete or abstract essential part of a larger system that relates in specific ways with all parts of the larger entity.

**suffering.** Pain in one of the human domains of physical, psychological, spiritual, or social.

**suicidal ideation** The experience of having unwanted, fleeting, and intrusive thoughts of being dead or wanting to be dead. Suicidal ideation may or may not be accompanied by a suicidal plan. Individuals with suicidal ideation without a plan can be at high risk for suicide.

**suicidal plan.** A vision of how one would attempt suicide, that is, what means would be used to kill oneself, such as with pills, a gun, and so on. A person with a suicidal plan is considered to be at very high risk. The lethality of the suicidal plan can be an indication of the seriousness of the intention of the individual to commit suicide. It should be noted however that individuals who choose a means of suicide with lower lethality risk could also be at high risk for suicide.

**suicide.** The conscious choice of a personal action to kill oneself.

**suicide prevention.** The therapeutic process that is initiated when a client indicates one or more risk factors outlined in the preceding that indicate a risk for suicide.

**suicide risk.** The assessment of the presence of specific factors that make a person more vulnerable to death by suicide.

**summarizing.** A skilled form of verbal communication that occurs at the end of a session or interview, in which the nurse briefly describes the important affective and intellectual experiences that occurred.

**sundowning.** A decrease in orientation at night to which clients with cognitive disorders are susceptible.

**supersystem.** A large complex made up of many systems, essential for an entity to function.

**support group.** A group in which members explore feelings and thoughts related to a particular subject, such as women's issues or being discharged from the hospital.

**suppression.** A defense mechanism that stores thoughts or memories in the subconscious mind where they are easily retrievable.

**sympathy.** A situation in which the caregiver adopts the same feelings as the client and loses objectivity.

**synergism.** The effect of separate entities that, when combined, have a greater effect than the sum of their individual actions.

**system.** A collection of working parts that, when combined, make up a more complex working object or entity.

**tangentiality.** A disturbance in thought process characterized by frequent digression until the initial reason for beginning a discussion is forgotten.

**tardive dyskinesia.** Severe, usually irreversible side effect associated with long-term use of typical antipsychotic agents, characterized by involuntary movements of the mouth, tongue, and face. It may also progress to involve the client's fingers, arms, trunk, and respiratory muscles.

**team communication.** The basis of effective care planning; each team member provides specific information based on his or her training and skills, providing a comprehensive picture of client needs, which can then be incorporated into a care plan that meets the unique and specific needs of each client.

**termination.** The ending of the therapeutic relationship.

**therapeutic index.** The dosage range within which medications are effective but above which they are toxic.

**therapeutic milieu** The concept of treatment based on the premise that an individual's current "here and now" behavior reflects his or her current reality and normal social interactions; this reflection provides insights into why the individual is having difficulty in his or her internal reality and social interactions with others.

**therapeutic relationship.** A caring relationship that uses professional knowledge and skills in a way that is constructive to the well being and adaptation of the client.

**thought content.** What a person thinks.

**thought disorder.** A mental state in which the normal cognitive processes are altered and there is a change in mental status.

**thought process.** How a person thinks.

**token economy.** A therapeutic approach that reward clients with tokens for positive behaviors; clients can then redeem tokens for desired privileges or activities.

**transformation.** The process of working through experiences; the constant state of change or growth that is characteristic of human beings.

**traumatic coma.** A state in which an individual is unconscious or has lost consciousness owing to a blow to the head or other sudden unexpected injury.

**traumatic delirium.** A condition that may follow emergence from a traumatic coma or stupor. If the delirium is mild, the client acts more or less bewildered, irritable, and restless. If it is severe, the client may be noisy, belligerent, demanding, and verbally abusive.

**triage.** The process by which an individual with a health problem is assessed by a health care provider to determine the type(s) of illness present and immediate health care needs.

**triangle.** A social dynamic that begins with a conflict between two people. Instead of communicating directly, one of these people engages a third, uninvolved, person in the conflict. This creates a communication pattern called triangulation.

**triggering or precipitating event.** An event or situation that precipitates a psychological crisis in a person.

**trust.** The ability of one person to rely on another, to experience consistent and reliable interactions, and expect to be treated with dignity.

**unconditional positive regard.** Accepting a client without negative judgment about his or her basic worth.

**undifferentiated type schizophrenia.** Less severe psychotic symptoms that cannot be classified in the other schizophrenia subtypes or symptoms that meet the criteria for more than one of the other schizophrenia categories.

**unknowing.** The perspective of a listener who understands that he or she does not know the experience of the other.

**values.** Deeply held beliefs that a child acquires during the formative years as the result of exposure to people, objects, or ideas that are important to him or her.

**vascular dementia.** A condition caused by small thromboses in small intracranial blood vessels that results in a series of minor strokes. Symptoms are confusion, speech difficulties, memory dysfunction, and sometimes a small degree of muscular paralysis.

**violence.** An unjust or unwarranted exertion of power that is fueled by anger.

**visual hallucinations.** False sensory perceptions characterized by seeing object(s) not present in reality.

**volume of speech.** A way to evaluate a person's speech, indicates the quietness or loudness.

**voluntary hospitalization.** A client's decision to enter the hospital for treatment.

**waxy flexibility.** A pathologic condition in which the body maintains the position in which it is placed. Seen in some forms of schizophrenia.

**withdrawal.** A progressive shutting out of the world.

**withdrawal sickness.** This occurs when a person addicted to an abused substance stops using the drug. Symptoms include sweats, shakes, chills, diarrhea, vomiting, and sharp stomach pain.

**wisdom.** The understanding of what is true or right; insight, common sense, or good judgment.

**word salad.** A jumbled mixture of words and phrases that have no meaning and are illogical in their sequence. Seen most often in schizophrenia (eg, "Backter dyce tonked up snorfel blend.")

**work therapy.** A form of therapy whose function is to provide a working environment where a person can re-enter the work force within a supportive environment.

# Assessment Tools: Barry Psychosocial Assessment

This comprehensive assessment tool uses Gordon's functional health patterns to facilitate the data-gathering process and promote the identification of corresponding nursing diagnoses.

The assessment categories include the following patterns:

- Health perception–health management
- Nutritional-metabolic
- Elimination
- Activity-exercise
- Sleep-rest
- Cognitive-perceptual

- Self-perception–sell-concept
- Role-relationship
- Sexuality-reproductive
- Coping–stress tolerance
- Value-belief

These categories help the nurse focus on specific aspects of assessment and identify problem areas. Problem areas are identified through a focused assessment.

Assess all boxed questions subjectively, rather than asked of the client directly. Bold italic statements advise the nurse how to proceed.

## ADMITTING INFORMATION

Name _____ Age _____ Date of admission _____
Marital status S_____ M_____ W_____ D_____ How long? _____
Occupation _____ Years of education completed _____
Date of assessment _____ Admitting diagnosis _____

## HEALTH PERCEPTION-HEALTH MANAGEMENT

### Patient's Perception of Illness

What was the original problem that caused you to come to the hospital?
_____

On what date did you first become ill? _____
What caused this illness? _____
How do you feel about being in a hospital? _____
How can the physician's and nurses help you most? _____
How will this illness affect you when you are out of the hospital? _____
_____

Do you think it will cause any changes in your life? _____
How will it affect your family?_____

| | | |
|---|---|---|
| Potential for noncompliance? Yes _____ No _____ Possible _____ | | |
| Related to: _____ Anxiety | _____Unsatisfactory relationship with care-giving environment or care-givers | |
| _____Negative side effects of prescribed treatment | _____Other | |
| Explain: | | |
| Potential for injury? Yes _____ No _____ Possible _____ | | |
| Explain: | | |

## NUTRITIONAL-METABOLIC

How does your current appetite compare with your normal appetite?

Same _____    Increased _____    Decreased _____

How long has it been different? _____

How your weight fluctuated by more than 5 lb in the last several weeks?

Yes _____    No _____    How many pounds? _____

What is you normal fluid intake per day? ml* _____ Your current intake? ml _____

**\*Nurse can substitute estimate of milliliters for client's reported fluid intake.**

---

Aspects of client's illness or condition that could contribute to organic mental disorder?

No _____    Yes _____

Delirium type _____            Dementia type _____

Possible cause:

_____ Metabolic                      _____ Infectious disease

_____ Electrolytes                   _____ Neoplastic disease

_____ Other metabolic or endocrine   _____ Nutritional disease

condition                            _____ Degenerative (chronic) brain

_____ Arterial disease                     disease

_____ Mechanical disease             _____ Drug toxicity

_____ Electrical disorder

---

## ELIMINATION

What is your current pattern of bowel movements?

Constipated _____    Diarrhea _____    Incontinent _____

How does this compare to normal?

Same _____    Different _____

Explain:


What is your current pattern of urination? _____

How does this compare to normal?

Same _____    Different _____

Explain:


---

Possibility that emotional distress may be contributing to any change?

High _____    Moderate _____    Low _____

---

## ACTIVITY-EXERCISE

What is your normal energy level?

High _____    Moderate _____    Low _____

Has it changed in the past 6 months?   Yes _____    No _____

To what do you attribute the cause?_____

How would you describe your normal activity level?

High _____    Moderate _____    Low _____

How may it change following this hospitalization? _____

What types of activities do you normally pursue outside the home? _____

_____

What recreational activities do you enjoy? _____

Do you anticipate your ability to manage your home will be changed following your
 hospitalization?_____
Explain:

---

Current self-care deficits?
Feeding _____    Bathing _____    Dressing _____    Toileting _____
Anticipated deficits following hospitalization? _____
Current impairment in mobility? _____
Anticipated immobility following hospitalization?_____
Alterations in the following?
Airway clearance   How? _____
Breathing patterns   How?_____
Cardiac output   How? _____
Respiratory function   How? _____
Potential for altered tissue perfusion as manifested by altered cognitive-perceptual
patterns?

---

## SLEEP-REST

### Normal Sleeping Pattern
How many hours do you normally sleep per night?
From what hour to what hour? _____ to _____

### Changes in Normal Sleeping Pattern
Do you have difficulty falling asleep? _____
Do you awaken in the middle of night?_____
Do you awaken early in the morning? _____
Are you sleeping more or fewer hours than normal? _____    How many? _____

## COGNITIVE-PERCEPTUAL
Are you feeling pain now? _____    How severe? _____    How often? _____
What relieves the pain?_____

---

What information does this client need to know to manage this illness or health
 state?
Ability to comprehend this information?
Good _____    Moderate _____    Poor _____
If poor, explain:

### Mental Status Exam
Level of awareness and orientation_____
Appearance and behavior _____
Speech and communication _____
Affect (mood) _____
Thinking process_____
Related to: Inability to evaluate reality _____    Aging _____    Other _____
Explain:

**If there is a distortion of the thought process, a focused assessment is indicated.**
Perception_____
Abstract thinking _____
Social judgment_____
Memory _____
Impairment in short-term memory _____    Long-term _____
Is there evidence of unilateral neglect?   Yes_____   No____   Does not apply _____

### Self-Perception
Does the client describe feelings of anxiety or uneasiness?_____
Is he able to identify a cause?   Yes _____    No _____
Cause?_____
**If the client feels anxious but cannot identify a cause, assess for the major coping risks of physical illness below.**

Is there anything you are frightened of during this hospitalization or illness?
Yes _____No ____What is it? _____
How will this illness affect your future plans? _____
Normally, do you believe that you control what happens to you (internal locus of control) or do you believe that other people or events control what happens (external locus of control)?
Will this illness affect the way you feel about yourself? _____
How about your body? _____

Internal locus of control _____
External locus of control _____

### Psychosocial Risks of Illness
What are the major issues of this illness for this client? _____
For this family?_____
Use the following space to record client and family comments illustrating how they are coping with these issues.

| | |
|---|---|
| Trust | Client_____ |
| | Family_____ |
| Self-esteem | Client_____ |
| | Family_____ |
| Body image | Client_____ |
| | Family_____ |
| Control | Client _____ |
| | Family _____ |
| Loss | Client_____ |
| | Family_____ |
| Guilt | Client_____ |
| | Family_____ |
| Intimacy | Client_____ |
| | Family_____ |

Could one or more of these issues be contributing to feelings of anxiety, hopelessness, powerlessness, or disturbance in self-concept?   Yes _____    No _____
Possible _____
If so, explain which ones and proceed with a focused assessment.

## ROLE-RELATIONSHIP

What is your occupation? _____

How many years have you been in this occupation? _____

Do you anticipate that this illness will have an effect on your ability to work?

Yes _____   No _____   How?_____

With whom do you live? _____Are they supportive? _____

Who are the most important people in your life?_____

Do you ever feel socially isolated?   Yes_____No _____

Explain:

---

Is there any indication in this history of social isolation or impaired social interaction?

Yes _____   No _____

Explain:

Ability to communicate

Within normal limits _____   Impaired _____

Describe:

---

## FAMILY HISTORY

Who are the members of your immediate family? What are their ages and how are they
related to you? Please include deceased members and when they died.

Name of family member _____

Relationship to you _____ Age _____ Date of death _____

Name of family member _____

Relationship to you _____ Age _____ Date of death _____

Name of family member _____

Relationship to you _____ Age _____ Date of death _____

Name of family member _____

Relationship to you _____ Age _____ Date of death _____

Name of family member _____

Relationship to you _____ Age _____ Date of death _____

What is your position in relation to your brothers and sisters? For example, are you the
second oldest, the youngest...? _____

How often do you see your immediate family members? _____

What goes on in your family when something bad happens? _____

What do most of the members do? _____

Have any of your relationships within your immediate and extended family changed
recently?_____

Which ones? _____

How have they changed?_____

Is there any change in the way you parent your children?

Yes _____No _____

Is so, to what do you attribute the cause?

_____ New baby

_____ Death of family member

_____ Illness in other family member

_____ Change in residence (describe reason for change)

_____ Other (describe)

What is your normal role within your family?_____

What role do the significant other people in your family play? _____

Potential for disruption of these roles by this illness?
High _____    Moderate _____    Low _____
Explain:

While the client is describing the family, is there any indication of uncontrolled anger or rage?
Yes _____    No _____
Related to a specific issue or person?

Explain:
Open (trusting) or closed (untrusting) communication style in family? (Can be initially determined by statements and emotional expression of client.) _____

Development stage of family
_____ Early married
_____ Married with no children
_____ Active childbearing
_____ Preschool or school-age children
_____ Adolescent children and children leaving home

_____ Middle-aged, children no longer at home
_____ Elderly, well-functioning
_____ Elderly, infirm

Is there any other aspect of your family or the way your family normally operates that you think should be added here? What is it?

**If any item discussed in this section appears to be a current stressor for this client or family, it can be assessed using a focused approach with the other items under coping-stress tolerance pattern.**

**Interpersonal Style**
_____ Dependent
_____ Controlled
_____ Dramatizing
_____ Suspicious
_____ Self-sacrificing

_____ Superior
_____ Uninvolved
_____ Mixed (usually two styles predominate)
_____ No predominant personality style

Write a brief sentence explaining your choice.

Response to you as the interview.    Guarded? _____    Open? _____
Is the client able to maintain good eye contact?

## SEXUALITY-REPRODUCTIVE
Have you experienced any recent change in your sexual functioning?
Yes _____ No _____
How? _____
For how long? _____
Do you associate your change in sexual functioning with some event in your life?
_____

Do you think this illness could change your normal pattern of sexual functioning? _____

How? _____

---

Is this change in sexuality patterns related to:

_____ Ineffective coping

_____ Change or loss of body part

_____ Prenatal or postpartum changes

Changes in neurovegetative functioning related to depression

Explain:

**Use focus assessment if necessary.**

---

## COPING-STRESS TOLERANCE

### Level of Stress During Year Before Admission

How long have you been out of work with this illness? _____

Have you experienced any recent change in your job? _____

Have you been under any unusual job stress during the past year? _____

What was the cause?

_____ Retirement _____ Same job, but new boss or working relationship

_____ Fired

_____ Other. Explain: _____ Promotion or demotion

Do you expect the stress will be present when you return to work? _____

**The preceding questions should be adapted for students to a school situation.**

Have there been changes in your family during the last 2 years?

Which family members are involved? Include dates.

Death_____

Was this someyou you were close to? _____

Divorce _____

Child leaving home _____

Cause?_____

Other _____

Has there been any other unusual stress during the last year that is still affecting you?

Describe:

Any unusual stress in your family?

Describe

### Normal Coping Ability

When you go through a very difficult time, how do you handle it?

_____ Talk it out with someone     _____ Get angry and yell

_____ Drink     _____ Get angry and clam up

_____ Ignore it     _____ Get angry and hit or throw something

_____ Become anxious     _____ Other (explain)

_____ Withdraw from others     _____ Become depressed

How often do you experience feelings of depression? _____

In the past, what is the longest period of time this feeling has lasted? _____
Have you felt depressed during the past few weeks?    Yes _____    No _____
To what do you attribute the cause? _____
_____

**If rape trauma is the cause of this admission, do not explore the psychological reaction with the client until reading the report of the rape crisis counselor, who should have met with the client within an hour of arrival at the emergency department. Either follow the recommendations on the report for ongoing assessment or proceed with gentle questioning about current feelings.**
What is the most serious trauma you have experienced? _____
What was the most difficult time you have experienced in your life? _____
How long did it take you to get over it? _____
What did you do to cope with it? _____  _____

## Potential for Self-Harm
**This part of the assessment should be included if moderate to severe depression is present.**
Have you ever thought of committing suicide?    Yes _____    No _____
**If yes, continue on.**
What would you do to end your life?    No plan _____    Plan _____
Describe:


What would prevent you from committing suicide? _____

## Substances That May Be Used as Stress Relievers
*Smoking history*
Do you smoke? _____        How long have you been smoking? _____
How many packs per day? _____
*Alcohol use history*
Do you drink? _____        How often? _____        How much? _____
Is there a history of alcoholism in your family? _____    Who? _____
*Drug use*
What prescribed medications are you currently using?
Name of medications _____
Dose or schedule _____ Prescribing physician _____
Are you currently using any other drugs?    Yes _____    No _____
What are they? _____
How long have you been using them? _____
What is the usual amount?        _____        How often? _____
Have you ever been treated for substance abuse? _____

## VALUE-BELIEF
What is your religious affiliation? _____
Do you consider yourself active or inactive in practicing your religion?
Active _____    Inactive _____
Is your religious leader a supportive person?    Yes _____    No _____
Explain:


What does this illness mean to you? _____
Are you experiencing spiritual distress?    Yes _____    No _____
Explain:

What would you consider to be the primary cause of this spiritual distress (actual, possible, or potential)?

_____ Inability to practice spiritual rituals

_____ Conflict between religious, spiritual, or cultural beliefs and prescribed health regimen

_____ Crisis of illness, suffering, or death

_____ Other (explain)

Do you expect there will be any disparity in your care-givers' approach that could present a problem to you? _____

Any problems in the areas of

| | |
|---|---|
| _____ Spiritual rituals | _____ Communication |
| _____ Cause of illness | _____ Problem solving |
| _____ Perception of illness and sick role | _____ Nutrition |
| _____ Family response | |
| _____ Health maintenance | |

Explain:


How has this illness affected your relationship with God or the supreme being of you religion?

Explain:


The 11 functional health patterns were named by Marjorie Gordon (1987) in *Nursing diagnosis: Process and application.* New York: McGraw-Hill.

From Barry, P.D. (1996). *Psychosocial nursing: Care of physically ill patients and their families* (3rd ed.). Philadelphia: J.B. Lippincott.

# B North American Nursing Diagnosis Association (NANDA) Nursing Diagnoses: Definitions and Classification

Note: NANDA nursing diagnoses that are most frequently used in mental health/psychiatric settings are preceded by the following symbol: ♦ The categories listed below are general categories, many of which have sub-categories related to the general category. For further information about these categories, the reader is referred to Carpenito, L. (2000). *Nursing diagnosis: Application to clinical practice* (8th ed.). Philadelphia: Lippincott Williams & Wilkins.

In addition to those diagnoses that have active mental health implications, there are several categories listed below that include physical changes in functioning that are related to mental disorders. The following list includes the names of NANDA nursing diagnoses associated with physical disorders that may have mental health etiologies. If the physical problem has a possible mental health etiology, the type of mental disorder that may contribute to the change in physical functioning is included in parentheses.

♦ Activity intolerance (related to mental disorder, such as depression)
♦ Adjustment
♦ Airway clearance
♦ Anxiety
♦ Aspiration
♦ Attachment
♦ Autonomic dysreflexia
♦ Bed mobility
♦ Body image
♦ Body temperature
♦ Breastfeeding
♦ Breathing pattern (related to anxiety disorders)
♦ Cardiac output (related to anxiety or other type of mental disorder)
♦ Caregiver role strain
♦ Confusion
♦ Constipation (related to side effect of psychotropic medication)
♦ Coping
♦ Death anxiety
♦ Decisional conflict
♦ Denial
♦ Dentition
♦ Development
♦ Diarrhea
♦ Disuse syndrome (related to immobility associated with mental disorder)

- ◆ Diversional activity (related to mental disorder)
- ◆ Elimination (related to mental disorder)
- ◆ Energy field
- ◆ Environmental interpretation (related to mental disorder)
- ◆ Failure to thrive (related to mental disorder)
- ◆ Falls (related to mental disorder, such as delirium or dementia)
- ◆ Family processes
- ◆ Fatigue
- ◆ Fear
- ◆ Fluid volume (related to mental disorder, such as delirium or dementia)
  Gas exchange
- ◆ Grieving
- ◆ Growth (related to mental disorder, such as delirium or dementia; mood disorder; schizophrenia, substance abuse disorder, and so on)
- ◆ Growth and development (related to mental disorder, such as delirium or dementia; mood disorder; schizophrenia, substance abuse disorder, and so on)
- ◆ Health maintenance (related to mental disorder, such as delirium or dementia; mood disorder; schizophrenia, substance abuse disorder, and so on)
  Health-seeking behaviors
- ◆ Home maintenance (related to mental disorder, such as delirium or dementia; mood disorder; schizophrenia, substance abuse disorder, and so on)
- ◆ Hopelessness
  Hyperthermia
  Hypothermia
- ◆ Incontinence (related to mental disorder, such as delirium or dementia)
- ◆ Identity disturbance
  Infant behavior
  Infant feeding pattern
  Infection
  Intracranial adaptive capacity
- ◆ Knowledge
  Latex allergy response
- ◆ Loneliness
- ◆ Management of therapeutic regimen (related to mental disorder, such as delirium or dementia; mood disorder; schizophrenia, substance abuse disorder, and so on)
- ◆ Memory
- ◆ Nausea
- ◆ Noncompliance (related to mental disorder, such as delirium or dementia; mood disorder; schizophrenia, substance abuse disorder, and so on)
- ◆ Nutrition (related to mental disorder, such as delirium or dementia; mood disorder; schizophrenia, substance abuse disorder, and so on)
  Oral mucous membrane
  Pain
- ◆ Parenting (related to mental disorder, such as delirium or dementia; mood disorder; schizophrenia, substance abuse disorder, and so on)
  Perfusion
  Perioperative-positioning injury
- ◆ Physical mobility
- ◆ Poisoning
- ◆ Post-trauma
- ◆ Powerlessness
- ◆ Protection
- ◆ Rape-trauma syndrome

- ◆ Relocation stress
- ◆ Role conflict
- ◆ Role performance
- ◆ Self-care
- ◆ Self-esteem
- ◆ Self-mutilation
- ◆ Sensory perception
- ◆ Sexual dysfunction
- ◆ Sexuality patterns
- ◆ Skin integrity
- ◆ Sleep deprivation
- ◆ Sleep pattern
- ◆ Social interaction
- ◆ Social isolation
- ◆ Sorrow
- ◆ Spiritual distress
- ◆ Spiritual well-being
  Spontaneous ventilation
- ◆ Suffocation
- ◆ Suicide
- ◆ Surgical recovery (related to mental disorder, such as delirium or dementia; mood disorder; schizophrenia, substance abuse disorder, and so on)
  Swallowing
  Thermoregulation
- ◆ Thought processes
  Tissue integrity
  Transfer
- ◆ Trauma
  Unilateral neglect
  Urinary retention
  Ventilatory weaning response
- ◆ Verbal communication
- ◆ Violence
  Walking
- ◆ Wandering
  Wheelchair mobility

## NEW NURSING DIAGNOSES, APRIL 2000
Note: The nursing diagnoses associated with these new nursing diagnoses are included in the prior list.

- ◆ Risk for Falls
- ◆ Risk for Powerlessness
- ◆ Risk for Relocation Stress Syndrome
- ◆ Risk for Situational Low Self-Esteem
- ◆ Risk for Suicide
- ◆ Self-Mutilation
- ◆ Wandering

# C DSM-IV Classifications

## DISORDERS USUALLY FIRST DIAGNOSED IN INFANCY, CHILDHOOD, AND ADOLESCENCE

### Mental Retardation
| | |
|---|---|
| 317 | Mild Mental Retardation |
| 318.0 | Moderate Mental Retardation |
| 318.1 | Severe Mental Retardation |
| 318.2 | Profound Mental Retardation |
| 319 | Mental Retardation, Severity Unspecified |

### Learning Disorders
| | |
|---|---|
| 315.00 | Reading Disorder |
| 315.1 | Mathematics Disorder |
| 315.2 | Disorder of Written Expression |
| 315.9 | Learning Disorder NOS |

### Motor Skills Disorder
| | |
|---|---|
| 315.4 | Developmental Coordination Disorder |

### Communication Disorders
| | |
|---|---|
| 315.31 | Expressive Language Disorder |
| 315.31 | Mixed Receptive-Expressive Language Disorder |
| 315.39 | Phonological Disorder |
| 307.0 | Stuttering |
| 307.9 | Communication Disorder NOS |

### Pervasive Developmental Disorders
| | |
|---|---|
| 299.00 | Autistic Disorder |
| 299.80 | Rett's Disorder |
| 299.10 | Childhood Disintegrative Disorder |
| 299.80 | Asperger's Disorder |
| 299.80 | Pervasive Developmental Disorder NOS (including Atypical Autism) |

### Attention-Deficit and Disruptive Behavior Disorders
*Attention-Deficit/Hyperactivity Disorder*
| | |
|---|---|
| 314.01 | Combined Type |

### 314.9 Attention-Deficit/Hyperactivity Disorder NOS
| | |
|---|---|
| 314.00 | Predominantly Inattentive Type |
| 314.01 | Predominantly Hyperactive-Impulsive Type |
| 314.9 | Attention-Deficit/Hyperactivity Disorder NOS |
| 312.8 | Conduct Disorder |
| 313.81 | Oppositional Defiant Disorder |
| 312.9 | Disruptive Behavior Disorder NOS |

### Feeding and Eating Disorders of Infancy or Early Childhood
| | |
|---|---|
| 307.52 | Pica |

307.53    Rumination Disorder
307.59    Feeding Disorder of Infancy or Early Childhood

## Tic Disorders
307.23    Tourette's Disorder
307.22    Chronic Motor or Vocal Tic Disorder
307.21    Transient Tic Disorder
307.20    Tic Disorder NOS

## Elimination Disorders
787.6    Encopresis with Constipation and Overflow Incontinence
307.7    Encopresis without Constipation and Overflow Incontinence
307.6    Enuresis (Not Due to a General Medical Condition)

## Other Disorders of Infancy, Childhood, or Adolescence
309.21    Separation Anxiety Disorder
313.23    Selective Mutism
313.89    Reactive Attachment Disorder of Infancy or Early Childhood
307.3    Stereotypic Movement Disorder
313.9    Disorder of Infancy, Childhood, or Adolescence NOS

### DELIRIUM, DEMENTIA, AND AMNESTIC AND OTHER COGNITIVE DISORDERS

## Delirium
293.0    Delirium due to [indicate the General Medical Condition]
—    Substance-Induced Delirium (refer to specific substance for code)
—    Substance Withdrawal Delirium (refer to specific substance for code)
—    Delirium Due to Multiple Etiologies (use multiple codes based on specific etiologies)
780.09    Delirium NOS

## Dementia
*Dementia of the Alzheimer's Type*
## With Early Onset: If Onset at Age 65 or Below
290.11    With Delirium
290.12    With Delusions
290.13    With Depressed Mood
290.10    Uncomplicated

## With Late Onset: If Onset After Age 65
290.3    With Delirium
290.20    With Delusions
290.21    With Depressed Mood
290.0    Uncomplicated
—    With Behavioral Disturbance (can be applied to any of the above subtypes)

## Vascular Dementia
290.41    With Delirium
290.42    With Delusions
290.43    With Depressed Mood
290.40    Uncomplicated
—    With Behavioral Disturbance (can be applied to any of the above subtypes)

## Dementia Due to Other General Medical Conditions
294.9    Dementia Due to HIV Disease (Code 043.1 on Axis III)

294.1    Dementia Due to Head Trauma (Code 854.00 on Axis III)
294.1    Dementia Due to Parkinson's Disease (Code 332.0 on Axis III)
294.1    Dementia due to Huntington's Disease (Code 333.4 on Axis III)
290.10   Dementia Due to Pick's Disease (Code 331.1 on Axis III)
290.10   Dementia Due to Creutzfeldt-Jakob Disease (Code 046.1 on Axis III)
294.1    Dementia Due to Other General Medical Condition
—        Substance-Induced Persisting Dementia (refer to specific substance for code)
—        Dementia Due to Multiple Etiologies (use multiple codes based on specific etiologies)
294.8    Dementia NOS

### Amnestic Disorders
294.0    Amnestic Disorder Due to a General Medical Condition
—        Substance-Induced Persisting Amnestic Disorder (refer to specific substance for code)
294.8    Amnestic Disorder NOS

### Other Cognitive Disorders
294.9    Cognitive Disorders NOS

### MENTAL DISORDERS DUE TO A GENERAL MEDICAL CONDITION NOT ELSEWHERE CLASSIFIED
293.89   Catatonic Disorder Due to a General Medical Condition
310.1    Personality Change Due to a General Medical Condition
293.9    Mental Disorder NOS Due to a General Medical Condition

### SUBSTANCE-RELATED DISORDERS
### Alcohol-Related Disorders
*Alcohol-Induced Disorders*
303.90   Alcohol Dependence
305.00   Alcohol Abuse
303.00   Alcohol Intoxication
291.8    Alcohol Withdrawal
291.0    Alcohol Withdrawal Delirium
291.0    Alcohol Intoxication Delirium
291.2    Alcohol-Induced Persisting Dementia
291.1    Alcohol-Induced Amnestic Disorder

*Alcohol-Induced Psychotic Disorder*
291.5    With Delusions
291.3    With Hallucinations
291.8    Alcohol-Induced Mood Disorder
291.8    Alcohol-Induced Anxiety Disorder
291.8    Alcohol-Induced Sexual Dysfunction
291.8    Alcohol-Induced Sleep Disorder
291.9    Alcohol-Related Disorder NOS

### Amphetamine (or Amphetamine-like)—Related Disorders
*Amphetamine Use Disorders*
304.40   Amphetamine Dependence
305.70   Amphetamine Abuse

*Amphetamine-Induced Disorders*
292.89   Amphetamine Intoxication

292.0      Amphetamine Withdrawal
292.81     Amphetamine Intoxication Delirium

### Amphetamine-Induced Psychotic Disorder
292.11     With Delusions
292.12     With Hallucinations
292.84     Amphetamine-Induced Mood Disorder
292.89     Amphetamine-Induced Anxiety Disorder
292.89     Amphetamine-Induced Sexual Dysfunction
292.89     Amphetamine-Induced Sleep Disorder
292.9      Amphetamine-Related Disorder NOS

### Caffeine-Related Disorders
305.90     Caffeine Intoxication
292.89     Caffeine-Induced Anxiety Disorder
292.89     Caffeine-Induced Sleep Disorder
292.9      Caffeine-Related Disorder NOS

### Cannabis-Related Disorders
*Cannabis Use Disorders*
304.30     Cannabis Dependence
305.20     Cannabis Abuse

### *Cannabis-Induced Disorders*
292.89     Cannabis Intoxication
292.81     Cannabis Intoxication Delirum

*Cannabis-Induced Psychotic Disorder*
292.11     With Delusions
292.12     With Hallacinations
292.89     Cannabis-Induced Anxiety Disorder
292.9      Cannabis-Related Disorder NOS

### Cocaine-Related Disorders
*Cocaine Use Disorders*
304.20     Cocaine Dependence
305.60     Cocaine Abuse

*Cocaine-Induced Disorders*
292.89     Cocaine Intoxication
292.0      Cocaine Withdrawal
292.81     Cocaine Intoxication Delirium

*Cocaine Psychotic Disorder*
292.11     With Delusions
292.12     With Hallucinations
292.84     Cocaine-Induced Mood Disorder
292.89     Cocaine-Induced Anxiety Disorder
292.89     Cocaine-Induced Sexual Dysfunction
292.89     Cocaine-Induced Sleep Disorder
292.9      Cocaine-Related Disorder NOS

### Hallucinogen-Related Disorders
*Hallucinogen Use Disorders*
304.50     Hallucinogen Dependence
305.30     Hallucinogen Abuse

## HALLUCINOGEN-INDUCED DISORDERS
292.89   Hallucinogen Intoxication
292.89   Hallucinogen Persisting Perception Disorder (Flashback)
292.81   Hallucinogen Intoxication Delirium

*Hallucinogen-Induced Psychotic Disorder*
292.11   With Delusions
292.12   With Hallucinations
292.84   Hallucinogen-Induced Mood Disorder
292.89   Hallucinogen-Induced Anxiety Disorder
292.9    Hallucinogen-Related Disorder NOS

## Inhalant-Related Disorders
*Inhalant Use Disorders*
304.60   Inhalant Dependence
305.90   Inhalant Abuse

*Inhalant-Induced Disorders*
292.89   Inhalant Intoxication
292.81   Inhalant Intoxication Delirium
292.82   Inhalant-Induced Persisting Dementia

*Inhalant-Induced Psychotic Disorder*
292.11   With Delusions
292.12   With Hallucinations
292.84   Inhalant-Induced Mood Disorder
292.89   Inhalant-Induced Anxiety Disorder
292.9    Inhalant-Related Disorder NOS

## Nicotine-Related Disorder
*Nicotine Use Disorders*
305.10   Nicotine Dependence

*Nicotine-Induced Disorder*
292.0    Nicotine Withdrawal
292.9    Nicotine-Related Disorder NOS

## Opioid-Related Disorders
*Opioid Use Disorders*
304.00   Opioid Dependence
305.50   Opioid Abuse

*Opioid-Induced Disorders*
292.89   Opioid Intoxication
292.0    Opioid Withdrawal
292.81   Opioid Intoxication Delirium

*Opioid-Induced Psychotic Disorder*
292.11   With Delusions
292.12   With Hallucinations
292.84   Opioid-Induced Mood Disorder
292.89   Opioid-Induced Sexual Dysfunction
292.89   Opioid-Induced Sleep Disorder
292.9    Opioid-Related Disorder NOS

## Phencyclidine (or Phencyclidine-like)-Related Disorders
*Phencyclidine Use Disorders*

304.90    Phencyclidine Dependence
305.90    Phenyclidine Abuse

*Phencyclidine-Induced Disorders*
292.89    Phencyclidine Intoxication
292.81    Phencyclidine Intoxication Delirium

*Phencyclidine-Induced Psychotic Disorder*
292.11    With Delusions
292.12    With Hallucinations
292.84    Phencyclidine-Induced Mood Disorder
292.89    Phencyclidine-Induced Anxiety Disorder
292.9     Phencyclidine-Related Disorder NOS

## Sedative-, Hypnotic-, or Anxiolytic-Related Disorders
*Sedative-, Hypnotic-, or Anxiolytic Use Disorders*
304.10    Sedative-, Hypnotic-, or Anxiolytic Dependence
305.40    Sedative-, Hypnotic-, or Anxiolytic Abuse

*Sedative-, Hypnotic-, or Anxiolytic-Induced Disorders*
292.89    Sedative-, Hypnotic-, or Anxiolytic Intoxication
292.0     Sedative-, Hypnotic-, or Anxiolytic Withdrawal
292.81    Sedative-, Hypnotic-, or Anxiolytic Intoxication Delirium
292.81    Sedative-, Hypnotic-, or Anxiolytic Withdrawal Delirium
292.82    Sedative-, Hypnotic-, or Anxiolytic-Induced Persisting Dementia
292.83    Sedative-, Hypnotic-, or Anxiolytic-Induced Persisting Amnestic Disorder

*Sedative-, Hypnotic-, or Anxiolytic-Induced Psychotic Disorder*
292.11    With Delusions
292.12    With Hallucinations
292.84    Sedative-, Hypnotic-, or Anxiolytic-Induced Mood Disorder
292.89    Sedative-, Hypnotic-, or Anxiolytic-Induced Anxiety Disorder
292.89    Sedative-, Hypnotic-, or Anxiolytic-Induced Sexual Dysfunction
292.89    Sedative-, Hypnotic-, or Anxiolytic-Induced Sleep Disorder
292.9     Sedative-, Hypnotic-, or Anxiolytic-Related Disorder NOS

## Polysubstance-Related Disorder
304.80    Polysubstance Dependence

## Other (or Unknown) Substance Use Disorders
304.90    Other (or Unknown) Substance Dependence
305.90    Other (or Unknown) Substance Abuse

*Other (or Unknown) Substance-Induced Disorders*
292.89    Other (or Unknown) Substance Intoxication
292.0     Other (or Unknown) Substance Withdrawal
292.81    Other (or Unknown) Substance-Induced Delirium
292.82    Other (or Unknown) Substance-Induced Persisting Dementia
292.83    Other (or Unknown) Substance-Induced Persisting
    Amnestic Disorder

*Other (or Unknown) Substance-Induced Psychotic Disorder*
292.11    With Delusions
292.12    With Hallucinations
292.84    Other (or Unknown) Substance-Induced Mood Disorder
292.89    Other (or Unknown) Substance-Induced Anxiety Disorder

292.89     Other (or Unknown) Substance-Induced Sexual Dysfunction
292.89     Other (or Unknown) Substance-Induced Sleep Disorder
292.9      Other (or Unknown) Substance-Related Disorder NOS

## SCHIZOPHRENIA AND OTHER PSYCHOTIC DISORDERS

### Schizophrenia

295.30     Paranoid Type
295.10     Disorganized Type
295.20     Catatonic Type
295.90     Undifferentiated Type
295.60     Residual Type
295.40     Schizophreniform Disorder
295.70     Schizoaffective Disorder
297.1      Delusional Disorder
298.8      Brief Psychotic Disorder
297.3      Shared Psychotic Disorder (Folie à Deux)

### *Psychotic Disorder Due to a General Medical Condition*

293.81     With Delusions
293.82     With Hallucinations
—          Substance-Induced Psychotic Disorder (refer to specific substance for codes)
298.9      Psychotic Disorder NOS

## MOOD DISORDERS

### Major Depressive Disorders

296.2x     Single Episode
296.3x     Recurrent
300.4      Dysthymic Disorder
311        Depressive Disorder NOS

### Bipolar Disorders

*Bipolar I Disorder*

296.0x     Single Manic Episode
296.40     Most Recent Episode Hypomanic
296.4x     Most Recent Episode Manic
296.6x     Most Recent Episode Mixed
296.5x     Most Recent Episode Depressed
296.7      Most Recent Episode Unspecified
296.89     Bipolar II Disorder (Recurrent Major Depressive Episodes with Hypomanic Episodes)
301.13     Cyclothymic Disorder
296.80     Bipolar Disorder NOS
293.83     Mood Disorders Due to a General Medical Condition
—          Substance-Induced Mood Disorder (refer to specific substances for codes)
296.90     Mood Disorder NOS

## ANXIETY DISORDERS

300.01     Panic Disorder Without Agoraphobia
300.21     Panic Disorder With Agoraphobia
300.22     Agoraphobia Without History of Panic Disorder
300.29     Specific Phobia

| 300.23 | Social Phobia |
| 300.3 | Obsessive-Compulsive Disorder |
| 309.81 | Posttraumatic Stress Disorder |
| 308.3 | Acute Stress Disorder |
| 300.02 | Generalized Anxiety Disorder (Includes Overanxious Disorder of Childhood) |
| 293.89 | Anxiety Disorder Due to a General Medical Condition |
| — | Substance-Induced Anxiety Disorder (refer to specific substances for codes) |
| 300.00 | Anxiety Disorder NOS |

## SOMATOFORM DISORDERS
| 300.81 | Somatization Disorder |
| 300.81 | Undifferentiated Somatoform Disorder |
| 300.11 | Conversion Disorder |
| 300.7 | Hypochondriasis |
| 300.7 | Body Dysmorphic Disorder |
| 300.81 | Somatoform Disorder NOS |

### Pain Disorder
| 307.80 | Associated with Psychological Factors |
| 307.89 | Associated with Both Psychological Factors and a General Medical Condition |

## FACTITIOUS DISORDERS

### Factitious Disorder
| 300.16 | With Predominantly Psychological Signs and Symptoms |
| 300.19 | With Predominantly Physical Signs and Symptoms |
| 300.19 | With Combined Psychological and Physical Signs and Symptoms |
| 300.19 | Factitious Disorder NOS |

## DISSOCIATIVE DISORDERS
| 300.12 | Dissociative Amnesia |
| 300.13 | Dissociative Fugue |
| 300.14 | Dissociative Identity Disorder |
| 300.6 | Depersonalization Disorder |
| 300.15 | Dissociative Disorder NOS |

## SEXUAL AND GENDER IDENTITY DISORDERS

### Sexual Dysfunctions
*Sexual Desire Disorders*
| 302.71 | Hypoactive Sexual Desire Disorder |
| 302.79 | Sexual Aversion Disorder |

*Sexual Arousal Disorders*
| 307.72 | Female Sexual Arousal Disorder |
| 302.72 | Male Erectile Disorder |

*Orgasmic Disorders*
| 302.73 | Female Orgasmic Disorder |
| 302.74 | Male Orgasmic Disorder |
| 302.75 | Premature Ejaculation |

*Sexual Pain Disorders*
| 302.76 | Dyspareunia (not due to a general medical condition) |
| 306.51 | Vaginismus (not due to a general medical condition) |

*Sexual Dysfunctions Due to a General Medical Condition*

| | |
|---|---|
| 625.8 | Female Hypoactive Sexual Desire Disorder Due to a General Medical Condition |
| 608.89 | Male Hypoactive Sexual Desire Disorder Due to a General Medical Condition |
| 607.84 | Male Erectile Disorder Due to a General Medical Condition |
| 625.0 | Female Dyspareunia Due to a General Medical Condition |
| 608.89 | Male Dyspareunia Due to a General Medical Condition |
| 625.8 | Other Female Sexual Dysfunction Due to a General Medical Condition |
| 608.89 | Other Male Sexual Dysfunction Due to a General Medical Condition |
| — | Substance-Induced Sexual Dysfunction (refer to specific substances for codes) |
| 302.70 | Sexual Dysfunction NOS |

*Paraphilias*

| | |
|---|---|
| 302.4 | Exhibitionism |
| 302.81 | Fetishism |
| 302.89 | Frotteurism |
| 302.2 | Pedophilia |
| 302.83 | Sexual Masochism |
| 302.84 | Sexual Sadism |
| 302.3 | Transvestic Fetishism |
| 302.82 | Voyeurism |
| 302. | Paraphilia NOS |

**Gender Identity Disorders**

| | |
|---|---|
| 302.6 | Gender Identity Disorder In Children |
| 302.85 | Gender Identity Disorder In Adolescents or Adults |
| 302.6 | Gender Identity Disorder NOS |
| 302.9 | Sexual Disorder NOS |

**EATING DISORDERS**

| | |
|---|---|
| 307.1 | Anorexia Nervosa |
| 307.51 | Bulimia Nervosa |
| 307.50 | Eating Disorder NOS |

**SLEEP DISORDERS**

**Primary Sleep Disorders**

*Dyssomnias*

| | |
|---|---|
| 307.42 | Primary Insomnia |
| 307.44 | Primary Hypersomnia |
| 347 | Narcolepsy |
| 780.59 | Breathing-Related Sleep Disorder |
| 307.45 | Circadian Rhythm Sleep Disorder |
| 307.47 | Dyssomnia NOS |

*Parasomnias*

| | |
|---|---|
| 307.47 | Nightmare Disorder |
| 307.46 | Sleep Terror Disorder |
| 307.46 | Sleepwalking Disorder |
| 307.47 | Parasomnia NOS |

**Sleep Disorders Related to Another Mental Disorder**

| | |
|---|---|
| 307.42 | Insomnia Related to [Axis I or Axis II Disorder] |
| 307.44 | Hypersomnia Related to [Axis I or Axis II Disorder] |

## Other Sleep Disorders

*Sleep Disorders Due to a General Medical Condition*

780.52     Insomnia Type
780.54     Hypersomnia Type
780.59     Parasomnia Type
780.59     Mixed Type
—          Substance-Induced Sleep Disorder (refer to specific substances for codes)

## IMPULSE-CONTROL DISORDERS NOT ELSEWHERE CLASSIFIED

312.34     Intermittent Explosive Disorder
312.32     Kleptomania
312.33     Pyromania
312.31     Pathological Gambling
312.39     Trichotillomania
312.30     Impulse-Control Disoder NOS

## ADJUSTMENT DISORDERS

### Adjustment Disorder

309.0      With Depressed Mood
309.24     With Anxiety
309.28     With Mixed Anxiety and Depressed Mood
309.3      With Disturbance of Conduct
309.4      With Mixed Disturbance of Emotions and Conduct
309.0      Unspecified

## PERSONALITY DISORDERS

### Cluster A Personality Disorders

301.0      Paranoid Personality Disorder
301.20     Schizoid Personality Disorder
301.22     Schizotypal Personality Disorder

### Cluster B Personality Disorders

301.7      Antisocial Personality Disorder
301.83     Borderline Personality Disorder
301.50     Histrionic Personality Disorder
301.81     Narcissistic Personality Disorder

### Cluster C Personality Disorders

301.82     Avoidant Personality Disorder
301.6      Dependent Personality Disorder
301.4      Obsessive-Compulsive Personality Disorder
301.9      Personality Disorder NOS

## OTHER CONDITIONS THAT MAY BE A FOCUS OF CLINICAL ATTENTION

### Psychological Factors Affecting Medical Condition}

316        [Specified Psychological Factor;] Affecting; [indicate the general medical condition]

Mental Disorder Affecting General Medical Condition
Psychological Symptoms Affecting General Medical Condition
Personality Traits or Coping Style Affecting General Medical Condition

Maladaptive Health Behaviors Affecting General Medical Condition
Stress-Related Physiological Response Affecting General Medical Condition
Other or Unspecified Psychological Factors Affecting General Medical Condition

## Medication-Induced Movement Disorders
| | |
|---|---|
| 332.1 | Neuroleptic-Induced Parkinsonism |
| 333.92 | Neuroleptic Malignant Syndrome |
| 333.7 | Neuroleptic-Induced Acute Dystonia |
| 333.99 | Neuroleptic-Induced Acute Akathisia |
| 333.82 | Neuroleptic-Induced Tardive Dyskinesia |
| 333.1 | Medication-Induced Postural Tremor |
| 333.90 | Medication-Induced Movement Disorder NOS |
| 995.2 | Adverse Effects of Medication NOS |

## Relational Problems
| | |
|---|---|
| V61.9 | Relational Problem Related to a Mental Disorder or General Medical Condition |
| V61.20 | Parent-Child Relational Problem |
| V61.1 | Partner Relational Problem |
| V61.8 | Sibling Relational Problem |
| V62.81 | Relational Problem NOS |

## Problems Related to Abuse or Neglect
| | |
|---|---|
| V61.21 | Physical Abuse of Child |
| V61.21 | Sexual Abuse of Child |
| V61.21 | Neglect of Child |
| V61.1 | Physical Abuse of Adult |
| V61.1 | Sexual Abuse of Adult |

## Additional Conditions That May Be a Focus of Clinical Attention
| | |
|---|---|
| V15.81 | Noncompliance with Treatment |
| V65.2 | Malingering |
| V71.01 | Adult Antisocial Behavior |
| V71.02 | Child or Adolescent Antisocial Behavior |
| V62.89 | Borderline Intellectual Functioning |
| 780.9 | Age-Related Cognitive Disorder |
| V62.82 | Bereavement |
| V62.3 | Academic Problem |
| V62.2 | Occupational Problem |
| 313.82 | Identity Problem |
| V62.89 | Religious or Spiritual Problem |
| V62.4 | Acculturation Problem |
| V62.89 | Phase of Life Problem |

## ADDITIONAL CODES
| | |
|---|---|
| 300.9 | Unspecified Mental Disorder (nonpsychotic) |
| V71.09 | No Diagnosis or Condition on Axis I |
| 799.9 | Diagnosis or Condition Deferred on Axis I |
| V71.09 | No Diagnosis on Axis II |
| 799.9 | Diagnosis Deferred on Axis II |

Diagnostic Criteria from DSM-IV. Washington, DC: American Psychiatric Association.

# Index

Note: Page numbers followed by *f* indicate figures; those followed by *t* indicate tables; and those followed by *b* indicate boxed material.